Public Health
in
America

This is a volume in the Arno Press series

PUBLIC HEALTH IN AMERICA

Advisory Editor

Barbara Gutmann Rosenkrantz

Editorial Board

**Leona Baumgartner
James H. Cassedy
Arthur Jack Viseltear**

See last pages of this volume
for a complete list of titles.

ESSAYS

ON

STATE MEDICINE

HENRY WYLDBORE RUMSEY

ARNO PRESS

A New York Times Company

New York / 1977

Editorial Supervision: JOSEPH CELLINI

Reprint Edition 1977 by Arno Press Inc.

Reprinted from a copy in the Library of the
  College of Physicians of Philadelphia

PUBLIC HEALTH IN AMERICA
ISBN for complete set: 0-405-09804-9
See last pages of this volume for titles.

Manufactured in the United States of America

Library of Congress Cataloging in Publication Data

Rumsey, Henry Wyldbore, 1809-1876.
    Essays on state medicine.

    (Public health in America)
    Reprint of the 1856 ed. published by J. Churchill,
London.
    1. Public health--Great Britain. 2. Medicine,
State--Great Britain. I. Title. II. Series.
[DNLM: WA R939e 1856a]
RA485.R93   1977   362.1'0941   76-40641
ISBN 0-405-09829-4

ESSAYS

ON

STATE MEDICINE.

ESSAYS

ON

STATE MEDICINE.

BY

HENRY WYLDBORE RUMSEY.

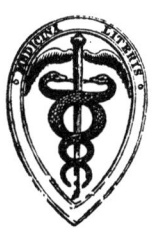

LONDON:
JOHN CHURCHILL, NEW BURLINGTON STREET.
MDCCCLVI.

[*The right of Translation is reserved by the Author.*]

TO

JOHN AYRTON PARIS, M.D., D.C.L., V.P.R.S.

ETC. ETC.

PRESIDENT OF THE ROYAL COLLEGE OF PHYSICIANS,
AND CHAIRMAN OF THE MEDICAL COUNCIL CALLED TOGETHER BY THE PRESIDENT
OF THE GENERAL BOARD OF HEALTH FOR AID AND ADVICE DURING
THE LAST VISITATION OF CHOLERA,

AND TO

THE OTHER LEARNED AND DISTINGUISHED MEMBERS
OF THAT COUNCIL,

WITH A DEEP SENSE OF THE IMPORTANCE OF THE PRINCIPLE RECOGNISED BY THE
GOVERNMENT IN THEIR APPOINTMENT, A CONVICTION OF THE VALUE OF THEIR
LABOURS AND THE WISDOM OF THEIR COUNSEL, AND A HOPE THAT THE LATE
DEMAND FOR THEIR TEMPORARY AND GRATUITOUS SERVICES MAY LEAD TO A
MORE JUST VIEW OF THE NATURE AND OBJECTS OF STATE MEDICINE,

THESE ESSAYS

ARE RESPECTFULLY

Inscribed

BY THE AUTHOR.

"THE Medical Council . . . . express their satisfaction at science having at length been recognised by the State as the ally of civil jurisprudence, and as the guide to a more enlightened code of Medical Police. They trust that this propitious movement may be regarded as the inauguration of a system ultimately destined to carry its ameliorating influence through all the ramifications of our sanitary institutions; and that the present fragmentary and imperfect application of medical knowledge in several departments of the State, may give place to a complete and comprehensive new system under the sole direction and control of one central department."

Report of Medical Council, 1855.

PREFACE.

So many Parliamentary inquiries have been lately instituted, and so many measures have been proposed, on subjects relating to the Public Health, and affecting either the agency of the Medical Profession for State purposes or the qualification of its members,—and the importance of these matters has become so generally acknowledged,—that any one who has thought much on them may, perhaps, be excused for endeavouring to reduce to some degree of order this accumulating mass of materials.

Parliament is now called upon to legislate respecting medical education and organization. It is required not only to constitute suitable authorities, central and local, for regulating sanitary measures, but also to define the localities to which such measures are to be applied. It is asked to enact special hygienic laws (for instance, on public vaccination);—to regulate trades and occupations, with reference to the health both of the community and of the operatives;—to prevent the adulteration of food and drugs;—to arrest the sale of poisons;—to regulate the practice of pharmacy;—and to carry into effect certain reforms in the administration of medical relief to the poorer classes.

There are Bills and Committees almost without end for these objects;—but, strange to say, they are treated as perfectly independent questions, and as having no connexion with each other, nor any common aims or bearings; while special sanitary regulations are to be enacted before any competent authorities have been constituted for carrying them into execution.

Hence we are threatened with the perpetuation of one of the

principal errors of English sanitary legislation, of all the administrative embarrassments which it causes, the conflicting jurisdictions which it creates, and the innumerable "Amendment Acts" to which it leads.

If individuals are slow to learn wisdom by misfortunes, nations are said to be still slower. May we then indulge the hope that Parliament will profit by the failure of past shortcomings? For example:—A few years ago, it became notorious that people were being poisoned in considerable numbers by arsenic. A specific law was forthwith enacted to control the sale of this article alone, as though there were no other poisons in or out of the Pharmacopœia. If precedent is to be followed, recent tragical events will probably lead to an Act for prohibiting the sale of Strychnine, another for Chloroform, and so on.

Our insular method might have been thought to undergo a *reductio ad absurdum*, when in the session of 1853 an Honorable Member brought in a " Bill for the Prevention of Glanders." But beneath every depth there is still a lower deep, for in 1854 both Lords and Commons—having been occupied for several days in devising a law to amend (as usual) an imperfect and impracticable measure respecting public vaccination passed in the previous year—agreed only upon a solitary clause (which however did not become law) to the effect that the vaccinated subject should appear on the seventh instead of the eighth day for inspection. Surely a Council of State Medicine, competent to settle such a question in half-an-hour, might relieve Parliament from so preposterous a waste of time, speech, and printing.

Perhaps it may be replied, that no harm was done;—but, in an age when everybody feels himself at liberty to ask—*Cui bono?* about everything, one may be forgiven for questioning whether any particular advantage is likely to result from this method of legislating on details, to any class, profession, or order of society.

With regard to future administration, a ray of hope glimmers in the fact, that the able sanitarian, who last year pithily described our Public-Health arrangements as " little dabs of doctoring done by several departments of Government,"*—is now appointed one of that body, which is called, and aspires to become, a General Board of Health.

The extraordinary course which has been taken within the last few years by the Legislature and Government, will astonish our descendants as it has already puzzled our European contemporaries. Who would have thought that in the last decade of advancing civilization, and in a nation boasting of its intellectual and material resources, of its administrative energy and efficiency, the whimsical experiment should have been actually tried of appointing three non-medical authorities—two Lords and a Barrister,—to preserve the health of the living; and then, after a year or so of doubtful success, calling in a Physician to bury the dead!†

For efficient sanitary protection, and for the promotion of their physical well-being, the people do not require a Central Board of sanitary amateurs, bent on forcing crude and impracticable schemes upon those reluctant and resisting municipalities which have been unwisely authorized to administer laws, of the first principles of which they are necessarily, though pardonably, ignorant. The real public want is a Board or Council, representing the administrative skill and ability of a great nation, aided by its physicians, and enlightened by its philosophers; a body invested with sufficient power to regulate, amend, and perfect the willing efforts to be made in every locality by judiciously-constituted district authorities, and by a trained and scientific corps of officers.

———

Three years ago, after an interview with a Minister of State, I prepared a Memorandum on the natural and essential connexion between the various branches of State Medicine, and on the necessity of keeping in view that connexion, in the progress of sanitary legislation.

* *Minutes of Evidence on Adulteration of Food*, &c., 806 (1855).

† Few readers will need to be told that I refer to the appointments made under the Public Health Act of 1848, and the Metropolitan Interments Act of 1850.

This Memorandum gradually expanded into a series of articles,—and these again have been amplified (and, I hope I may add, illustrated and rendered more likely to be useful) by historical and statistical details which had been long accumulating.

The original design of this Work comprehended (as might be inferred from the outline of a Sanitary Code in the First Essay) a final article on the formation of a Central Board or Council of State Medicine in this country, with suggestions respecting its sphere of action and extent of power,—its duties of superintendence, deliberation, and control,—its constitution, its comprehension of existing departments, and its relation to the supreme Government,—including also some notice of the establishment and operations of the "General Board of Health." In such an article it would be important to consider the bearings of Preventive Medicine upon the several questions of general legislation,—as Education, Public Works, Popular Representation, Agriculture and Commerce, &c.,—and to inquire how far hygienic principles had been, or might be, recognised in the framing and execution of various measures of national economy and reform.

But I found the subject so vast, and the rough materials so numerous,—yet requiring so much collation, arrangement, and indeed further investigation than I could bestow upon them in a short time and at a distance from the Metropolis,—that I had to decide between—the immediate publication of those articles which I had prepared, and which seemed to be presently called for—and the indefinite postponement of the whole work.

I resolved, therefore, to omit the last portion of my scheme in this publication,—and with the more readiness, as it seemed probable that important changes might soon be made in the existing central authority; and I thought it better to reserve to myself an occasion for future remark, than to commit myself by premature suggestion.

I have also avoided all allusion to the War department of State Medicine; firstly, because I had reason to believe that our national deficiencies in this respect were already under consideration by some whose long study and experience in Military Hygiéne qualify them specially for the task of criticism and advice; and, secondly, because I would fain hope that the recent publication of an authentic Report—showing that thirty-five per cent. of our forces in the Crimea perished in ~~about six~~ *seven* months, owing chiefly (as it appears) to gross neglect of the most obvious precautions for the preservation of health and life, and to want of power in the Medical Department to enforce attention to its recommendations—may convince the most sceptical that the success of a campaign depends as much upon the completeness and efficiency of the medico-sanitary organization of the army as upon the strategic skill of its Generals or the heroism of its soldiers, and may thus impel the nation and the Government to make permanent provision against a recurrence of late errors and calamities.

The publication of these Essays has been deferred much longer than I intended; and I may perhaps state, as the main cause of the delay, that the greater part of the work has been written during the brief, uncertain, and weary intervals of an active professional life,—and that, for months together, I have been unable, from various causes, even to look at the manuscript. I have also laboured under the disadvantage of being out of reach of any good library of reference; such literary accommodation being as yet supplied in very few of our provincial towns.

These circumstances are mentioned, not with the object of deprecating all fair criticism, but in the hope of encouraging others, more favourably situated, to pursue the subject more carefully and successfully.

The few who may be acquainted with my former writings, especially the *Health and Sickness of Town Populations*, may observe that I have often referred to them, and sometimes quoted from them without acknowledgment. If the authority of a great example be considered a sufficient justification for taking such a liberty with oneself, I may offer the following extract from the Editor's preface to *Coleridge's Table Talk* (2nd Ed., 1836):—

"Mr. Coleridge's prose works had so very limited a sale, that although published in a technical sense, they could scarcely be said to have ever become *publici juris*. Hence, in every one of his prose writings there are repetitions, either literal or substantial, of passages to be found in some other of his writings, and there are several particular positions and reasonings which he considered of vital importance, reiterated in the *Friend*, the *Literary Life*, the *Lay Sermons*, *Aids to Reflection* &c."

ADDENDUM.

Since the Essay on Medical Education has passed through the press, another edition of the Bill for regulating the Medical Profession has appeared. The alterations it contains are not important. If any portion of the measure should perchance become law, the new clause (29) which empowers any one of the several colleges to procure the erasure of names from the National Register of legally qualified practitioners, will scarcely be allowed to pass. Another and more serious alteration is for the worse. According to the scheme of constituting the proposed Medical Council in the first version of this Bill, an undue, or at least disproportionate share of influence was to be conceded to the Scotch Colleges and practitioners (see p. 79). This preponderance is now to be made more remarkable, for out of the total number (twenty-four) not fewer than nine members of Council are awarded to Scotland, not more than nine to England, and only six to Ireland.

One is curious to know whence this amended scheme of representation proceeded.

CHELTENHAM, *April 2nd*, 1856.

CONTENTS.

ESSAY I.

INTRODUCTORY—OUTLINE OF A SANITARY CODE.

CHAP. FIRST.—PRELIMINARY.—*Unity of State Medicine:* Scheme of State Agenda, 3—6.

CHAP. SECOND.—DIV. I. STATE INVESTIGATION:
Subdiv. A. *Statistics.*—§ 1. ... of Population, 7. § 2. ... of Mortality, 8. § 3. ... of Reproduction, 8. § 4. ... of Sickness and Accidents, 9. § 5. ... of Dwellings, 10. 6. ... of Food, 10. 7. ... of Animal Life, 11. *Subdiv.* B. *Topography, Climate, &c.*—§ 1. Physical Geography, 12. § 2. Chemical Analysis. § 3. Meteorological Observations, 13. *Subdiv.* C. *Jurisprudence.*—§ 1. Death-inquests, 13. § 2. Personal Disqualifications. § 3. ... other Legal Questions, 14.

CHAP. THIRD—DIV. II. SANITARY REGULATIONS:
Subdiv. A. *Preventive Measures.*—§ 1. Localities, 15. § 2. Construction of Towns and Buildings, 16. § 3. Purification of the same,—viz., Nuisances, —Water-supply,—Drainage and Sewerage,—Pavements,—Smoke, 18—20. § 4. Healthy progeny, physical education, 21. § 5. Sale of food, 22. § 6. Sale of medicines and poisons, 24. § 7. Trades and occupations,— protection of operatives and of public, 24—26. § 8. Locomotion, 27. § 9. Recreations and places of public resort, 27—29. § 10. Public establishments, 29. § 11. Burial, 31.
Subdiv. B. *Palliative Measures;—firstly, ordinary.* § 1. Medical attendance, 32. § 2. medicines and dispensaries, *ib.* § 3. Hospitals, &c., 33. § 4. Medical officers, 34. *Secondly, during Epidemics.*—§ 5. Preparatory measures, 35. § 6. domiciliary visitations, &c., 36. § 7. Quarantine, 37. § 8. Vaccination, 38. § 9. Animal diseases, 39.

CHAP. FOURTH.—DIV. III. ADMINISTRATIVE MACHINERY:
Subdiv. A. *Education of Agents.*—§ 1. Medical education, 40. § 2. Licence and Registration, 41, 42. § 3. District faculties, 42. § 4. Rights and immunities, 43. § 5. Education and licence of other therapeutic agents, 44. § 6. Veterinarians, 45.
Subdiv. B. *Official Authorities,—Councils and Boards.*—§ 1. Metropolitan Sanitary and Medical Council, 46,—its sections, 47. § 2. Local Boards, 48. *Territorial Divisions.*—§ 3. Sanitary districts, 49. § 4. *Officers.*—A. of Central Council, B. of District Boards, C. of parishes, 50—53.

CHAP. FIFTH.—SUPPLEMENTARY, 55.
Postscript—Humboldt and centralization, 57.

ESSAY II.

EDUCATION IN THE HEALING AND HEALTH-PRESERVING ARTS.

§ 1. Introductory, 61. § 2. "Medical Reform," *ib.* § 3. Conflict of Colleges, *ib.* § 4. Protection to practitioners, 62. § 5. Heterodoxy, 63. § 6. Prohibition of ignorant pretenders, *ib.* § 7. Varieties of empiricism, 64. § 8. Protection to public, 65. § 9. State intervention in medical education, 66. §§ 10 and 11. Professorships of Medical Jurisprudence and Hygiéne, 67. § 12. Council of State Medicine, 69. §§ 13 and 14. Subjects for medical studies and Regulations of Council, 70. § 15. Final examinations, 71. § 16. Limitation of numbers admitted to practise, *ib.* § 17. Examination for civil appointments, 73. § 18. Age for licence to practise, 74. §§ 19 and 20. State and Collegiate qualifications, 75. § 21. Obstetric art, 76. § 22. Pharmacy, *ib.* § 23. Chemists and Druggists, 77. § 24. Last Medical Reform Bill, 78. § 25. Its "Council of Medicine," 79. § 26. Plea for legislation, 80. § 27. District Faculties, 81. § 28. Practitioners' fees, *ib.* § 29. Penalties against Irregulars, 82. § 30. Medicine and Literature, 83.

ESSAY III.
ON SANITARY INQUIRY.

CHAP. FIRST. — SOME OF THE CHARACTERISTICS OF ANCIENT AND MODERN INQUIRY.

§ 1. Early records, 87. § 2. Hippocrates, 88. § 3. Lord Bacon, 89. § 4. Principles of Inquiry, 91. §§ 5 and 6. Statistical errors, 92. § 7. Health of Towns' Inquiry—sanitary reports—interment reports, 94. § 8. medical evidence ... 97. § 9. recent official inquiries ... 98. § 10. Local inquiries, 99. § 11. indefinite results, *ib.*

CHAP. SECOND.—SUBJECTS ON WHICH PUBLIC SANITARY INQUIRY NEEDS EXTENSION AND PERMANENCE IN ENGLAND.

§ 1. Neglect of duty by Government, 101. § 2. General register office, *ib.* §§ 3 and 4. Certification of causes of deaths, 102. § 5. Statistics of Sickness, 106. §§ 6 and 7. Medical relief returns—England and Ireland, *ib.* § 8. ... from hospitals and dispensaries, *ib.* § 9. ... from medical clubs, 108. § 10. ... from undefined classes, *ib.* § 11. ... from friendly societies, *ib.* § 12. ... from labourers in civil service, 109. §§ 13 and 14. Influence of trades upon health and life, 110. § 15. "Industrial Pathology," 111. § 16. Effects of "great-town" system, 112. "Flats" and cottages, 113. § 17. Inquiry as to food, 114. § 18. Agricultural statistics, 115. § 19. Climate and meteorology, 116. § 20. Voluntary meteorological returns, 118. § 21. Local publication of sanitary reports, 119. § 22. ... necessary to remove current fallacies, 120.

CHAP. THIRD.—INVESTIGATION OF EPIDEMICS.

§ 1. Our ignorance thereon, 122. §§ 2 and 3. Certain conditions of inquiry and qualifications of inquirers—course taken by Board of Health, 123.

§ 4. Effects of pestilence upon research, 125. § 5. Board-of-Health inquiry in 1849, *ib.* § 6. Registrar-General and Dr. Farr—law of altitude, 126. § 7. College of Physicians and Dr. Baly, 127. § 8. law of aggregation, 128. ... not affected by a late observation, 129. § 9. Personal communicability of cholera, 130. § 10. Board of Health refuted, *ib.* § 11. Course adopted in 1854, better, yet incomplete, 131. § 12. Want of registration of sickness, ... 132. § 13. Objects of Epidemiological Society, ... 133. § 14. ... intended to supersede State action—mistakes and failures, 134. § 15. International Congress at Paris—its programme for inquiry, 135. § 16. Need for verification of facts, 136. § 17. Existence of three orders of investigators, 137. § 18. Sir John Herschel's rules, *ib.*

ESSAY IV.

MEDICAL CARE OF THE POOR. PART I.—HISTORICAL.

CHAP. FIRST.—FROM THE REFORMATION TO 1827.

§ 1. Mediæval provision, 141. § 2. Separation of medicine from the ecclesiastical office, 142. § 3. Legislation under Henry VIII.—Diocesan medical licences, 143. § 4. Establishment of College of Physicians, 144. § 5. Diminished number of practitioners, and their higher demands, 145. § 6. No public medical provision, 147. § 7. Statute of Elizabeth, 148. § 8. Plan of John Bellers, 149. § 9. Institution of Hospitals, T. Guy, 150. § 10. Statute of 1790, 151. § 11. Rise of parish medical contracts, 153. § 12. Growth of pauperism, 154. § 13. Efforts of Kerrison and Burrows, 155. § 14. Plans of Dunn, Yeatman, &c., 156. § 15. Warwickshire committee of inquiry, 157.

CHAP. SECOND. — RISE AND PROGRESS OF SELF-SUPPORTING SCHEMES OF MEDICAL RELIEF.

§ 1. Mr. H. L. Smith and the Warwickshire committee, 158. § 2. Benefit society arrangements, *ib.* § 3. Self-supporting dispensaries ...... 160. § 4. their defects and results, 161.

CHAP. THIRD.—FROM 1838 TO 1842.

§ 1. Limited scope of government inquiries, 163. § 2. ... and of official views, 164. § 3. Aggravation of former evils—i. tenders—ii. large districts—iii. reduction of medical staff—iv. diminution of aid—v. medical clubs, 165—169. § 4. Defence of Commissioners, 170. § 5. Reasons for noticing controversy, 171. § 6. Parliamentary inquiry, 1838, Mr. Wakley, 172. § 7. Counter inquiry by Commissioners, 173. § 8. Sir T. N. Talfourd, 175. § 9. ... his measure, 176. § 10. General medical order of 1842—its provisions and their deficiencies, 177—180.

CHAP. FOURTH.—PROSPECTS OF SANITARY LEGISLATION UNDER THE POOR-LAW BEFORE 1844.

§ 1. Causes of committal of sanitary functions to Poor-Law Boards, 181. § 2. Vaccination Acts—1840 and 1841—dilemma of authorities, 182. § 3. "General Sanitary Report"—1842—official recommendations of a poor-law machinery, 185. § 4. Prospects not fully realized, 187.

CHAP. FIFTH.—FROM 1842 TO 1850.
§ 1. Mr. Guthrie's movement—Lord Ashley, 188. § 2. Parliamentary inquiry, 1844, 189. § 3. weak points in the mover's case, 191. § 4. Plan of provincial delegates, 192. § 5. Dilemma of Committee and the results, 193. § 6. Sir R. Peel's measure, 1846, 194. § 7. General order, 1847, 195. § 8. Renewed agitation—Lord Shaftesbury's propositions, 196. § 9. Medical inspectors, 197. § 10. Convention of Medical Officers, 198. § 11. Spread of larger views, 200. § 12. Second cholera visitation—administrative difficulties—medical sacrifices, 201.

CHAP. SIXTH.—RISE, REVOLUTION, AND PRESENT POSITION OF THE MEDICAL CHARITIES IN IRELAND.
§ 1. Official inquiries before 1851, 204. § 2. acknowledged defects in dispensaries—discussions about their reform, 206. § 3. Views of dispensary surgeons—their support of the Act of 1851—their sufferings in the fever epidemics, 207. § 4. Improvements in administration, 209. § 5. Inconvenient districts—their enormous size, 210. § 6. Grievances of Medical Officers, 212. Dispensary committees, 213. § 7. Supply of nutriment and cordials, 214. § 8. unsuccessful attempts to define the class for relief, 265; and to check its indiscriminate supply, 216. § 9. Mr. Ellis's protest, ib. § 10. Conclusions from the discussion, 217. § 11. Attempt to pauperize the County Infirmaries, 218. § 12. opposition of infirmary surgeons, 219. § 13. Dr. Little's arguments, 220. § 14. Attempts upon fever hospitals, 221. § 15. Danger to independence of poor from official measures, 222. § 16. method of dealing with founders and benefactors, 224. § 17. Failure of last attempt in 1854—threatenings for the future, 225. § 18. Dublin Hospitals, 226. § 19. Parliamentary Committee, 1854— evidence of English surgeons, 227.

CHAP. SEVENTH.—FROM 1853 TO 1855.
§ 1. Medical provision for Bristol poor, 229. § 2. Cholera in 1854 — Dr. Wallis's pamphlet, 230. § 3. Mr. Miles's motion in Parliament, 1853, ib. § 4. Third parliamentary inquiry, 1854, 231. § 5. Report of Committee, 232—234.
Postscript.—Sir G. Nicholl's History of the Poor Laws, 235.

PART II.—THE PRESENT CONDITION AND REQUIREMENTS OF MEDICAL RELIEF—ITS RELATIONS TO POLITICAL ECONOMY AND SANITARY MANAGEMENT.
§ 1. Introductory, 239. I. *Statistics.*—§ 2. Number of officers and size of districts, 240. § 3. salaries, *ib.* § 4. cases of sickness, 241. § 5. comparison with Ireland, 242. § 6. variations, *ib.* II. *Social economy of a Poor-Law provision.*—§ 7. Cotemporaneous fall and rise in pauperism and medical relief, 243. § 8. ... confirmed by local observations, 244. § 9. difference in town and rural districts, 245. § 10. abolition of pauperizing condition, inconsistent with poor-law control, 246. § 11. public healing and teaching, 247. III. *Methods by which the poor obtain the right to medical aid.*— § 12. Orders, recommendations, and tickets objectionable, ... 248.— § 13. danger to life and independence, 249. § 14. defence of orders, &c., 250. —recipient class undefinable, 251. IV. *Proportion of population requiring a public provision.*—§ 15. A more extensive grant safe under a different

system, 252. § 16. moiety of population requires a public provision, 253 ; especially in epidemics, 254. § 17. Safety of a State provision on certain conditions, 255. V. *Self-provision by working classes.* — § 18. primary objects of mutual insurance, 256. § 19. failure of benefit and medical clubs, 257. § 20. Barham Downs' Society, 258. § 21. self-provision to follow the establishment of a State provision, *ib.* VI. *Power of ordering dietetic tonics and personal comforts in sickness.* — § 22. present system, a source of altercation, 259. § 23. ..provision of medical relief to be separated from grant of other relief, 260. § 24. ... present practice, a cause of pauperism, 261. VII. *Provision of medicines.*—§ 25. supply by medical officers, leads to difficulties ... 261. § 26. official discrepancies ... 262. § 27. authorities for a reform ... 263. § 28. precedents for it ... 265. § 29. practicability of a dispensary system, 266—drugs in rural districts, *ib.* § 30. cost of a dispensary provision ... 267. VIII. *Workhouses.* — § 31. a separate provision—sanitary management, 268.—workhouse dispensaries, cost of in-door medical relief ... 269. IX. *Medical charities.*— ¿ 32. ... called upon to diminish the Poor-Law supply, 270. ¿ 33. defects of charitable institutions, 271—conflicting sources of aid, 272. ¿ 34. Want of organization, 273. X. *Inspection of public medical aid.*—¿ 35. Incapacity of present managers, 274—official opinions thereon, 275. ¿ 36. Medical inspection in Ireland ... 276. XI. *Sanitary duties and reports.* — ¿ 37. need of a registration of sickness, 277—waste of skilled labour, 278. ¿ 38. ... preventive duties ... 279. ¿ 39. ... sanitary visitation ... 280. XII. *Medico-Sanitary Officers.*—¿ 40. their qualifications and age, 282. ¿. 41. their number ...... 283 — union with private practice ...... 284. ¿ 42. their remuneration ...... 285 — endowment of districts ...... 286. ¿ 43. payment from a national fund ...... 287. ¿ 44. composition for fees — midwifery .... *ib.* ¿ 45. mode of appointment .... 288. XIII. *Dispensary Committees.* ¿ 46. ... their fourfold constitution ... 289. ¿ 47. their business, 291. *Conclusion.*—¿ 48. Origin of misconceptions, 292. —analogies of medical aid, 293—real cure for present evils, 294.

ESSAY V.

LOCAL SANITARY ADMINISTRATION.

CHAP. FIRST.—OFFICERS OF HEALTH, THEIR PRIMARY DESIGN AND FUNCTION.

§ 1. Recent appointments in England peculiar, 297. § 2. Ancient Health-officers, *ib.* § 3. Roman organization, 298. § 4. Mediæval iatrarchy, 299. § 5. German *Stadt-Arzt*, 300. § 6. Office of *Kreis-physicus*, 301. § 7. *Officiers de Santé*, 303. § 8. Mr. Chadwick's propositions, *ib.* § 9. Clause in Bills of 1845 and 1848, 304 ; General Order of 1851, 305. § 10. Author's "Remarks" in 1848, *ib.*; his inquiry in 1854, 306. § 11. number of provincial Health-officers, *ib.* § 12. their districts, 307. § 13. their means of information, *ib.* § 14. assistance afforded them, 308. § 15. their salaries, *ib.* § 16. duties, 309. § 17. opinions as to separation of duties from private practice, 310. § 18. results of inquiry, 312. § 19. two orders of local officers necessary, 313. § 20. recent legislation for metropolis, 314—questions for M.P.s, 315. § 21. impending difficulties, 316.

CHAP. SECOND.—LOCAL BOARDS. (A). *As they have been and are.*
§ 1. English system of local administration, 317. § 2. *Boards of Guardians.*— Evidence in 1854, *ib.* § 3. official evidence in 1850, 318. § 4. no amendment in 1854, 320. § 5. official evidence; precautionary measures, 321; Houses of Refuge, ib.; house-to-house visitation, 322; medical relief, 323. ¿ 6. causes of defects, *ib.* ¿ 7. original design of these Boards, 324. ¿ 8 replies of provincial Health-officers, *ib.* ¿ 9. claims of Union Boards to consideration, 325. ¿ 10. *Local Boards of Health*, 326; instances of mal-administration, 327. ¿ 11. Composition of Town Boards, 328. ¿ 12. obstructive elements, 329. ¿ 13. Boards of Health in 1831-2, 330. ¿ 14. Town Improvement Commissioners, *ib.* ¿ 15. Limited areas of jurisdiction, 331. ¿ 16. excluded population, 332. ¿ 17. an instance, 334. § 18. restriction of sanitary reform to places with excess of mortality, 334. ¿ 19. New Metropolitan Boards, 335. ¿ 20. division of administrative powers, 336. ¿ 21. defects of Act, 337. ¿ 22. "Nuisances Removal Act," 1855, 338; new local sanitary authorities, 339. ¿ 23. defective legislation, *ib.* ¿ 24. misapprehensions about centralization ... 340. ¿ 25. failure of present system, 341.
(B). *Local Boards as they might be.*—¿ 26. necessity for new bodies, 341. ¿ 27. difficulties created by existing jurisdictions, 342. ¿ 28. Suggestions; districts, 343. ¿ 29. constitution of new bodies, 344. ¿ 30. medical faculties, 345. ¿ 31. duties of proposed courts, 346.

ESSAY VI.

CERTAIN DEPARTMENTS OF HEALTH-POLICE, IN THEIR RELATIONS WITH LOCAL SANITARY ADMINISTRATION.

CHAP. FIRST.—REGISTRATION OF BIRTHS AND DEATHS.
¿ 1. Registrars a class of sanitary agents, 349. ¿ 2. Early view of office, *ib.*; diminished number of medical registrars, 350. ¿ 3. application of registration to sanitary reports, *ib.* ¿ 4. scientific certification ... 351. ¿ 5. scientific superintendence; Officers of Health, 352.

CHAP. SECOND.—MEDICAL EVIDENCE IN FORENSIC INQUIRIES:
§ 1. Characteristic feature of English inquests, 354. § 2. Medical Witnesses Act, 355. § 3. indiscriminate call for medical evidence, *ib.* ¿ 4. unskilful medical testimony, 357. ¿ 5. *Medical Coroners*, 358. ¿ 6. reform of forensic inquiries, 359. § 7. Officer of Health, 360. § 8. minute chemical analyses, *ib.*

CHAP. THIRD.—ADULTERATION OF FOOD, DRINKS, AND MEDICINES.
§ 1. The "Lancet"—Dr. Arthur Hassall, 362. § 2. Parliamentary inquiry, 1855—its origin, 363. § 3. propositions of witnesses, 364. § 4. domestic causes of the evils, untouched ... 365. § 5. Patent medicines ... 366. § 6. application of sanitary machinery, 367.

CHAP. FOURTH.—PUBLIC VACCINATION. A.—*Historical.*
§ 1. Establishment of National Vaccine Board, 368. § 2. Its officers, duties, and reports, 369. § 3. Parliamentary inquiry, 1833, 370. § 4. Present duties of Vaccine Board, 371. § 5. Provincial arrangements, 372. § 6. Lord

Ellenborough's Act, 372. § 7. inconsistency of poor-law connexion, 373.
§ 8. Epidemiological Society, 374. § 9. Lord Lyttelton's Act, 375.
§ 10. its defects, 376. § 11. neglect of providing for supply of lymph, 377.
§ 12. "Three-months" clause, *ib.*—its unpopularity and danger, 378.
§ 13. Vague notions of compulsory vaccination, 379. § 14. proposed exemption from penalty, *ib.* § 15. Registrar's returns .... 380.
B. *Suggestive.*—§ 16. demands for fresh legislation 382. § 17. Epidemiological Society's Bill,—Official Bill, *ib.*—proposed changes of management, 383. inspection, 384. combination with medical care, 385. other clauses, 386. Want of comprehensive legislation, 387. § 18. Objects of Vaccine Board, *ib.* supply of lymph, 388. § 19. London supply insuficient, 389. § 20. two main objects of future legislation ...... 390.
§ 21. provincial vaccine institutions, *ib.* § 22. inspection by Officers of Health, 391. § 23. adaptation of other sanitary machinery ... 392.
§ 24. amended regulations, *ib.* § 25. Registrars of Births, 393.

CHAP. FIFTH.—LOCAL ORGANIZATION OF A CIVIL MEDICO-SANITARY SERVICE.
§ 1. Appointment of Health Officers—defective legislation—recent abuses, 394.
§ 2. Suggestions for the future—competitive examinations ...... 395.
§ 3. objections thereto, 396. § 4. official connexion of Health Officer with medical officers, 397. § 5. cost of organization, *ib.* § 6. National expenditure, 398.

CHAP. SIXTH.—CIRCUIT INSPECTION.
§ 1. Position, numbers, and official relations of Inspectors unsettled—precedents, 399. § 2. duties, 400. § 3. Visitation of medical charities, 401.
§ 4. Conflicts in their management, 402. Public objects of hospitals—need of State interference, 403. § 5. Visitation of Hospitals for the Insane—Commissioners in Lunacy, 404. § 6. Private Asylums .... 405.
§ 7. Visitation by County Magistrates, *ib.* § 8. ... its ill effects, 406.
§ 9. substitution of circuit inspection, 407. § 10. Quarterly reports, *ib.*
§ 11. Number of Inspectors, 408. § 12. Waste of official inspection, 409.
Completion of staff, 410.

SUPPLEMENTARY NOTES.

A. Nurses for the sick Poor, 411.
B. Sir G. C. Lewis's comments on plans for medical aid, 412.
C. Application of mutual assurance to medical aid, 414.
D. Charitable Dispensaries, 415.
E. Medical aid in France and Belgium, 417.
F. Expulsion of Greek physicians from Rome, 420.
G. Conseils d'Hygiène publique, 422.
H. Mr. Estlin and the National Vaccine Board, 423.

ESSAY I.

INTRODUCTORY.

THE OUTLINE OF A SANITARY CODE.

Πολιτικὸν, ἔφη, λέγεις Ἀσκληπιόν. Δῆλον, ἦν δ' ἐγώ . . . . . . Ἆρ' οὐκ ἀγαθοὺς δεῖ ἐν τῇ πόλει κεκτῆσθαι ἰατρούς ; εἶεν δ' ἄν που μάλιστα τοιοῦτοι, ὅσοι πλείστους μὲν ὑγιεινοὺς, πλείστους δὲ νοσώδεις μετεχειρίσαντο.—PLATO. *De Repub.* lib. iii.

INTRODUCTORY ESSAY.

CHAPTER FIRST.

PRELIMINARY.

HAD it been my intention, in the following pages, to treat methodically of all the various matters pertaining to the care of the Public Health, for which either the enactment of special laws, or the delegation of discretionary power to constitutional authorities, has been found necessary in this and other countries,—I should, both as regards matter and arrangement, have drawn more or less from some of the most approved treatises, chiefly German and French, which have been published within the last eighty years* on the continent; for, to say the truth, this subject has never been systematically† written upon in England.

Or, had I wished to describe in detail the most successful methods of effecting a few sanitary objects, special in kind and limited in application, I should have examined the measures now in progress in certain cities and towns, at home and abroad; I should have compared these, not merely with some of the public works and municipal regulations of ancient times, but also with those other more appropriate and practicable

---

* Johann Peter Frank's classical work on *Medicinische Polizei*, commenced publication in 1779.

† The nearest approach to a system of Medical Police—and the first attempt, I believe of the kind—in this country, was the large work on *Medical Jurisprudence*, by Dr. Paris and Mr. Fonblanque, in 1823. But by far the larger portion of that treatise is occupied with that department of Medical Police, to which we now restrict the term—Medical Jurisprudence.

projects, suggested in the many pamphlets and reports on sanitary affairs, which have deluged this country during the last twenty years.

My design is, however, of a more elementary character, as regards this introductory Essay; and, in some respects, of a more temporary nature, as regards the subjects considered in the following Essays.

In the first place, I wish to draw attention to the UNITY OF STATE MEDICINE; and to point out the connexion, legislative and administrative, which ought to exist between its several departments; and partly, also, to induce those whose leisure, scholarship, and opportunities for research, qualify them specially for such a task, to bring before English readers a correct account of the rise, progress, and present condition of medical and sanitary police in Europe.*

Secondly and mainly, I am anxious to show the singular absence of comprehensive design which has characterized all attempts at legislation in this country, whenever circumstances or events have imposed on Government and Parliament the necessity of adopting measures, either for preserving the health and diminishing the sickness of the people, or for regulating the education and duties of the medical profession.

"Medical polity," said Niemann,† "is a necessity for every State. Hence, in some nations, laws and regulations for the improvement of the Public Health were in existence *before those nations brought the principles of such laws into scientific combination.*"

England is almost the only great European State still in this anomalous position.

So little indeed have our countrymen considered the subject as a whole, that in the rare event of its being referred to, the

---

* Have any of the Travelling Fellows of our old Universities employed their ample means and opportunities thus usefully?

† *Taschenbuch der Staats-Arzneiwissenschaft.* Leipzig, 1828, § 7.

question is probably asked, "What is the meaning of State Medicine?"

To this question, which has often been put to myself, I would now reply; not by endeavouring to define State Medicine with logical accuracy, and in a sentence or two, but by stating in order what appear to me to be its principal constituents, and their mutual relationships.

Without following any of the systems of arrangement which are to be found in French works on *Hygiène Publique*, or in German systems of *Medicinal Polizei*, or *Staats-Arzneikunde*; without attempting to make a philosophical classification of the details of State Medicine; and without professing even to specify every requisite particular, I venture to offer a new scheme of STATE AGENDA, for promoting the physical welfare of the people at large.

This scheme may show, I hope, the intimate, and not safely separable, connexion of its several divisions.

It is almost needless to explain, that many English expressions, relating to places, territorial areas, institutions, office and regulations, are often used in what follows, although the sanitary arrangements which they are intended to designate, may not exist in this country at the present time.

This introductory Essay is, in fact, but little more than a *catalogue raisonné* of Public Hygiene. It may, I fear, prove somewhat dry and insipid to the literary Sybarite, who cannot relish a grave and difficult subject, unless it be served up in dainty style, seasoned with Attic salt, and garnished with illustrative anecdote. But, it is my earnest hope, that all who take a real and hearty interest in this, the most momentous subject of the day, as regards the internal policy of the nation, will not hesitate to follow me through these details, nor have reason to regret the time devoted to their perusal, even though they may sometimes differ from the opinions of the writer.

The outline of a Sanitary Code, traced in the succeeding chapters of this Essay, may also serve as a normal project, a theoretical standard, by which to test some of those errors, anomalies, and short-comings of English sanitary legislation and management, which will have to be noticed in subsequent Essays.

The Agenda of a State with regard to the Public Health may, I believe, be advantageously comprised in three great divisions :—

I. In relation to subjects concerning which the State should direct INVESTIGATION.
 Whether these be—
   A. Statistical.
   B. Topographical.
   C. Jurisprudential.

II. In relation to PRACTICAL ARRANGEMENTS for the personal safety and health of the people, requiring for their enforcement either direct or legislative enactments, or local institutions and regulations.
 These may be subdivided into—
   A. Preventive, and
   B. Palliative, measures.

III. In relation to the establishment by law, of an ORGANIZED MACHINERY for carrying into effect the aforesaid inquiries, for deliberation and advice on special arrangements and emergencies, and for the administration of existing laws.
 And this would comprehend—
 A. The education of medical men, and the qualification of other technical, scientific, and administrative agents.
 B. The institution of official authorities—Boards and Offices—for central and local superintendence and action.

Before proceeding, I would explain that, in the following scheme, the terms *law* and *legislation* are used, not only for the enactments of a constitutional legislature, and the decrees of a monarchy, but, also, for such decisions and orders of central, provincial, and local authorities, as are invested, by the supreme Civil power, with the force of law.

CHAPTER SECOND.

DIVISION I. — SUBJECTS CONCERNING WHICH THE STATE SHOULD DIRECT INVESTIGATION.

Subdivision A.—Statistics.

§ 1. *Statistics of Population.*—A CENSUS of the people may be either annual or triennial, as in Austria and Prussia; or quinquennial, as in France; or decennial, as in the British Isles: but it should be taken at uniform intervals, and always on the same day of the year. It should distinguish the sexes: it should show the distribution of the inhabitants, in territorial divisions, whether in provinces, counties, districts, parishes, towns, or public institutions: it should note the precise increase or decrease of the population in each and all of these divisions: it should inquire into the alleged or apparent causes of such changes: it should record as accurately as possible the ages of the inhabitants: it should distinguish strangers or immigrants from the natives of each locality or district: it should be the medium of information relating to the civil or conjugal condition of all adults: it should show the occupations of all engaged in business, in bodily labour, or in strictly mental pursuits: it should record the number of families and of persons dependent for support on the heads of families: it should state the number of sick persons at home or in hospitals; also of the infirm, blind, deaf, dumb, insane, idiotic, or permanently helpless: it should report the number of persons maintained or secluded by the State (paupers and prisoners) with the age and sex of each: and it should distinguish, as far as possible, that class of the community which, while just able to procure the necessaries of existence, is incapable of providing against casualties, or for the prevention and relief of disease, or for the instruction of their children, or for the maintenance of public religious worship.

§ 2. *Statistics of Mortality.*—In collecting and recording facts relating to mortality, the duties of the State are threefold.

First,—A correct registration should be made of the time, the place, and, according only to medical certification, the cause of death; together with the age, sex, condition, occupation, and birthplace* of each deceased person.

Secondly,—The facts thus obtained should be compiled, abstracted, and published in the form of mortality tables. In crowded districts these tables should be issued weekly or monthly; in provinces and kingdoms, quarterly or annually. Local mortality returns should always refer to precisely the same districts of territory as are adopted for the census returns and for sanitary administration.†

Thirdly,—The conclusions to be drawn from these tables should be stated systematically, in a report, showing the rates of mortality in regard to sex, age, occupation, or position in society; and in regard to locality, as modified by climate, natural position, and density of population, during successive seasons, and especially during times of prevalent disease or of famine.

§ 3. *Statistics of Reproduction.*—Under this head the law should enforce and regulate—

First,—The registration of every *marriage*, with the ages, position in life, and birthplaces* of the persons married:

Secondly,—The registration of every *birth*, stating the place and time of birth, and the sex of the infant, distinguishing illegitimate births; and with regard to all legitimate births, recording the residence, age, occupation, and birthplace* of both parents. Still-born children should be registered separately:

Thirdly,—The compilation, abstract, and publication of the records of marriages and births, in connexion with the before-named mortality tables, in the same territorial divisions and at the same times.

* Birthplace where practicable. † See B. I. p. 12.

Considered physically, the main object of a correct civil registration of births, deaths, and marriages is, to aid in disclosing *the causes of disease*. Considered legally, the object is to provide the means of tracing descent and proving personal identity. And considered politically, it is to assist the Government in arriving at correct conclusions with regard to measures of internal economy, taxation, employment, and commerce.

As the world no longer affords an instance of the unanimous agreement of the people of any one country for one form of religion, Governments can no longer prudently leave the registration of births, deaths, and marriages solely to the ministers of the State religion, if there be one. But, the greatest care should be taken, in carrying out a merely civil registration, to avoid anything like disrespect towards those sacred rites and solemnities, which, however varied the forms in different Christian countries, hallow alike man's entrance upon this stage of existence, his departure from it, and his fulfilment of the divinely appointed condition for the succession of his race.

§ 4. *Statistics of Sickness, Accidents, and Infirmity.*—It has been assumed, somewhat too hastily, that facts of this kind cannot be collected, fully and accurately, by public authority without infringing on private rights and social proprieties.

But, at all events, the census of population would show the total number of the sick, the hurt, and the infirm; whilst more precise information on the subject could at all times be obtained amongst those classes of society, which owe, as it were, such information to the public. And as the numerical ratio which these classes bear to the whole population is known, some estimate, with the aid of mortality returns, might be formed respecting the sanitary state of the entire population.

Moreover, by placing the members of the Medical Faculty in a more correct relation with the State, a still nearer approximation to truth might readily be obtained, especially in times of unusual sickness.

The public registration of diseases and injuries should include particulars respecting their connexion, in different cases, with occupation, social neglect, or mismanagement, personal habits, natural and artificial peculiarities of locality; with climate, weather, and season; and with the density, grouping, and migration of the population.

This department of registration should also contain full and correct details relating to epidemic visitations, noting all the circumstances connected with the origin, advent, propagation, and decline of zymotic diseases.

§ 5. *Statistics of Dwellings.*—Each census of the population should record the number of inhabited and uninhabited houses in every territorial subdivision; the number of connected and of isolated dwellings; the annual rated value of each house; its construction, height, cubic space, state of drainage and water-supply.

A public registration should be kept of all buildings in a state of dilapidation, dangerous or incommodious to the public; and should note every instance of the injury or destruction of houses by fire.

§ 6. *Statistics of Food.*—Under this head, the law should enforce inquiries of various kinds.

First, *as regards produce*, the subject connects itself with agriculture, and includes the periodical record of facts relating to the nature and amount of vegetable products, whether in field or garden, and whether intended for the nourishment of man, or of animals, or for the facture of fermented drinks.

These agricultural statistics should also contain accurate information respecting all morbid conditions of grains, roots, and other important parts of plants; the invasions of what may be called *Epiphytic* diseases;* and the prevalence of destructive or pestiferous insects.

---

* The word "*Epiphytic*," in botany, has hitherto been applied to those insects which attach themselves temporarily to plants, as distinguished from those which are *parasitic*, and which feed on the structures they inhabit.

But the word may be very properly applied to that class of diseases of the vege-

Secondly, *the consumption of food** bears more directly on the health and nutrition of the people. Accurate information respecting the quantity, the nature, and the quality of the food sold for consumption in every district, should be collected and registered at all times; inasmuch as on particular and unforeseen occasions, such statistics are exceedingly important. The effects of different kinds of aliment on large masses of the population, especially on the inmates of all public establishments, should be carefully observed and recorded in every district.

Measures—hereafter to be noticed†—are necessary for the scientific inspection of whatever is sold for human food or beverage, and for the detection of falsification and deterioration in various alimentary substances.

On this point, statistical inquiries also should be invariably carried on, and the results published, in order to show the extent to which articles of food, which are more or less unfit for use, are offered for sale in each district.

§ 7. *Statistics of Animal Life.* — For obtaining accurate statistics relating to animal life, a periodical census should be taken of all the more important domestic or gregarious animals which are bred, either for labour or for human food, and which are as a general rule included in the agricultural term,—" live stock."

The condition and growth of these animals, their increase or decrease, and their diseases of all kinds (sporadic and epizoötic) should be accurately registered in every district.

The effects of different kinds of food, whether cereal, vegetable, or manufactured, upon the nutrition of these animals, should be also recorded, especially with reference to the development of

table kingdom, which resembles the *Epizoötics* of the lower animals, and the *Epidemics* of the human race.

Since the above was written, I observe that the word *Epiphytic* has been used in the sense I propose, by the Statistical Congress lately held at Paris.

* As the quantity of food consumed in the country equals the sum of the quantities produced and imported, minus that exported, the *total* consumption of the State is easily reckoned.

† See II. A. 5. pp. 22, 23.

their osseous, fibrous, and fatty tissues. Such observations—if carried on systematically in different districts, where the soil, the temperature, and the climate are more or less varied—would form a very important element of sanitary investigation; but they could be conducted only by those who are thoroughly instructed in comparative physiology and pathology, and should therefore be entrusted solely to the more scientific members of the veterinary profession.*

Subdivision B.—*Topographical Inquiries and Meteorological Records.*

§ 1. As the physical geography of a district is intimately connected with the health, vigour, and longevity of its inhabitants, correct topographical data should form the basis of all local inquiries.

Certain permanent features of each district should be recorded, after a thorough scientific survey, under Government direction.

The elevation of every portion of the surface should be shown, by contour-lines, on a large and clear map, together with the current, fall, and average volume of brooks and rivers; and the various stratifications and composition of the soil.

A copy of this tabular record should be accessible for reference in every town and parish of the district it describes.†

The extent of surface comprised in each map should depend mainly on the natural features of the locality, but partly on its population, area, and legal divisions.

Hills and valleys, lakes and fens, rivers and coasts, are nature's landmarks, and to these man should adapt the limits of his local efforts at self-preservation.

* "A watchful and considerate Government, provident for the future, never allows sweeping Epidemics, or infectious diseases, among our domestic animals, to devastate the land without accurate scrutiny; and to the aid of Government come well educated veterinary surgeons, bringing to the task sagacity and experience."—On the Variola Ovis, *Companion to British Almanack*, 1849, p. 87.

† The popular uses of *Parish Maps* have been well described in a pamphlet under this title, by the late Mr. C. R. Walsh.

The boundaries of cities and boroughs, parishes, districts, and counties, are secondary considerations.

§ 2. Chemical analysis of the various soils, and of the water-springs, wells, and rivers, belonging to each district, should be made and recorded, at certain intervals, by scientific officers.

Still more frequent notice and report would be required in regard to the condition of small streams, stagnant waters, and marshes, and their periodical variations; the impediments, always on the increase, to natural drainage; the progress of artificial drainage, the recovery of waste and marsh lands, and the conservation and improvement of watercourses.

§ 3. The changes of climate, seasons, and weather—(meteorological observations), should be recorded in every district by Government authority and regulation.

It is utterly impossible to draw any satisfactory conclusions respecting either epidemic visitations, or variations in the rate of sickness and mortality, without constant registration of the temperature, pressure, tension, elasticity, humidity, motion, electricity, and ozone of the atmosphere. These conditions should therefore be carefully registered, together with notices of storms, quantity of rain, force and direction of winds, and the rarer cosmical phenomena.

Subdivision C.—Judicial Investigations—Forensic Medicine.

§ 1. In all civilized communities, certain institutions or ordinances are necessary for the purpose of instituting legal inquiries into the causes of deaths occurring under doubtful circumstances. These institutions will vary according to national character and habits; but a well ordered and complete system of mortality registration will always render important aid in such inquiries.

Whatever may be the form or constitution of the legal court, provision should always be made, for securing scientific evidence from medical officers of superior skill and experience in the following events. (*a*) In cases of apparent death. (*b*) In instances of suspected poisoning, with further provision for scientific analyses, chemical and microscopical, when required. (*c*) In cases of death by drowning, hanging, or suffocation, by the inhalation of noxious gases, by lightning-stroke, by starvation, or by cold. (*d*) In cases of death from wounds, injuries, burns, and scalds. (*e*) In cases of supposed infanticide. (*f*) In cases of alleged rape. (*g*) In cases where the loss of life is attributed to the severity of corporal punishment inflicted on offenders under legal sentence.

§ 2. Judicial inquiry is often required in questions relating to *personal disqualification*.

These investigations should always be aided by competent medical evidence, of an official, rather than of a casual character.

Persons may be disqualified—either for self-control, or for social, civil, or military duties—by mental, moral, or physical infirmities, by extreme youth or old age. In certain cases, such disqualification may be feigned by healthy and qualified persons.

Insanity and bodily incapacity may, in ordinary cases, be determined by medical examination, and pronounced upon by medical certificate. But for such inquiries, legal directions and selected inquirers are necessary.

§ 3. Questions of *succession* to property, of *survivorship*, of *personal identity*, and of *pregnancy*, often involve medical and obstetrical evidence, for which legal provision should be made. All these matters of inquiry need specially trained and experienced medical referees.

CHAPTER THIRD.

DIVISION II.—ON THOSE ARRANGEMENTS FOR THE PERSONAL SAFETY AND HEALTH OF THE PEOPLE, WHICH REQUIRE, FOR THEIR ENFORCEMENT, DIRECT ENACTMENTS OR LOCAL REGULATIONS, WITH THE INFLICTION OF PENALTIES FOR THEIR NON-OBSERVANCE.

Subdivision A.—Measures for the Prevention of Disease.

IN the first division of State *Agenda*, contained in the preceding chapter, vital statistics were placed before topographical records.

But in detailing and defining practical measures of prevention, I propose to reverse that order, and to consider, in the first place, those arrangements which apply to localities and dwellings.

§ 1. *Localities.*—Whenever it may be proved that any place or district is destructive to the life and health of its inhabitants—that no public works for its improvement have availed or are likely to avail to render it safely habitable, and that its occupation is not indispensable either for national defence or for securing the necessaries of life—the law should peremptorily interfere, and compel the abandonment of such locality.

In districts also where permanently unhealthy influences are confined to a very limited area, the erection of dwelling-houses should be prohibited; and the extension of towns in the direction of sources of malaria should be strictly forbidden.

At the same time, the law should enforce all known expedients for improving the natural condition of those malarious spots, the pernicious influence of which may be perceptible at great distances, especially during the prevalence of certain winds.

The straightening and deepening of the channels of navigable rivers, especially at their deltas and mouths; the drainage of low lands, marshes, and swamps in the vicinity of towns and navigable rivers, and the removal of all impediments, whether natural or artificial, to the course of streams, are duties imperative on all communities.

Where, in obedience to general and inevitable laws for the welfare of society, man is compelled to inhabit unhealthy districts and small areas of local poison,—and where all possible means have been adopted for the removal of natural defects; certain palliative measures, to be described hereafter, should be brought into full action.

§ 2. *Construction of Buildings.*—The construction of houses and the choice of dwelling-places, whether in towns or villages, cannot be safely left either to mere caprice or to the commercial theory of supply and demand.

It has been truly said that, in crowded districts, where the lower orders are neglected and life is cheaply estimated, if tubs were ticketed "to be let," they would soon be tenanted by the most wretched.

Legal interference is therefore necessary on the following points:—

(*a*) The occupation of such cottages, huts, cellars, or parts of houses, as are ruinous or otherwise unsafe to the inmates or neighbours, or as are incompatible with habits of common decency, should be absolutely *prohibited*.

With reference to the external form and position of dwelling-houses:—

(*b*) Builders should be required to take precautions against exhalations of the soil, by providing for the removal of its natural moisture and for the circulation of air through the foundations of the structure built upon it.

(*c*) The height of houses should be limited with relation to the width of the thoroughfares which they face.

(*d*) On no pretext whatever should houses be permitted to join on more than two of their sides.

(e) Regulations are necessary with regard to the materials of which houses are built; such only being permitted, in towns especially, as are not easily destructible, or hazardous to the inmates or neighbours.

With reference to the internal arrangements of buildings :—

(f) The law should prescribe a certain thickness of walls, according to their height, material, and contiguity with other property; a hard and level surface of cottage ground-floors, and their thorough under-drainage; a safe construction of fire-places, chimneys, and flues; a *minimum* of cubic space proportioned to the number of families or persons to be accommodated, and a *minimum* of height for dwelling-rooms.

(g) Plans for securing good ventilation, water supply, closet accommodation, and drainage should also be enforced in the erection of all new houses.

(h) The regulations named under heads *f* and *g*, are specially necessary in the case of cellars, or underground dwellings; which, indeed, should be prohibited in ground not at present built upon; and which should be permitted in existing towns and buildings, only on condition that a surrounding area of proper dimensions should be sunk below the under-ground floor.

As regards streets and open places :—(i) a *minimum* width should be invariably required for all new streets, together with a *minimum* extent of open space within blocks of houses, proportioned to the number, size, and height of the buildings enclosing it.

(k) The law should facilitate the opening of thoroughfares through closed courts and alleys; the clearing away of buildings in ill-contrived, neglected, and filthy neighbourhoods; and the removal of all impediments to street-ventilation.

(l) Open spots in or near to towns should be preserved free from the intrusion of building speculators, and should be set apart for the growth of vegetation, and as spaces for exercise.

(m) In all old towns, provisions should be made for distributing the population more widely.

(n) Special regulations, varying according to the nature and objects of each establishment, require to be enforced in the construction of all buildings intended to be inhabited by communities, whether for the gain of a proprietor or for objects of public utility.

Careful structural arrangements are especially demanded in lodging-houses, whether for vagrants and poor travellers, or for bodies of resident artisans ; in asylums, almshouses, workhouses, prisons, and schools.

§ 3. *Purification of Buildings and Towns.*—The chief features of a permanent and legalized system of local purification are as follows :—

(a) *Removal of Nuisances.*—The law should interfere to secure the speedy removal, from towns and houses, of all animal and vegetable refuse—all that we understand by the expressive term "nuisances."

It may be often important to decide whether a particular matter of complaint be really a "nuisance." For this decision, in doubtful cases, official medical inspection and certificate are necessary ; but in ordinary cases, the information of intelligent surveyors or policemen would suffice.

In removing nuisances, and in abolishing or clearing out ancient receptacles of animal remains, or any kind of refuse, the law should enforce provisions for safety, by regulating the times and modes of conducting such operations, and the scientific application of deodorizers and disinfectants.

Some specific "nuisances" would come under the head of insalubrious occupations.*

The powers vested in local authorities, with respect to removal of nuisances, should be ample, and their execution prompt. The cost should be speedily recoverable from either the occupier or the owner of the premises on which the nuisance exists ; but where this proceeding would be oppressive, the charge should be made on the public fund of the place or district.

(b) *Water-supply.*—Provision should be made for a constant

* See p. 25, II. A. 7, *f.*

MEASURES OF PURIFICATION.

supply of fresh and pure water, to be derived from the least objectionable source in the neighbourhood,—careful scientific analysis being required in all cases before the selection of a source.

When their purity can be scrupulously preserved, rivers will generally be found the best sources of water-supply.*

The current of water through aqueducts and service-pipes, should be always flowing at a pressure sufficiently high to raise it above the tops of the houses to be supplied.

The house-supply of water should not be permitted to be retained in cisterns, nor to run to waste so as to sop and drench the soil by a worse than useless profusion.

The town-supply should also be sufficient for other public purposes, as the cleansing of pavements, the extinction of fires, and the demands of industrial enterprize.

(c) *Drainage and Sewerage.*—A well-ordered system of house-closets and sinks should be instituted for connecting the pure-water house-pipes with the foul-water house-drains; in analogy with the structure of the human body, where the capillaries connect the arteries with the veins.†

The main sewerage of towns, in connexion with the drainage of houses, should be planned and conducted by skilful and experienced civil engineers, on the principle of combining strength and impermeability of structure with a scientific adaptation of the capacity, shape, and fall of drains and sewers to the volume of fluid, which they are intended to convey, in a rapid and equable current.

The law should enforce such a prolongation of main sewers, as

---

* The English Board of Health has, however, adduced excellent reasons for "gathering grounds" in proper soils, of sufficient extent for the formation of reservoirs large enough to hold the required amount of water.

† In some communities, especially on the continent, there exist different plans and regulations for accomplishing the objects of town and house drainage. I have been struck with the advantage of some arrangements of this kind, including the application of town refuse to agricultural purposes, which exist in a few of the larger towns of Belgium. I have, however, recommended in the text that system only, which, in this country, has met with most approval.

would carry their contents to depôts at a safe distance from human habitations, without contaminating rivers and water-courses. No system of town purification should be sanctioned by law, which does not admit of the products of sewerage being ultimately applied to agriculture.

(*d*) *Pavements.*—Uniform regulations for securing the smooth and hard pavement of all foot-ways and alleys, and for maintaining an even and durable surface in all carriage-ways and streets, are indispensable to an efficient system of town-cleansing.

All surface water should be directed into subterranean channels large enough to carry off the most copious and sudden rain-falls. These channels, wherever possible, should be carefully separated from the system of drains connected with the houses.

(*e*) *Smoke Nuisance.*—Defilement of the atmosphere by smoke should be prevented in towns where coal is the staple fuel. Such prohibition should at once apply to all public, commercial, and industrial establishments;[*] and scientific invention may soon justify legal interference with regard to the products of coal consumption, even in private houses.

Many of the public improvements and sanitary arrangements, mentioned in the preceding sections, are of a permanent character, and require for their completion a large outlay of capital.

When the beneficial effects of any such improvements are not confined to the owners of the property improved, the cost should be borne by national or public funds. And where the benefits of such improvements are strictly local, the cost should be distributed over many years.

For the most durable and expensive works of this class—aqueducts and water-works especially[†]—a century is probably not too long a period to be allowed to proprietors of land and inhabitants of towns, for the ultimate repayment of the original

---

[*] This subject will again be mentioned under the head of "occupations."

[†] The term of thirty years, allowed by the English Public Health Act, is by no means sufficient. It has doubtless tended greatly to impede the execution of the law.

outlay; and this might be advanced either out of State funds or by capitalists on legal security. As a general rule, the nation can bank most profitably for itself.

§ 4. *Healthy Progeny.*—Legislation is required for the purpose of promoting the healthy succession and development of the human race.

1. (*a*) The question has been raised, whether the wilful transmission of personal or hereditary disease by marriage, should be made an illegal and therefore a punishable act. I venture no opinion on so doubtful a point. The people should, at all events, be supplied with able advisers on this and on other matters hereafter to be mentioned.

(*b*) There can be no doubt, however, that the State should do its utmost to ensure the safety of mothers and their offspring, especially during the period of parturition, by requiring that all practitioners in midwifery, and nurses, be thoroughly educated and properly qualified.

(*c*) The State should also provide for the care of indigent parturient women and new-born children; firstly, by promoting the establishment of *Lying-in-Hospitals*, and *Orphan Asylums*, and, to a limited extent, *Foundling Institutions;* and secondly, by appointing, at the public cost, competent midwives for attendance on the poorest class of women, at their own houses.

(*d*) In all such matters, the State should avail itself, as far as possible, of private and associated benevolent efforts: not omitting its duty, at the same time, as the trustee and guardian of all public institutions, even when charitably founded.

2. The intervention of legal authority is of the greatest importance in promoting the healthful training of the young:—

(*e*) By checking, if not prohibiting, the employment in factories of mothers having young children;

(*f*) By limiting strictly the age at which children can be engaged or indentured in factories and workshops;

(*g*) By regulating the number of hours during which they can be employed, according to their age;

(*h*) By frequent and independent medical inspection and report concerning their physical condition and growth, whilst so employed;

(*i*) By forbidding absolutely the employment of children in mines, chimney sweeping, and other equally injurious occupations;

(*k*) By restrictions upon mental exercise, long confinement, and vehement competition, in schools;

(*l*) By securing, under legal compulsion, the proper site, construction, ventilation, drainage, and water-supply of all buildings occupied by young people of every grade;

(*m*) By special regulations as to the diet, clothing, education, and general management of those children who are under the immediate guardianship of the public.

§ 5. *The Sale of Food.*—(*a*) All manufactories and places for the sale of articles intended for aliment or refreshment, should be legally liable to visitation, without previous notice, by properly qualified persons, holding office in every district: and legal provision should be made for the chemical and microscopical analysis of all suspected articles. When any such articles are proved to be detrimental to life and health—should the evil arise from decay, decomposition, or adulteration—they should be destroyed; and penalties should be inflicted on the vendors.

(*b*) The production, importation, and manufacture of those articles which are known to be injurious, even in their purest state, unless taken in very small quantities (but which cannot and ought not to be wholly prohibited), should be subjected to rigorous control and inspection; and their consumption would be rightly checked by taxation.

(*c*) A well-organized system of sanitary police is required for the prevention and detection of abuses, especially in the following transactions:—

> The sale of adulterated bread or biscuits, whether home-manufactured or imported.
> The sale of diseased or tainted meat, fish, game, and poultry.
> The sale of damaged grain, flour, and farinaceous food of all

kinds; as well as of decayed or diseased vegetables, roots, and fruits, whether of home production or imported.

The manufacture of confectionary, preserves, perfumery, sauces, pickles, sausages, &c.

The importation and sale of all groceries of foreign produce, as tea, coffee, sugar, &c.

(*d*) The mode of feeding animals intended for the butcher, and the condition of the places in which they are kept before slaughter, are matters of deep concern to the community.

To secure the purity and wholesomeness of milk, the stabling of cows in populous districts should be subject to regulations as to cleanliness and ventilation; and the health of the animals should be watched. In these inquiries, also, skilled inspection is necessary.

(*e*) In a rightly organized and educated community, legislation would be directed to the prevention of intemperance generally; and prohibition of a more positive and summary kind would apply to the needless use of ardent spirits.

Some provision, too, would be made for the surveillance and control of habitual drunkards, by whom the peace and safety of society are, in fact, endangered, as much as by insane persons and certain other offenders, with whose personal liberty the laws of every civilized country interfere.

(*f*) By a wise adjustment of indirect taxation, it is both practicable and expedient, on the one hand, to check the use of such articles of food and drink as are proved to be decidedly injurious; and, on the other hand, to promote the consumption of those articles which are known to be most conducive to the health and vigour of man.

But fiscal regulations of this kind ought to vary according to the different conditions of life, the multifarious employments, and the varieties of locality, season, and climate, to which the people are subject.

(*g*) Certain notions of political economy, prevalent in some countries, seriously interfere with correct legislation on this question. But no theoretical views should be allowed to release any State from a duty incumbent on all governments—namely, to provide for the instruction of all classes, working people especially, in those maxims of health preservation which relate to the choice and preparation of food.

§ 6. *The Sale of Medicines and Poisons.**—(*a*) Imported drugs should be subjected to inspection and analysis before their delivery to manufacturing and wholesale druggists.

Certain articles intended for medicine, whether herbs grown and collected in the country, or its animal or mineral productions, should be subjected to a similar process of inspection and verification, before being offered to the public.

The purity and genuineness of both these classes of medicines should be certified by a legal stamp.

(*b*) Pharmaceutical laboratories and shops should be liable to visitation at all times by scientific inspectors; and those who keep establishments of this kind, should be required to be properly educated, examined, and licensed.†

(*c*) The sale of secret remedies should be prohibited, unless their composition has been revealed to competent authorities, and approved of by them.

(*d*) The retail sale of powerful medicines or poisons, not prescribed by a medical practitioner, should be either forbidden, or controlled by the strictest regulations.

(*e*) Advertisements of remedies, except in an authorized form, should be absolutely prohibited. The publishers of all newspapers or hand-bills, containing descriptions of symptoms and modes of cure, should be liable to penalties, which should be specially severe if the advertisements be of an indecent or demoralizing tendency.

§ 7. *Other Trades and Occupations.*—All industrial processes and establishments require the control of public law for the

---

* It is worth remembering, that the Greeks applied the same word—φάρμακα—to both medicines and poisons.

† See III. A. 5, p. 44.

safety, not only of those employed, but also of the neighbouring community.

I. (a) In trades and employments connected with building and engineering; workmen and others should .be protected against injuries from sudden accidents caused by defective construction of scaffolding, vaulting, and shoring.

(b) In factories, mines, and workshops; the hours of labour need limitation according to the sex and age of the persons employed. In mines and collieries, no female of any age should be allowed to work.

(c) Workpeople should also be protected against maiming by machinery; against injuries to the eyes; against gaseous emanations and explosions; against the cutaneous absorption and the inhalation of irritating or poisonous particles; against damp; against injuries to particular organs, or undue stress on particular parts of the body.*

(d) Thorough ventilation and purification should be enforced in all work-rooms, mines, and manufactories; and extremes of temperature prevented as far as possible.

(e) The law should insure frequent medical inspection and report, and the provision of prompt surgical aid for accidents, in all factories and mines.

II. (f) Certain arts and manufactures, chemical processes, and commercial establishments, cannot be carried on, in populous districts, without endangering the life and health of residents in the immediate neighbourhood, or at least causing serious public annoyance and inconvenience. Such trades and occupations should, therefore, be banished to prescribed distances from towns, as nuisances of the worst description.†

In this class may be named, manufactories and stores of com-

---

* See a good article on this subject in the *Med. Times and Gaz.*, May 6, 1854.

† A three-fold classification of insalubrious occupations was first made by State authority in France, under Napoleon I.

The regulations were carried into effect by local *conseils de salubrité* and *préfets*, with the sanction of the central government. Dr. Waller Lewis's valuable Report of 1855 gives full information respecting these *ordonnances* in France.

bustible or explosive materials; establishments for the preparation of various substances from animal remains; knackers' yards; collections of town refuse; lay-stalls, and the like.

If it be found impossible to condense or decompose the noxious fumes arising from metallic or mineral-acid works, these establishments should also be classed with the most dangerous processes, and prohibited within such distance from human habitations, as may be legally defined, upon scientific advice.

(*g*) Other factories and trades, although highly objectionable, if recklessly conducted, admit of sufficient modification to justify their being tolerated within the limits of towns, under inspection and regulation, and with proper guarantees that the most approved precautions shall be taken to prevent injury and annoyance.

Slaughter-houses, as a general rule, should be expelled from towns; and *abattoirs* of proper construction established extramurally. All such establishments, especially intramural slaughter-houses, should be subject to constant inspection and control, as regards their water-supply, ventilation, and deodorization, the speedy removal of their offal, and the careful protection of meat for sale.

(*h*) The erection of water-mills and the formation of other mechanical and industrial obstructions to rivers and streams, should not be permitted within inhabited districts; and the law should facilitate the purchase and removal of existing obstructions of this kind.

The owners of factories, and of steam-engines generally, should be compelled either to use fuel which does not discharge smoke, or to take measures for securing the consumption of the products of coal-combustion in their furnaces.

(*i*) The extent to which existing establishments should be subjected to new laws; the modes of procedure against these, and in particular against fresh manufacturing or commercial undertakings of a noxious or offensive character; and the degrees of preventive or corrective power to be vested in local and central authorities, are matters for careful yet decisive legislation.

§ 8. *Locomotion.*—All means of artificial locomotion, both on land and water—whether by steam, or by older mechanical expedients—need the intervention of law, in order to secure the safety and health of voyagers and travellers.

Hence the making and repairing the roads of a country,—the erection and maintenance of bridges, — the construction and ventilation of public conveyances, and especially, arrangements for personal security in railway carriages, — are by no means remotely connected with sanitary police.

Hence, also, the absolute necessity of legal enactments for the safety of navigators and emigrants. The proper sanitary condition of ships should be secured by regulations against overcrowding,—by enforcing a perpetual supply of fresh air between decks, a thorough purification of the hold, a sufficient provision of pure water and wholesome food (vegetables and fresh meat), an adequate supply of medicines and other remedial appliances; and the appointment of qualified medical officers.

§ 9. *Public Amusements and Recreations.* — The pursuits of the people during the intervals of labour or business, affect most deeply the welfare of the State.

If wisely chosen and conducted, they may conduce greatly to the public health, recreating the physical energy, and elevating the moral tone, of the working-classes especially.

If, however, those portions of time, which may be thus usefully spent, are abandoned to the natural operation of degrading influences and debasing associations,—popular sports and pastimes sink in character, causing the degeneration and demoralization of the finest race, and shaking the foundations of good government, civil order, and social happiness.

A wise Legislature will, therefore, studiously interpose on the following points:—

(*a*) Those public amusements, which involve cruelty to man or animals, and are abhorrent to humanity and public decency, are also incompatible with public health and longevity, and should therefore be promptly and vigorously suppressed.

(b) All places of public entertainment require legal control and the enforcement of well-considered regulations, under official supervision.

When they are situated in crowded or unhealthy localities, and during the prevalence of epidemics, sanitary precautions become more urgently necessary; and particularly with reference to the sale, in these places, of unwholesome refreshments and liquors, and the occurrence of sudden alternations of temperature.

(c) Together with a system of scientific ventilation in theatres, provision should be made against casualties, first, by a fire-proof construction of the building; secondly, by securing ample means of egress in cases of accidents or alarm; and thirdly, by limitation of the hours of entertainment.

It will be observed that these suggestions apply with equal force to places of public worship.*

(d) The Government should not only control popular amusements, but should take care to furnish opportunities to the people for innocent and beneficial relaxation.

Parks and gardens, open to the working classes for air and exercise, should be formed in or near all crowded districts. Gymnasia should be established to promote the healthful development of their bodily frames.

Libraries, museums, exhibitions of art, and schools of music, open to the poorer classes, although not directly bearing on physical health, are indirectly of great importance, and should always be promoted by the rulers of a State.

(e) In order to complete administrative arrangements on the subjects mentioned in this and previous sections, it is necessary to organize a proper staff of medical officers, as sanitary visitors, as instructors of the poorer classes in all matters relating to hygiéne, and as detectors of the threatenings as well as of the causes of disease.†

---

* Churches, &c., are not included in the heading of this section, on account of their distinct and sacred character.

† See II. A. 5, h, p 24. II. B. 1, p. 32.

(*f*) Before entering upon another section of this scheme, I cannot altogether omit to notice a delicate and painful subject, regarding which sanitary regulations exist in most civilized countries.

So long as a class of women live by the wages of prostitution, they should be considered as offenders against society and public morality, whom it is proper to place under surveillance;* and this involves systematic inspection and control, both of which are of great importance, not only for the prevention of diseases† of which this unfortunate class are the propagators, but for the diminution and detection of other crimes of which they are often the abettors.

Legal inspection in their case is also humane and expedient, as affording them the means of escape from the perils of their miserable lives.

§ 10. *Public Establishments.* — All institutions in which numbers of people are maintained, demand the most carefully-considered and the best applied sanitary regulations.

Establishments thus requiring legal interference and supervision, may be either—(*a*) Sanative; such as public baths, hospitals, and *sanatoria*:‡ (*b*) Eleemosynary; as almshouses, or *hospitia* for the aged, infirm, and incurable, lodging-houses for poor travellers, orphan and foundling refuges: (*c*) Industrial or reformatory; as workhouses, houses of industry, and penitentiaries: (*d*) Educational; as boarding-schools of different kinds for the various classes of society: (*e*) Penal; as houses of correction, and prisons.

It is almost needless to specify the points on which all these institutions need sanitary regulation; but to obviate any charge of slurring over an important item of this scheme, I would say

---

* See p. 23, II. A. 5, *f*.

† "A disease which a mock morality makes it a very crime to name, but which leaves its base imprint more or less marked on every hundredth babe, at least, born in this great metropolis, and which engrafts a host of maladies on half our Saxon race. This, of all diseases, is most preventible by coercive legislation."— *Journal of Public Health,* 1855, p. 204.

‡ Hospitals for the sick, the hurt, the insane, the infected, and the convalescent, will be noticed more particularly in the next subdivision.

that in addition to general rules as to site,* construction, and means of purification,† provision should be made and enforced for *scientific ventilation*, by an equable and not too rapid circulation of dry, fresh (and in cold weather and cold climates, of warmed) air through every dwelling room, with a continuous withdrawal of the used and impure air; for regulated *exercise* to be taken by the inmates where active employments are not provided; for *diet* adapted to the moral and physical circumstances‡ of the inmates; for *clothing* regulated according to climate, season, and the nature of the building ; for *medicines* of good quality, with trustworthy dispensers ; for *nurses* properly trained and of good character; for *physicians* and *surgeons* to visit the establishment regularly, and to superintend its general sanitary condition.

In all these institutions, the medical superintendents should be skilled in the detection of "malingering," or feigning of disease; and the whole arrangements should be subject to superior medical inspection.

The ARMY and NAVY are not mentioned in this category of national establishments; because they constitute distinct departments of the State, and their health is protected by special medico-sanitary codes.

* The following note has been kindly placed at my disposal, in illustration of this point :—

"The Millbank Penitentiary is, perhaps, as lamentable a specimen as any in England, of the neglect of sanitary precaution in selecting a site for a costly public building. Thirty thousand pounds were laid out in the construction alone of the foundation of this prison. The site is a low marsh, on the banks of the Thames, separated from the river by a narrow causeway. The foundation of the prison is below high-water mark.

"Diarrhœa and dysentery have for years been the pests of the establishment, until at last, after the loss of many lives, injury to the health of a still larger number, and pardon of maimed prisoners, this expensive building is admitted to be unfit for anything but the detention of prisoners for a very short term of confinement. It can no longer be used strictly as a penitentiary."

† See II. A. 1, 2, 3, pp. 15—19.

‡ Whenever classes of persons are taken out of the general population, and congregated in separate establishments, the regulation of diet becomes a more important and difficult question. Food, on which the cottager may work and thrive, will starve the caged pauper and prisoner.

But since we owe the principles and details of many preventive and palliative measures, besides much useful information on general hygiéne—especially as regards climate, foreign and colonial topography—to the war medical departments, the State may at all times derive great advantage from bringing military and naval experience to bear, officially, upon civil sanitary administration.

§ 11. *The Burial of the Dead.*—(*a*) Mortuary interment should be prohibited within the limits of towns; and in or near churches and public buildings of every description, except in rare and specified cases, and under safe and approved precautions.*

(*b*) The right periods and methods of retaining corpses in the dwellings of the living, should be prescribed, and their observance enforced. Reception-houses should be provided, in dense and poor populations, for closed coffins, previous to interment.

(*c*) Special regulations are necessary, as to sites and soils; as to the plans, arrangement, inclosure, surface, and planting of all new cemeteries;—as to the size and depth of graves in every place of burial, varying according to difference of soil and elevation;—together with positive limitations (according to population) as to the number of coffins to be deposited in any one grave. The requirement of a fixed period for the non-disturbance of the ground is likewise necessary, and this would also vary with the nature of the soil.

(*d*) The law should provide decorously for the burial of those who have no means or friends to bear the cost; and should promote simple and cheap, yet reverential, methods of conveying the remains of the poor from towns and crowded districts to extra-mural or rural cemeteries.

(*e*) The families and survivors of the dead often need counsel and protection (especially in deaths from epidemic and contagious

---

* See an able article on the practical application of charcoal to the purposes of burial, in No. 2, *Journal of Public Health*, 1855. The scientific author believes, that, by this expedient, judiciously used, the dissolution of the body may be promoted; and the interment of the dead in greater numbers and frequency, near the habitations of the living, be rendered comparatively innocuous.

disease) as to the disposal of the remains, the use of disinfectants, and the purification of houses.

(*f*) For carrying into effect, or for superintending these regulations, sanitary visitors, before mentioned, are necessary.

Division II.

Subdivision B.—Measures for the Arrest and Palliation of Disease.

Notwithstanding the most efficient application of the most judicious measures of prevention, a certain amount of sickness will ever remain, as the lot of man, to be relieved and mitigated by his fellows.

Certain curative measures should therefore be prescribed and enforced by law.

Firstly:—Under Ordinary Circumstances and at all Times.

§ 1. Medical and surgical attendance should be everywhere supplied, at the cost of a national fund (if there be no local endowments for this purpose), in districts limited as to population and area, and at their own homes, to those classes of the community, which are unable to provide adequately for themselves in this respect.

It may also be deemed expedient to extend the supply of public medical aid to inferior officials* in the civil service.

§ 2. Legal provision for sickness at the houses of the poor, should include a supply of medicines and other remedial appliances from public dispensaries or appointed *pharmaciens ;*† also for the poorest class, efficient nursing, proper diet, cordials, bedding, and clothing, under careful regulation against fraud.

The cost of these provisions should be defrayed by the district or parish ; *i. e.*, by local taxation.

* See III. B. 4, *i.* p. 52.
† The English language supplies no word for a mere scientific compounder of medicines. "Apothecary" has now a larger signification.

§ 3. (*a*) The medical officers appointed for the sanitary superintendence of any of the public institutions before mentioned, (p. 29) should be also responsible for the treatment of the diseases occurring among their inmates.

(*b*) Hospitals and infirmaries are necessary in large towns—and in other places where the extent and population of the district is great—for the care of those sick and injured people whom it may be desirable, for various reasons, to treat collectively.

(*c*) Special hospitals ought to be established in or near metropolitan and first-class cities, for the reception and treatment of certain contagious or specific disorders, for ophthalmic affections, for skin diseases, for consumption, for sick children, and for local deformities or defects.

(*d*) Sea and mineral bathing establishments, and houses of recovery situated in salubrious places, are also needed for the working classes.

(*e*) Hospitals for the correct and humane treatment of the insane belonging to various classes of society, should be established in districts containing from 300,000 to 400,000 of population. If any such institution be intended wholly for the poor, it should be maintained at the public cost. If, on the other hand, suitable accommodation be provided in it for patients from the independent and middle classes of society, their payments would aid the general fund of the establishment.*

A special code is required for the management of hospitals for the insane. They should be visited by scientific inspectors; and a highly qualified medical superintendent should reside in each.

(*f*) Asylums for idiots, cretins, the deaf and dumb, are also worthy of a civilized State.

* The main reasons for combining different classes in one establishment, are—that the medical superintendents have the advantage of thus observing a wider range of morbid phenomena; and that the insane poor participate in all the benefits of the most scientific treatment, and the most able and liberal management. Nevertheless, the great improvements which have been effected of late, in England, in the public treatment of the insane, tend, on the whole, to the separation of the classes. The English Pauper Asylums are Institutions of a very superior kind.

§ 4. (*a*) The numbers, qualifications, duties, and position of the physicians and surgeons appointed to the care of the districts and institutions mentioned in the preceding sections, are matters for national legislation. Nor should the State leave these important appointments to private or corporate patronage, to the arts of solicitation and cozenage, or to party cabals.

(*b*) For the establishment and support of these various sanative institutions, benevolent association and private charity should be encouraged to the utmost; *e. g.*, by legally exempting the establishments from direct taxation and local burdens, by the protection of charitable bequests, and by public grants, if needed.

The principle of voluntary aid should also be promoted by conferring on individual contributors a share in the management of the institution.

(*c*) Although laws and rules for the government of medical charities may be more zealously administered by those who act from benevolent motives, and whose cultivated intelligence may, in some instances, qualify them for the self-imposed task; yet, in general, the public interests are not so well promoted by leaving the management of sanative establishments, entirely and irresponsibly, to voluntary and local agency, which is often irregular and uncertain, and not always the most competent or the best informed.

(*d*) The site, distribution, and construction of hospitals of every kind, are matters of public concern, and should therefore be subject to national control.

The interference of public authority is necessary for the prevention of abuses in their administration, and for limiting their benefits to proper objects. For these reasons, the law should make all sanative institutions, of a public character, responsible to a central council of health, and subject to the visitation of a high order of inspectors.

(*e*) The cost, whether of original foundation or of maintenance —where it is not borne by the State, or met by philanthropic combination or private endowment—should be equitably charged, by law, upon the inhabitants and proprietors of the localities benefited.

Secondly:—On the Advent and during the Prevalence of any Important Epidemic or Pestilential Disease.

§ 5. Physicians, properly informed with respect to the leading phenomena of diseases of the zymotic class, are sometimes able to predict their invasion or outbreak, and frequently to detect their approach. Acting, therefore, on medical advice in anticipation of such visitations—measures which may be always in force for the prevention of disease, should at these times be still more carefully applied; and any defects in the ordinary arrangements more narrowly inquired into and remedied.

(*a*) Previous to a threatened outbreak of epidemic disease in any locality,—the houses, sewers, and drains should be thoroughly cleansed, cess-pools cautiously cleared out, and collections of refuse removed, disinfecting agents being always used in the process.

After the disease is established, however, it is undoubtedly safer to cover and close up foul accumulations caused by previous neglect, than to disturb them.

The proper season, temperature, and weather should be wisely selected for the removal of nuisances and execution of all measures of purification.

(*b*) In the houses of the poor and uncleanly, rules should be enforced for cleansing the furniture, lime-washing the walls, drying damp places and articles, and destroying or thoroughly disinfecting foul clothing and bedding.*

* "How else can we account for the revival of small-pox, scarlet-fever, and other contagions, after long cessation, but in the unpurified flock and feather beds, which contain the contagion, till *susceptible subjects* and *peculiar seasons* call it again into operation? In many parts of the continent they are subjected to annual purification. Here, at home, they often remain untouched for as long as they can hold together, no matter what diseased bodies may have lain upon them. Ventilation can never be made to visit, or the light to penetrate, their interiors. Can we, then, wonder that they should retain, *it may be for years*, the seeds of infection?" —Ferguson's *Notes and Recollections*, pp. 136-7.

Improvements in domestic ventilation, at these times especially, should be judiciously directed.

(*c*) Special instructions should be issued as to the choice and preparation of food and beverage, and as to clothing and personal cleanliness.

To the poorest class of sufferers, nutriment, clothing, and fuel should be supplied from public or charitable sources.

(*d*) All places of public resort should be more closely inspected; and assemblages of the people limited, both as to the numbers congregated, and as to the times and duration of meetings.

(*e*) Any crowding of inmates in public establishments should be strictly prohibited; even the average number may have to be reduced, and this especially in common lodging-houses, where, also, the personal conditions and habits of the lodgers should be subject to more stringent control.

(*f*) The numbers, the health, and the accommodation of cattle and domestic animals, in all populous localities, should at such times receive the special attention of local authorities.

Pernicious trades and unhealthy occupations, as well as nuisances of every kind, should be peremptorily removed or arrested.

§ 6. In order to carry into effect these measures, with the greatest promptitude and advantage, and to fix upon the places and houses most needing their application, the system of domiciliary visitation should be enforced much more frequently and minutely.

(*a*) Every house in a threatened district should be visited twice or thrice weekly, and in pressing emergencies, *daily*.

(*b*) The medical officers of districts should be supplied at such times with a sufficiently numerous staff of assistants; each district being so subdivided, that the several duties of house inspection, medical attendance, and sanitary advice, may be thoroughly performed.

(*c*) Dispensaries, or depôts of drugs and necessaries for the sick, in addition to the permanent establishments, should be opened in crowded and poor sub-districts.

* III. B. 4, *i*, p. 52.

(*d*) Temporary hospitals, properly located and arranged, are necessary for the reception of those portions of the sick which cannot be satisfactorily treated at their own miserable dwellings.

(*e*) "Houses of Refuge" in airy situations, are also needed for those not attacked, whom it may be desirable to remove from infected localities, and to classify according to their liability to attacks.

§ 7. Separation and isolation are principles of sanitary management requiring special enactments, which, for four centuries, have been known by the name of "quarantine" laws,* and the erroneous appellation has led to errors in practice.

Whilst, however, several diseases are propagated by human intercourse, certain regulations for controlling that intercourse are indispensable for preventing both the importation and transmission of such diseases from infected to comparatively healthy localities, and their extension in ports and populous districts, into which they may have entered.†

Without either creating panic, or depriving the sick of any needful attentions or visitations, well-considered restrictions may have to be imposed upon personal communication with those diseased, and upon the use or transfer of their apparel.

(*a*) In time of pestilence, the law should not permit the departure of any ship from an infected port, without the closest investigation of its sanitary condition, nor without a certificate based on satisfactory proof of its thorough purification and ventilation.

Passengers should also be limited to a number much less than would be permitted in ordinary times.‡

---

* The first code of Quarantine Laws established in Europe, was that of Venice, in the year 1448.—White *On the Plague*, 1846, p. 75. Hecker mentions a Council of Health for Quarantine, at Venice, in 1485.—*Epid. of Middle Ages*, p. 64.

The technical terms and phraseology of quarantine have been avoided as much as possible in this sketch.

† The long established, though imperfect rules of international quarantine were discussed and revised by the *Conférence Sanitaire*, at Paris, in 1851-2. It is to be hoped that the results will be published, and made the basis of a uniform and improved European system.

‡ See II. A. 8, p. 27.

The grant of certificates of health and non-infection, during certain pestilences, should depend on the result of rigid inquiry into the nature of the freightage, and into the existing conditions and antecedent circumstances of each passenger, his clothing and effects.

(*b*) If, notwithstanding these precautions, and a due medical provision on board, the pestilence should break out during the voyage, the passengers able to be removed should, on the arrival of the ship at a port free from the disease, be transferred to a healthy and isolated situation on land, for a reasonable period; no one being permitted to disembark without a supply of fresh clothing, nor any article of personal use to be brought into a crowded district until submitted to a cleansing and disinfecting process.

The ship, too, should not be moored near to any other vessel until after the lapse of a specified time, and the completion of proper measures for its purification.

(*c*) In a minor degree as to communications on land, regulations should exist with regard to the movements of trampers and vagrants from town to town,—for enforcing the cleanliness, ventilation, and dryness of public carriages, and preventing the general use of such as have been employed for the conveyance of the sick or dead.

Regulations are also necessary as to the transmission of unwashed articles of clothing, &c., which may have been worn or used by the patients and their attendants in infected localities.

(*d*) Lastly, water intended for drinking, or domestic use, as well as food of all kinds, should be carefully preserved from defilement by emanations or excretions from the sick.

It is scarcely necessary to add, that the measures recommended in this section are based on the theory of contagion or infection; the force of which is admitted, by all who hold that theory, to vary exceedingly in different diseases of the zymotic class.

§ 8. *Vaccination* is commonly called a preventive measure; but, as it is also the substitution of a mild and tolerably uniform animal disease for a severe and uncertain human one, I prefer, for this and other reasons, classing it among measures for the arrest of zymotic disease.

(*a*) The law should either make vaccination compulsory, or afford such encouragement to its universal adoption, and impose such disadvantages on its non-performance, as would practically (and in free countries more safely) lead to the desired result.

(*b*) Legislation should promote the performance of vaccination in infancy, without too strictly limiting the period.

(*c*) A central council of health should also provide for a proper national supply of genuine virus, by the establishment of vaccine stations or depôts in populous localities.

(*d*) To the medical officer of every district, remote from the stations, should be committed the duty of public vaccination at specified times.

(*e*) The law should secure both the reappearance of vaccinated subjects on certain days, and their inspection and certification by officers of health, or sanitary superintendents.

Finally, the State should demand from the proper authorities the construction or publication of reports, in relation to the performance, progress, and results of vaccination.

§ 9. The last section of this division of State Medicine relates to the prevention and palliation of *Diseases among Animals*. For this object there are required :—

1. Certain regulations for the scientific construction and management of stables, kennels, cowhouses, pigsties, &c.

2. Correct and scientific directions relating to the isolation, separation, and management of animals, during the prevalence of various epizootic diseases.

3. Careful observation, registration, and treatment of the animals affected.

4. Preventive measures or precautions to be observed by those who have the charge and attendance of animals suffering from disease.[*]

---

[*] See *Code Rural,* compiled by M. Verneil, 1810. Art. 227, 234.—*Correspondence with Board of Trade,* 1848. No. 689, p. 4.

CHAPTER FOURTH.

DIVISION III.—ON THE ESTABLISHMENT BY LAW OF AN ORGANIZED MACHINERY FOR CARRYING INTO EFFECT THE AFORESAID INQUIRIES AND REGULATIONS, FOR DELIBERATION AND ADVICE IN EMERGENCIES, AND FOR THE ADMINISTRATION OF EXISTING LAWS.

Subdivision A.—The Education of Medical and other Technical, Scientific, and Administrative Agents.

THE care of the public health cannot be safely committed to authorities, the majority of which are not educated and specially prepared for so weighty a charge.

Hence, before boards and officers can be judiciously constituted and appointed, the State must be assured that it can enlist the services of fully competent persons.

None but wild theorists, or ignorant and presumptuous meddlers, would suppose it possible that the public health can be properly superintended without the aid of highly-educated physicians or surgeons. A certain proportion of the members and officers of health councils and boards ought, therefore, to belong strictly to the Profession of Medicine, the highest duties of which consist in the prevention of disease, and the prolongation of active life.

The third principal division of this scheme of State *Agenda* includes, therefore, under its first subdivision,—institutions and laws relating to the instruction and examination, the authorization and registration, the organization, government, character, and duties, the rights and privileges, of medical men.

§ 1. The State is bound to take care that those intended for the medical profession are thoroughly prepared for it by a sound preliminary education—moral, scholastic, scientific; and by a sufficient amount of professional instruction and observation.

In order to secure this adequate preparation, the State ought to possess a superintending, or at least a visiting, authority, in all medical schools.

The choice and appointment of learned and efficient professors should be secured, and the nature and amount of clinical study, and of some other items of the educational curriculum, should be determined on by a state-council of medicine.

The remuneration of professors should not depend directly on the fees of students, who are not always capable of assigning the true relative value to different branches and modes of instruction, nor generally competent to decide on the respective merits of their instructors.

In the education of the medical student, the highest and the only true motives for the performance of sanative and sanitary duties should be carefully inculcated. His sense of responsibility to Divine and human laws, to the profession he is about to enter, and to the sick, should be sedulously cultivated. He should be taught to observe, to note, to collect, and arrange facts; to act promptly and prudently, both under medical authority, and on his own discretion in emergencies.

His competency, or proficiency, on the completion of the successive stages of his education, should be tested by examining boards, carefully constituted, under legal sanction; and the law should prescribe the minimum age at which each step is to be obtained.

§ 2. In authorizing or licensing those who, on examination, obtain a certificate of competency or proficiency, a public pledge or engagement* should be required of each candidate, to fulfil

---

* The ὄρκος, attributed to Hippocrates, has been for ages the basis of such engagements. As a piece of Heathen morality it is admirable; but the Christian physician has an infinitely more exalted precedent, and far nobler maxims to guide his deportment.

honestly and diligently the important duties for which he has prepared himself: and he should be required to furnish proof that he has an opportunity for professional employment, either of a public or private nature.

In registering those who have been legally licensed, the law should prescribe either—

(a) A simple *alphabetical* arrangement, either of all in one list, or of each class separately; or, (b) a *chronological* list, either of all, or of each class; or, (c) a *local* list, which is by far the most important.

A perfect registration would combine a general alphabetical index, with a chronological list of each class, and local lists of all the medical persons in each sanitary district, stating their offices and titles.*

Where two or more grades of private practitioners are recognised by the institutions of a country, the legal or State licence to practise should depend on the attainment of the lower degree; which should certify the competency of the holder to practise both medicine and surgery.

This primary "qualification" should be required of all who enter the profession.

The attainment of higher titles or degrees should be optional, though perhaps the law might connect them with higher official advantages; and thus the superior sanitary offices of the State would be looked upon as rewards for the acquisition of more extensive knowledge in ætiology, in prophylaxis, in psychology, in general science, or in the history and literature of medicine.

Practitioners in midwifery (*obstetricians*) may be either physicians or surgeons. Yet this, being a distinct branch of practice, requires special regulations as to education, licence, and registration.

* The system long prevalent throughout Europe, has been to distinguish between physicians and surgeons, and in some countries to divide one or both of these classes into two or more grades. But the tendency of advancing scientific acquirements is to make the licence and registration uniform, leaving subsequent distinctions to result from legal appointments, the attainment of professional honours, or public favour.

Wherever Colleges of Physicians, Surgeons (or obstetricians) are established by law, or charter, they should be subject to Government visitation. Unless such colleges be compelled to adapt their regulations concerning the preparation, examination, and admission of candidates, to the decisions and arrangements of a State Council of Health and Medical Education, they ought not to be entrusted with the power of deciding on the standard of qualifications necessary for the State-licence to practise.

§ 3. The law should promote, if not define, the local organization of the profession into *District Faculties*, to which, in connexion with a central or metropolitan council, might be committed the administration of local affairs requiring the collective deliberation and action of the medical body, the promotion of medical observation and science, and particularly the power of advising the District Courts of Health hereafter to be proposed.*

The moral and professional character of physicians and surgeons, and their general duties to their own order, to the public, and to the sick, without reference to any particular offices which they may hold, constitute "*medical ethics.*"

Regulations with regard to medical conduct, are in some countries left to the internal arrangements of the medical body; in some they are wholly neglected; in others they are directed by law.

For some offences against medical laws,—as the assumption of titles not legally obtained, the presentation of false certificates of age or competency, the use of medical position for dishonourable or immoral purposes, and very obvious malpractice—the State should provide a proper tribunal, and inflict penalties on convicted offenders.

Internal regulations or "bye-laws," should be few and simple, and capable of being carried into effect by district faculties, and sanctioned by public law.

§ 4. Certain rights and immunities have been conferred on the profession by the State, from the earliest times.

For the safety of those who need their aid, the law exempts,

* See III. B. 3, p. 49.

or should exempt civil physicians, surgeons, apothecaries, and obstetricians from military service; also from serving in certain civil offices, which would interfere with casual and urgent calls to professional duty.

The law should also protect them from interference, defamation, and libel, in the practice of their profession.

It should enable them to recover just remuneration for private personal services; and secure them adequate stipends for their public employments.

§ 5. Those who professedly devote themselves to ailments of particular parts of the human body, as dentists and chiropodists, should be registered accordingly; but should not be recognised as belonging to the profession, unless possessing the uniform primary qualification.

Practitioners in pharmacy are, in some countries, considered to belong to the medical profession, even though not allowed to practise as physicians or surgeons.

The law should require that all practitioners of pharmacy, whether included in the medical body or not, be regularly instructed, examined, licensed, registered, and required to fulfil the directions of physicians and surgeons, if not such themselves.

Inferior practitioners in mechanical surgery, as bleeders, cuppers, bandagers, bathers, and rubbers,* constitute a class of operatives, who, with surgical mechanicians, bear the same relation to surgeons as *pharmaciens* do to physicians.

They should therefore be subject by law to regular instruction, licence, registration, and inspection; and required to fulfil the directions of physicians and surgeons.

Other skilled persons are necessary for the relief and prevention of sickness and injury, under certain conditions of life; such as *female midwives*, who are preferred in some communities, and by some individuals in all countries; and *nurses*† of different

---

* These are called, in some countries, surgeons of the second class; and three centuries ago, in England, were united as barbers with the corporation of surgeons.

† See Supplementary Note, A.

OTHER SANITARY AGENTS.

classes, whether for the care of lying-in women and new-born infants,* or for attendance on the sick and hurt in hospitals and dwelling-houses.†

The law should therefore provide for the instruction, examination, and licence of both midwives and nurses, and should place them under medical direction.

§ 6. Referring, once more,‡ to the intimate relations naturally existing between the physiology and pathology of man and of animals; recollecting also the close connexion between epidemics and epizootics, as regards both ætiology and sanitary regulations; the conclusion is inevitable that the law should provide for the scientific education, as well as for the examination, licence and registration, duties and rights, of veterinary physicians and surgeons.‖

Again, other orders of highly-educated professional men are necessary for co-operation in sanitary inquiries, and for employment in public works; *e. g.*, analytical chemists for the former, civil engineers for both.

Where universities do not provide a special course of study, nor furnish testimonials in chemistry, physics, and civil engineering, such as the State can accept as satisfactory vouchers of competency; the law should promote the institution of colleges and examining boards for improving the education of those who seek employment in these departments of sanitary inquiry and action.

The curricula and standards of qualification adopted by such institutions as may be voluntarily formed, should be subject to Government approval—on fixed principles—before the diplomas can be admitted as tests of qualification.

---

* See II. A. 4, p. 21. † See II. B. 4, p. 33.
‡ See I. A. 7, p. 11; II. B. 9, p. 39.
‖ In this respect, England is far behind other civilized countries.

Subdivision B.—The Institution of Official Authorities—Boards and Offices for Central and Local Superintendence and Action.

The last subdivision of this project of State medicine—that which completes and crowns the whole—includes:—

Firstly and secondly, the institution of boards or councils, central and local;

Thirdly, the territorial division of a country into sanitary districts, each to have its own local board; and

Fourthly, the appointment of officers of various grades and functions, in connexion with the central and local boards.

The objects of the whole machinery should be to investigate and report on the various matters before mentioned, to deliberate upon and form projects of law, whether general and permanent, or local and temporary, and to administer and carry into effect, under Government authority, existing laws of both kinds.

The better constituted, the more influential, competent, and adequately empowered are these boards, and the more highly qualified and efficient their officers, the less necessity is there for loading the statute-book of the realm with a perplexing and endless variety of minute and precise details, most of which can be better dealt with by "orders," or "bye-laws," framed by competent central and local authorities.

The following suggestions might be supposed to apply to a country in which nothing had hitherto been settled as regards the administration of sanitary laws. But a system of constitutional government and territorial division, somewhat analogous to that of England, is assumed throughout.

The Institution of Councils and Boards, Central and Local.

§ 1. In the metropolis, or seat of government, the imperial legislature should establish a superior sanitary and medical council, either presided over by a minister of public health, or connected with the ministry of the Interior (Home Affairs.)

CENTRAL COUNCIL.

This council might consist of several *departments*, or sections.

(*a*) Under one of its sections might be placed the direction of the vital and medical statistics of the entire population, general meteorological and topographical inquiries, and perhaps the supervision of medical jurisprudence.

(*b*) Another section would be required for directing public works of sanitary engineering, town-cleansing, water-supply, and the execution of building-laws.

(*c*) A third section might direct preventive measures relating to the sale of food, drinks, and medicines; the regulation of trades and employments, factories and mines; personal safety in locomotion, especially as regards railways, navigation, and emigration; and the interment of the dead.

(*d*) One or more distinct committees of council might be advisable for the sanitary control of the following institutions and establishments, and the direction of public medical duties.

Educational establishments of all kinds, especially those for children under public guardianship; workhouses, industrial institutions, almshouses, and public charities; prisons, convict establishments, and penitentiaries; asylums or hospitals for the insane; general hospitals, infirmaries, and dispensaries; the medico-sanitary care of the poor in districts; public vaccination and other measures for the arrest of epidemics and pestilences; "quarantine" regulations; veterinary medicine and police; places of public amusement, gymnasia; baths and washhouses.

(*e*) A separate section or committee would be absolutely necessary for the general superintendence of medical education in all its branches; and probably for directing the preparation and qualification of all other persons to be employed in remedial or preventive duties, except civil engineers, whose education would be very properly directed by section (*b*).

(*f*) For deliberation in great national emergencies, and on all important measures of legislation affecting the public health, the whole council should be summoned; and on such occasions the aid and co-operation of the superior medical authorities of the War departments should be secured, by making them *ex-officio* members of council.

(*g*) The composition of the central council is indicated by a cursory view of its duties and departments.

It should consist, partly, of *ex-officio* members; partly of nominees of the crown or head of the State; partly of those recommended by certain learned and professional bodies; and lastly, of those who may be considered by the other three portions as specially qualified to render valuable assistance in the management of the public health. The section for medical education should consist wholly of the recognised heads of the medical profession.

The number and the precise qualifications of each description of members should be defined by law.

§ 2. A local board or court should be established in each of the sanitary districts to be described in the following section.

It should somewhat resemble the central council in constitution. A certain proportion of its members should be crown nominees (*e. g.*, in England, magistrates). Another portion should be elected, either directly or mediately, by the tax or rate paying inhabitants of such sanitary district. A third portion should consist of highly-educated persons, such as men of science, professors, parochial clergy, &c., to be selected by the two former portions, and united with them to complete the court itself.

The qualifications and relative number of each portion should be defined by law.

But the medical element of local government should be distinct, and should form, as before suggested,* a sort of auxiliary committee, or faculty, for deliberation, advice, and co-operation, in each sanitary district.

The duties of the local courts would relate to many of the subjects mentioned under the first four departments of central

* See III. A. 3, p. 43.

sanitary administration, beside attention to other matters strictly belonging to their own jurisdiction.

§ 3. *The territorial division of a country into sanitary districts* should be founded on certain acknowledged principles, such as the following:—

(*a*) A careful adherence, wherever it may be practicable, to scientific topography and to the physical geography of the country:

(*b*) A recognition of towns of a certain size as the centres and seats of local jurisdictions:

(*c*) An adaptation, as far as possible, to the ancient divisions of the country, supposing these to be at all uniform and consentaneous, or capable of readjustment for the purposes required:

(*d*) A respect for parochial or communal boundaries; combining a suitable number of parishes and townships in each district; not omitting a single place, however obscure, in distribution; and altering their limits only when plainly necessary:

(*e*) A recognition of the boundaries of cities and towns, only so far as to include them wholly in the sanitary district or districts to which they would naturally or reasonably belong; municipal boundaries for political purposes being often diametrically opposed to all sound principles of sanitary management:

(*f*) Identity of areas for statistical returns with those for sanitary management:

(*g*) Special regard to density of population; the number of inhabitants in any district varying from about 30,000 where the "specific population" is under (say) 200 on an English square mile, to about 60,000 where it is above (say) 300 on a square mile, and to a still higher amount of population where a first-class town or city is to be included in one district, or to be divided into more than one.

§ 4. *The appointment of Officers of various grades and functions.*

A. Under the metropolitan or central council, a permanent organization of inspectors or commissioners is necessary.

(*a*) *Medical Inspectors of Circuits,*—analogous to the *Proto-Medici* of Austria and Italy, the *Medicinal Räthe* of Prussia, and the medical inspectors of Ireland.

Each circuit might contain twenty or thirty sanitary districts.

The superintendence of the medical officers of health, and of the chemical and veterinary officers, in the several sanitary districts, as well as the visitation of hospitals and other chief medical and public institutions in their circuits, would devolve upon these inspectors.

A few medical inspectors, unconnected with circuits, might be at the disposal of the central board, for foreign or colonial service.

(*b*) *Engineering Inspectors*—such as are now employed by the General Board of Health of England, should also be permanently appointed to the same circuits.

By these officers, the topographical surveys of the district courts should be examined and verified, the plans of public works revised, and their progress superintended.

(*c*) *Chemical Inspectors* need not be appointed to circuits, but a sufficient staff, say three or four, should be attached to the central board, for special scientific investigations, wherever they may be necessary.

All these inspectors, of whatever description, should be debarred from private practice, and salaried by the State.

B. Every district court of health should be provided with the following official staff:—

(*d*) *An Officer of Health,* analogous to the *Kreis Physicus* of Germany.

He might be appointed jointly by the court of health and the medical faculty of his district; and if these bodies do not concur in the choice, the central council should decide the point.

He also should be debarred from private practice. The law

should define his qualifications, his terms of engagement with local and central authorities, his official relations with his colleagues and with the medical officers of parochial districts; his prophylactic duties as to epidemics and disease generally, and as to mortuary interment; his duties of inspection as to public institutions, census of population, registration of births and deaths, reports of sickness and injury, vaccination, and registration of medical persons; his forensic duties as regards cadaveric examinations and inquests, and evidence on medico-legal questions; and his periodical and occasional reports on these subjects as well as on the medical topography and general sanitary condition and requirements of his district.

(e) *A district Chemist,* for the analysis of waters, soils, and gases; for the inspection and examination of articles sold for food and beverage, of drugs and articles sold for medicine, and of all industrial and commercial processes suspected to be injurious to the public health; for reports on these matters; and for aid (if required) to the Officer of Health, in forensic inquiries and meteorological observations.

(f) *A district Veterinarian,* for statistical inquiries,* for carrying into effect measures of prevention and palliation, in epizoötics and other diseases among cattle and domestic animals generally;† for the inspection of carcasses with reference both to comparative pathology and to the wholesomeness of animal food; and for veterinary reports, which would also be in connexion with those of the other two previously mentioned officers.

(g) *A district Engineer,* or *Surveyor,* for statistical inquiries as to the towns and dwellings in his district; for general surveys, and for plans and directions on the following matters:—making and repairing of roads; land, suburban, and town drainage; conservation and improvement of streams and watercourses; water-supply of towns; and for attention to public works generally in his district.

* See I. A. 7, p. 11. † See II. B. 9, p. 39.

His reports should be made to the engineering inspector of the circuit; and in all important matters he should be required to submit his plans and proceedings for the approval of that inspector.

With the aid of the district chemist and the veterinary officer, he should compile and classify the returns of the agricultural statistics of the district.

(*h*) In every principal seaport, a *Medical Superintendent of Quarantine* should be appointed; unless the important duties of giving sanitary directions with regard to immigration and emigration, and the transport of goods and passengers, be committed to the officer of health of the district.

c. Every parish, township, commune, or sub-district, should be provided with the following officers:—

(*i*) *A Medical Officer*, or *Visitor*, for the general sanitary superintendence of the poor in their dwellings, and for attendance upon them in sickness and accidents; for the care of sick soldiers, police, or other public servants, who may not be otherwise provided for; for periodical visitation of the residences of the working classes, especially in unhealthy places and in times of epidemic sickness; for the prompt detection and removal of premonitory symptoms of disease; for counsel, advice, and instruction to the poor on matters affecting their health; for reporting circumstances which may be considered prejudicial to health and requiring the interference of the local authorities; for the registration of births and deaths,* where not performed by other persons; for public vaccination; for reporting on the sickness in his parish or subdistrict—quarterly in ordinary times, and daily or weekly in epidemics.

(*k*) Wherever, as in Ireland, a national system of dispensaries is organized, *apothecaries* or *dispensers*, thoroughly instructed and examined in chemistry, pharmacy, and the materia medica,

---

* The registration of marriages and the performance of merely civil marriages, are matters so distinct from sanitary administration that they are not here mentioned.

should be appointed in every dispensary district. In other countries, properly qualified *pharmaciens* should be appointed, to whom such poor as are considered fit recipients of medicine at the public cost should apply.

(*l*) *A Searcher for Nuisances,* whose duties are indicated by his official title.

In fulfilling the orders of the local court, he should act under the superintendence of the officer of health and the district surveyor, to whom he should systematically report.

(*m*) A staff of *Assistant Visitors,* medical and other, should be always ready for action, but salaried only when on duty.

(*n*) An *Obstetrical Officer,* thoroughly qualified, is required for important cases of midwifery among the poor, in every parochial district where this duty may not be committed—as it is generally and very properly in England—to the medical officer.

(*o*) One or more *Midwives,* duly qualified and licensed, should be appointed in each subdistrict, for attendance on destitute women, with instructions to call in the medical or obstetrical officer in every serious case. The midwives should report all their cases to that officer.

(*p*) Nurses, educated and licensed, should also be appointed in sufficient numbers, for attendance on the poorest class, under the control of the medical visitor.

If not supplied from religious or charitable institutions, as in most European countries, they should be properly paid out of local funds.

None of the officers or agents named under the last head, c, need be debarred from private engagements.

In fact, it is to the advantage of the public that the medical and other attendants upon the sick poor should perform their duties occasionally among all classes of society.

Medical officers of distinct institutions are not again mentioned in this section. Their appointments, salaries, and duties would for the most part come under the notice of special departments of the central council, and be superintended by the circuit inspectors.

It might be undesirable for the officer of health to act as inspector of the higher order of medical institutions situated in his district, except on emergencies, and as the deputy of the circuit inspector.

CHAPTER FIFTH.

SUPPLEMENTARY.

SUCH a scheme of State medicine and health police as I have now completed, has never, that I am aware of, been realized in all its parts in any nation. But its leading principles, as I premised, have been long in operation in Central Europe. That is to say, whatever statistical inquiries respecting life and health, and matters affecting both, have been undertaken by governments; whatever preventive measures have been adopted, either under ordinary circumstances or against particular zymotic diseases; whatever palliative and remedial expedients have been put in force, as, for instance, the medical care of the poorer classes in public institutions and in their own residences; and whatever laws have been enacted for the education and regulation of medical practitioners;—ALL have been executed and administered by an organized body of State authorities and officers; they have formed parts, however distinct, of ONE Government object.

By the medical laws and regulations, of Italian rather than of Teutonic origin, in force in the several German States, the general unity of these matters has been recognised to the fullest extent.

It is true that special enactments, particular offices of various grades, and territorial areas of jurisdiction, vary considerably in different German States, and for no very intelligible reason.

The want also of English capital and energy may generally have prevented the application of engineering skill to the execution of great works of purification. And in but very few towns are the particular sanitary measures so much talked of in England, carried into effect, even imperfectly.

But the mutual interdependence of the several Departments of public health guardianship, their connexions with the Departments of Justice, War, Agriculture, and Commerce, Public Instruction, and Public Works, and their general subordination to the supreme civil power, are maintained universally, I believe, with the utmost advantage and satisfaction to the people, and to the furtherance of the highest object of Government,—namely, the welfare and happiness of the governed. In these communities the care of the public health is nowhere abandoned to chance, or to the vagaries of individual philanthropy and voluntary association; although the State, in several places, avails itself of the regulated assistance of such agencies for the better fulfilment of the ends it has in view. Nowhere is the adoption of sanitary regulations left to the choice of isolated groups of the population or municipalities.

On the contrary, everything which affects the physical condition of the community is brought under the cognizance of a system of Councils;—central, provincial, and district, with their respective official staffs, in graduated subordination to the State Government.

Hence, when unforeseen events and circumstances arise, perilous to the lives and health of the people—when existing laws prove defective, insufficient for the emergency, or inapplicable to altered social conditions,—there exists a State machinery already in operation, to which the preparation and administration of the required enactments can at once be committed.

Plato's principle*—that the physician must form part of the polity of his commonwealth—is thus fully realized.

Some inconsiderate objectors have disputed the necessity for a complete medico-sanitary organization, because, in countries where such exists, neither the duration of human life, nor the execution of certain sanitary works, are equal to what we have in England.

So illogical an objection cannot be answered until the dan-

---
* See motto to this Essay.

gerous experiment has been tried of depriving Germany of her cherished sanitary codes.

In the meantime, we may reasonably inquire, what additional advantages might be secured to a country so highly favoured, naturally and socially, as England, by the introduction of a principle which has been applied with inestimable benefit to many European communities, although it may have failed in some instances to accomplish its full design, owing, in a measure, to the want of that practical force and those ample resources which so remarkably distinguish the English nation.

POSTSCRIPT.

SINCE the completion of the preceding Essay, my attention has been directed to the opinions of the late Wilhelm Von Humboldt, who held, " that the State is to abstain from all solicitude for the positive welfare of the citizens, and not proceed a step further than is necessary for their mutual security and protection against foreign enemies; and that with no other object should it impose restrictions on freedom."* Whether the wide and somewhat ambiguous, term " mutual security" in this passage, might not be so interpreted as to include all the objects for which State-medicine is instituted, may be left to each reader to decide for himself. But if Humboldt did not intend to include those objects, there seems to me to be no limit to the *individualism* to which so wild a theory would lead a nation. If small and isolated minorities are to be allowed to exempt themselves from the operation of general laws for the public good, so ought persons to be allowed to resist the decisions of these minorities. If not, what extent or degree of aggregation is to constitute a right of compelling the submission of the individual will?

* *The Sphere and Duties of Government*, translated from the German of Wilhelm V. Humboldt, by Joseph Coultard, Junr.

If the vigorous agriculturist of Surrey or Herefordshire is permitted to declare that he will not contribute to a tax which provides health-protection, and sanative management for the pale weaver of Spitalfields,—so may the comfortable little shopkeeper, perfectly satisfied with, and doing well in, his narrow impure street, refuse his contribution to an assessment for improvements which he fancies are merely intended to gratify the fastidious tastes of the inhabitants of the nearest square, or circus.

"Because the sages of Little Pedlington or Hockley-in-the-Hole (no doubt very worthy people in their way) deem it a patriotic duty to oppose the enactment, and resist the execution of laws of which they do not happen to perceive the fitness or necessity; it would be both unjust and absurd to withhold from an immense willing majority of the people those amendments in local management, which are only to be attained under the discriminative direction and unbiassed control of well-informed authorities at a distance."

A medical police may be said to afford the same protection to life and property against *chemical* injury, as an ordinary police or a constabulary force affords against *mechanical* violence; and the maintenance of the latter may as reasonably be left to the option of every individual in a community as might the former.

Time would be wasted in further attempts to demolish a speculation which is opposed to all the facts of social progress.

As mankind mingle more and more, and as railways are gradually converting nations into great cities (for it now takes no longer time to travel from Canterbury to York than our ancestors spent on the way from Hackney to Brentford), the interests of the entire population become more directly and immediately mutual, and the necessity for a judicious centralization, aided by local enterprise, becomes more imperative.

ESSAY II.

EDUCATION IN THE HEALING AND HEALTH PRESERVING ARTS.

Ἰητρικὴ τεχνέων μὲν πασέων ἐστὶν ἐπιφανεστάτη· διὰ δὲ ἀμαθίην τῶν τε χρεομένων αὐτῇ, καὶ τῶν εἰκῆ τοὺς τοιούσδε κρινόντων, πολύ τι πασέων ἤδη τῶν τεχνέων ἀπολείπεται. Ἡ δὲ τῶνδε ἁμαρτὰς τὰ μάλιστά μοι δοκέει ἔχειν αἰτίην τοιήνδε· πρόστιμον γὰρ ἰητρικῆς μούνης ἐν τῇσι πόλεσιν οὐδὲν ὥρισται, πλὴν ἀδοξίης· αὕτη δὲ οὐ τιτρώσκει τοὺς ἐξ αὐτέης συγκειμένους. Ὁμοιότατοι γάρ εἰσιν οἱ τοιοίδε τοῖσι παρεισαγομένοισι προσώποισιν ἐν τῇσι τραγῳδίῃσιν· ὡς γὰρ ἐκεῖνοι σχῆμα μὲν καὶ στολὴν καὶ πρόσωπον ὑποκριτοῦ ἔχουσιν, οὐκ εἰσὶ δὲ ὑποκριταί, οὕτω καὶ ἰητροί, φήμῃ μὲν πολλοί, ἔργῳ δὲ πάγχυ βαιοί.—

HIPPOCR. *Lex.*

"Medicine is of all arts the most noble; but owing to the ignorance of those who practise it, and of those who, inconsiderately, form a judgment of them, it is at present far behind all the other arts. Their mistake appears to me to arise principally from this, that in the cities there is no punishment connected with the practice of medicine (and with it alone) except disgrace, and that does not hurt those who are familiar with it. Such persons are like the figures which are introduced in tragedies, for as they have the shape, and dress, and personal appearance of an actor, but are not actors, so also physicians are many in title, but very few in reality."—*Adams's Translation of the Above.*

ESSAY II.

§ 1. It seemed desirable in the preceding normal project to assume a theoretical standard, by which to test various measures which have been proposed or carried into effect in this country for the attainment of one or other of the objects of State medicine.

Some of these objects must now be viewed in a more practical light, with special reference to our own necessities, our own institutions, and our own modes of legislation and administration.

Medical Police must be anglicized.

§ 2. The aspects of State medicine in the *educational department* have determined me to consider in the first place, the vexed question of "Medical Reform," which has now been before Parliament in one shape or another for twenty years.

For there seems no reasonable ground to expect that any administrative machinery for the protection of the public health can be constituted satisfactorily to the legislature, to the medical profession, and to the better informed portion of the community, until the ground-work be laid in an improved system of medical education and organization.

§ 3. The courses of study and preparation deemed necessary for entering upon the profession of medicine in its various departments, and the nature and amount of the qualifications (so far as these can be ascertained by examination) of those legally admitted to practise in England, Ireland, and Scotland, are still determined by various licensing bodies in each part of the kingdom.

These bodies appear to treat medical education on different principles, and to hold different views as to the minimum degree of preparation and acquirement necessary for each class of practitioners.

Thus, as might have been expected, the main obstacle to the adoption of any general scheme for the uniform training and examination of medical candidates throughout the British Empire, has consisted in the difficulty, hitherto insuperable, of reconciling the contending claims, the conflicting educational theories, and the rival pecuniary interests of the several universities, medical or surgical colleges, and quasi-medical corporations, to which the legislature has unhappily committed the power of authorizing persons to treat the sick.

§ 4. Another weighty, though more passive hindrance to legislation has consisted in the indifference of the majority of the profession to any measure which would not guarantee to them a monopoly of curative practice. Their cry is "Protection." So that even if the educational bodies could arrange their differences, we must not expect the general hearty acquiescence of the profession in any measure, unless it contain stringent penal clauses against irregular practitioners.

Now, if the Government should decide on waiting until the various medical bodies and the majority of practitioners shall have concurred in one bold and publicly useful measure, all legislation on the subject must be indefinitely postponed.

Nor is it likely that such concurrence would be obtained, unless by delegating to a representative medical council an amount of power, the surrender of which by the Crown and Parliament would be scarcely consistent with a due regard to the public interests.

For instance, the medical corporations and the body of practitioners might require that none should be admitted into the ranks of the profession, except those adhering to "orthodox" medical theories, and authorized modes of practice.

§ 5. Now, it cannot be denied that improvements in medical

science of great benefit to mankind, have now and then originated externally to the pale of the "regular" faculty, whilst many of those still more important reforms and discoveries, made within that pale, have been vehemently opposed, and the progress of truth for a time checked, by the heads and governing councils of the profession.

Any medical doctrine, not sanctioned by those authorities, has accordingly been accounted heterodox; and no discreet aspirant for medical honours has ventured to consider it even an open question.

Supposing, then, that the Legislature, beside conferring exclusive privileges upon persons duly accredited on this exclusive system, could be persuaded further to prohibit, under penalty of fine and imprisonment, all others from practising the medical arts; it must be clear to any one who does not shut his eyes to notorious facts, that numbers of the educated and intelligent portion of her Majesty's subjects would be deprived of those sources of advice and aid on which, however unwisely, they choose to depend for the relief of their disorders.

§ 6. Prohibition, under such a law, would not be confined to those grossly "ignorant persons, of whom," says the old statute of 1511, "the greater part have no manner of insight in the same [science], nor in any other kind of learning; some also can (*sic*) no letters in the book, so far forth that common artificers, as smiths, weavers, and women, boldly and accustomably take upon them great cures and things of great difficulty, . . . to the grievous hurt, damage, and destruction of many of the king's liege people, most especially of them that cannot discern the uncunning from the cunning."*

The prohibition sought for, would not apply specially to uneducated medicine-vendors,† who, notwithstanding their entire

---

* Willock—*Laws relating to the Medical Profession,* part ii. p. vi.

† It seems that some thirty-three petitions were presented to Parliament from medical botanists—*alias* Coffinites—against Mr. Brady's Bill of 1854.

These petitions came chiefly from individual quacks, but one was signed by 4180 ignorance of the merest elements of pharmacy and therapeutics, profess, without legal hindrance, to furnish infallible remedies for every ailment of the million hitherto unprovided with proper medical care and sanitary regulation.

Nor would it be simply "a declaratory act withdrawing expressly from the St. John Longs and other quacks, the protection which the law is inclined to throw around the mistakes and miscarriages of the regularly educated practitioner."*

Nor would such prohibition stop, after the enactment of justly severe restrictions upon the sale of pernicious if not poisonous drugs—every one knows how the children of English working-people are narcotized into brain-disease and atrophy.

§ 7. But, on the protective hypothesis most in favour with the medical profession, what would become of certain legally qualified practitioners who forsake the beaten path; as, for example, the disciple of Hahnemann, who relies on infinitesimally small doses of certain substances, which even in large quantities have been, hitherto and generally, believed to be wholly inert; or his ally, who follows another German original in treating all diseases, acute or chronic, by enormous draughts and curiously diversified applications of pure water; or a third, who would revive under a new name the ancient iatroleptic or gymnastic treatment; or a fourth, of the dietetic school; or a fifth, proclaiming his exclusive confidence in the natural forces of galvanism and electro-magnetism; or a sixth, who, by means of mesmerism and its kindred arts, brings more questionable and

---

inhabitants of the West Riding of Yorkshire; another by 1800 persons at Bradford; another had 368 signatures from a meeting at Freemasons' Hall, London.

The principal drug used by this sect seems to be lobelia. At an inquest held in November, 1853, on a person poisoned by an emetic of lobelia-seeds given by one of the above petitioners, Dr. Letheby (the eminent toxicologist, and now medical officer of health for the City of London,) stated that thirteen cases of poisoning from this drug had occurred within the last three or four years; and that in six the coroner's jury brought in a verdict of *manslaughter*. Adding two more recent cases, it appears that eight cases of proved manslaughter have resulted from this quackery in four years!—*Med. Times and Gaz.*, May 13, 1854.

* Coleridge's *Table Talk*, Jan. 2, 1833, p. 189, 2nd edit.

mysterious influences to bear upon the disordered frame and impaired will?

Let any of these—more especially if highly educated or keen witted, most certainly if skilful or successful in their empiricism—be found in the nominal ranks of the medical profession, and they would inevitably be expelled, forbidden to exercise their profitable occupation, probably punished severely on the repetition of their offence, and thus be turned into " martyrs for the truth," if our legislators should adopt and enforce the hasty claim of the majority of the regular faculty in this country.

As one who may be supposed to have an interest in the decision, I do not pretend to estimate the amount of real benefit which might accrue to the public from the realization of the protective theory, nor is it necessary to speculate further on this demand. It will not be granted.

§ 8. The practical question now forced upon the consideration of statesmen is, to what extent, and by what safe measures, a principle could be recognised which in the main is correct and reasonable; namely, that *the public* should be protected from fraudulent and ignorant pretenders to a knowledge of the healing art.

It appears that, on this point, there are two very distinct demands:—

First, that no one should be legally authorized to practise medicine, who does not avow that he is prepared to treat disease on principles and precedents approved by the most eminent professors and practitioners of the day; in other words, on the therapeutical systems sanctioned by the heads of the medical colleges:—

Secondly, that the State should grant its licence to practise medicine to those only (1) whose knowledge of anatomy, physiology, and pathology, and of the various branches of abstract and natural science, on which philosophical medicine rests, has been duly tested; (2) who can produce evidence, by certificates fairly earned and fairly granted, of having carefully observed, by clinical attendance, enough of the medical systems now in force, and who have sufficiently studied the history of those in past ages to preserve them from ignorant, precipitate, and fallacious conclusions; (3) whose preliminary education has been sound and liberal, and whose character, disposition, and habits are such as to fit them alike for the sterner requirements and the more scrupulous proprieties of their calling.*

One of these demands, it will be at once perceived, is for professional protection against irregularity, heterodoxy, and intrusion.

The other is for public protection against ignorance, incompetence, and what is worst of all, a low standard of professional morality.

Now I do not hesitate to assume that the second only of these demands would be acceded to by an enlightened Government.

A law carrying protection to this extent, and no further, is so essential an item of public health protection, that it can no longer be neglected in this country, with just regard to the safety of its inhabitants.

§ 9. Merely negative or prohibitory legislation, however, will not meet the requirements of the case. The State must grapple with the difficulty in its earliest stage.

To train and prepare youths for medical and sanitary employment is elsewhere acknowledged to be one of the most serious responsibilities of Government. It is one, which no nation has ever neglected without loss to the State and injury to the people. Yet it is one which English Governments and Parliaments have strenuously shunned, for it affects neither political influence nor party ascendency. A loud and importunate outcry for intervention must arise before they can be induced even to shift their own responsibilities, in this matter, upon medical corporations. But

---

* Hippocrates, or whoever was the author of the Νόμος, was of opinion that the medical student should possess the following advantages:—a natural disposition; instruction; a favourable position (or place) for the study; early tuition; love of labour; leisure.

to take the initiative, and especially to found professorships in various branches of the healing and health-preserving arts, has been considered a kind of political Quixotism, of which no sober-minded English minister could possibly be guilty.

§ 10. Even with regard to forensic medicine, which so plainly concerns the administration of justice, there was no public professor until the year 1806, when the Fox ministry instituted a Chair of Medical Jurisprudence in the University of Edinburgh, and committed its duties to the able hands of the late Dr. Andrew Duncan, to whose venerable father, " conspicuous for the possession of every quality that can adorn the professional character," there is reason to believe that this measure was due.*

But that ministry was turned out, within a year from their perpetration of so dire an offence; and the Tory party of the day pounced upon this Edinburgh professorship with exclamations of astonishment and virtuous indignation.

Mr. Perceval, in moving for the renewal of the finance committee (June, 1807), said:—

"He should not dwell in detail upon all the acts of the late administration, but he confessed himself at a loss to understand what they could mean by the appointment of a Professor of Medical Jurisprudence. He acknowledged that he was ignorant of the duty of that professor, and could not comprehend what was meant by the science he professed"!

On the same occasion, Mr. Canning is reported to have said:—

"He could alone account for such a nomination by supposing that after a long debate, in the swell of insolence, and to show how far they could go, they had said—We will show them what we can do—we will create a Professor of Medical Jurisprudence."†

§ 11. No ministry has hitherto confessed, if it has perceived, that the State is especially called upon to provide public technical

---

* Dr. Duncan, Senr., had, for many years after his appointment to the chair of medicine, given private lectures on forensic medicine and medical police.—Dr. Gordon Smith's *Principles of Forensic Medicine*, Introd. p. xviii.

† Stockdale's *Annual Register*, 1807, pp. 206—210.

instruction in those matters which no one can undertake to teach on his own risk with a prospect of adequate remuneration,* but of which a right knowledge is indispensable to the public safety.

Hence, to this day, we are without a public professor of hygiéne or sanitary police in any university or capital of the United Kingdom.†

Not only are the people at large destitute of teachers in that department of knowledge, which, beyond all other temporal or material subjects of information, concerns their welfare in mind, body, and estate; but even those who are training for medicine, are left to provide instruction for themselves, as best they may, in a branch of science and art, which it is not made their interest to cultivate and practise.

Medical students, acting on their own discretion, naturally follow professors in the bread-winning employments of practical medicine and surgery, especially where these are taught by distinguished leaders of practice. Popularity, however, is not always the safest test of professorial excellence, even in those arts and sciences which are most eagerly pursued.

For the last three or four centuries, the "curative" order of physicians and professors of the remedial art, has been permitted to supersede the "preventive" order of teachers which adorned a former æra. England never profited by the example‡ which

---

* Mr. J. S. Mill, in his *Political Economy* (book v. ch. xi. § 3—6), justifies the interference of the Government, "7. When acts generally beneficial cannot be made to remunerate those who perform them."

† I am aware that there are one or two lecturers on hygiéne in private medical schools.

Dr. Richardson very justly remarks:—"In every school of medicine there ought to be, and we have reason to believe there soon will be, a professor of hygiéne, holding a position as important as the professor of physiology, or of practical medicine. In every collegiate or university examination for licences and degrees, a knowledge of hygiéne should be demanded."—*Journal of Public Health*, 1855, p. 7.

‡ "Quod academiam Salernitanam maxime commendavit, et ejus gloriam transmisit posteris, opus est illud—*De Conservandâ valetudine*—Roberto Duci Normanniæ et Regni Anglicani hæredi consecratum; tum propter dignitatem ejus

was set in the school of Salernum, so early as the twelfth century, under the auspices of a Norman duke of our own royal race. In that celebrated University, a main department of instruction was the conservation of health; and its sanitary precepts and principles have been handed down to us, in the famous leonine verses of the *Schola Salernitana*.

§ 12. Surely it is now the time for Government to revert to more rational principles; and to discard the application of commercial theories and maxims to medical education.

The more reflective advocates of what is called "Medical Reform," seem to agree that a comprehensive scheme of preparation and qualification for the practice of medicine, in its widest sense, can be thoroughly carried into operation, only through the medium of one central council of health or State Medicine.

The whole bearing of my Introductory Essay, and indeed the tendency of all large measures of medical polity, are in favour of an excellent principle, supported by Sir James Graham in 1845, —namely, that while the functions of a council of health should not be limited to the superintendence of sanitary police, so neither should the functions of a council of medicine be limited to the education and organization of the medical profession.

The latter might well exist in the form of a committee or section of the former. It should embody a limited number of the most learned and able physicians and surgeons of the kingdom; men of large minds, high principles, and of known administrative capacity. Such only would be competent to direct the details of medical qualification and instruction; but the decisions of such a committee when bearing upon public arrangements, as they must so often do, should be subject to the approval of the whole council.

§ 13. The medical education committee[*] should be empowered

Principis, cui inscriptum est, tum propter utilitatem operis, et insolitum scribendi genus, utile simul et jucundum."—*Schola Salernitana*, Præfat. cap. ii. Roterodami. 1667.

[*] The constitution of this committee is treated of at the close of this Essay, pp. 79, 80.

to appoint boards of preliminary examination in each metropolis, for the purpose, in the first place, of testing, at the commencement of the professional *curriculum*, the general scholarship and acquirements of those students, who have not taken University degrees.

A certain amount of attainment should be required, under each of the following heads :—

(*a*) Grammar and composition ; Greek and Latin, and at least one of the modern European languages :—

(*b*) Mathematics, pure and mixed :—

(*c*) Elements of logic and moral philosophy.

(*d*) Some department of natural science should also be taken up for examination: either (*a*) elements of chemistry and physics, or (β) zoology and botany, or (γ) outlines of physical geography, and of history as bearing upon science.

(*e*) Perhaps, proficiency in the arts of drawing or modelling might be accepted as equivalent to a subject of natural science.

The board of preliminary examination should, once at least, during the course of medical studies, ascertain the progress of students in chemistry, physics, medical botany, human and comparative anatomy and physiology.

§ 14. The central committee should be further empowered to nominate professors at London, Dublin, and Edinburgh, in those branches of medical knowledge, for which no instruction is provided in the metropolitan universities.

The salaries of such professors should be paid by the State, and their appointment sanctioned by the Government.

The same body should also have authority to provide adequate means of instruction in practical anatomy. The inspector of anatomy would be one of its agents.

It would also impose a sufficient period of clinical observation in hospitals ; and require proofs of regular attendance at cadaveric inspections during that period.

If necessary, it would even take measures to supply additional opportunities of practical study, in hospitals of various kinds, exhibiting and testing various principles and methods of treatment.

It should also make due provision for collegiate discipline in schools which are not subject to university regulations; for instruction in medical ethics; and for training in the practical performance of technical duties.

§ 15. The committee of medical education should determine the nature and extent of the final examinations to be passed by candidates for the licence to practise. It would secure uniformity in the minimum of qualifications in England, Scotland, and Ireland.

It should commit these examinations to a general examining board, in each of the three capital cities of the kingdom. Every college of physicians and surgeons might with great propriety be authorized to nominate a portion or section of its respective metropolitan board;* while the central committee would appoint other sections at its discretion, and where needed, on special subjects.

§ 16. The central committee would be the proper authority for registering those who pass the final examinations; and for licensing them to practise, in specified places, in any part of the United Kingdom.

It would also protect and regulate all registered and licensed persons in the lawful exercise of their profession.

But, on this head, I have more to say.

It is not enough to lay down a uniform standard of qualification, which must ever be a *minimum;* and then to abandon the οἱ πολλοὶ thus admitted into the profession, to the chance of becoming either benefactors to the community, or useless and incapable burdens on society, or perhaps even its dangerous pests.

---

* In London, the Society of Apothecaries having had so great a share, since 1815, in regulating and testing the qualification of English practitioners, should be allowed to exercise a joint right with the two Royal Colleges in such nominations. In Scotland, the Faculty of physicians and surgeons at Glasgow has a still better founded claim for exercising a joint right with the Edinburgh Colleges.

By whom are the ranks of the vilest quackery in this country filled up? How often are the degraded initials of M.D., M.R.C.S., L.S.A., attached to the most atrocious handbills and advertisements?

And where the fall has not been so great, let me further ask—Of what public or private advantage is it, for a college of surgeons to admit members, who afterwards shuffle down into their more appropriate occupation of railway porters and policemen?

On the present system, good, bad, and indifferent may pass, in unlimited numbers, and without any marked distinction; none, at least, that is patent to the public: the real selection being made by a subsequent process of probation and experiment,—a process which is attended with no little risk to the community.

Hundreds of "legally qualified practitioners" are to be found, men either of inferior attainments and capacity, or of low principles;—the former ready to be victimized by their more powerful or sharper-witted neighbours, the latter (probably not a less numerous body) prowling about to victimize others.

These are disagreeable statements to make and to hear; but their truth is too generally known to require a reference to particular facts in proof.

Is it not, then, desirable that the State should regulate the number of admissions into the profession by the demand for medical employment?

Is it safe or right to leave the rush of thoughtless youths into this body, to cure itself by a perilous glut on the labour-market of medical skill or medical ignorance, probity or laxity, as the case may be? Are the extraordinary variations of supply —injurious scarcity alternating with useless or mischievous superabundance—of the least benefit to society?

German systems are not at present in favour with us; but there are some, wide minded enough to lay aside national prejudices, who would admit that a State regulation—requiring direct correlation between the number admitted to practise, and the number of vacant or contingent spheres of employment—is infinitely preferable to the chance scramble for work, or for patronage, permitted in this country.

These considerations, long and carefully weighed, lead me to suggest that after conferring the "uniform primary qualification," available for every part of the kingdom, the acts of registration and licence should invariably apply to certain spheres of duty. They should, indeed, depend on proof, given by the candidates, that such opportunities for employment are actually open to them.

§ 17. This very necessary connexion between the State licence and the opportunity for using it, either in the civil service, or independently in places where the number of "unattached" is within a certain proportion to the population, leads to an inquiry whether the existing standard of medical qualifications is adequate to the growing requirements of State medicine.

A negative answer will be given at once by every one, who candidly observes the operation of arrangements now in force, with regard to the public health.

Here, then, is shown a most important particular in which medical reform bears upon sanitary legislation.

As the medical boards of the army and navy have instituted special examinations for their medical officers, in addition to the ordinary diploma, so I would suggest that at least all candidates for, or expectants of, the civil appointments mentioned in the Fourth and Fifth Essays, should be required to furnish proof of having studied, and should be examined upon the following subjects:—

(*a*) The elements of vital and sanitary statistics.

(*b*) The ætiology of disease—*e. g.*, the origin, outbreak, and propagation of zymotic diseases, and the causes and effects of malaria.

(*c*) Climate, locality, soil, and water.

(*d*) Food and diet of different kinds; their composition and liability to adulteration; clothing, exercise, and habitation; all these in relation both to health and sickness, and in connexion with the various circumstances included under the last head.

(e) Principles of ventilation and purification; preventive management in epidemics; protection of persons from disease or infection under various insalubrious conditions.

(f) Morbific effects of different trades and occupations, and the protection of the operatives.

(g) Sanitary regulations for aggregated communities, in workhouses, schools, factories, prisons, asylums, and ships.

§ 18. Another most objectionable feature in the recognised standards of qualification, is the *age* at which the licence to practise is granted—namely, twenty-one years.

It may be safely asserted that—with the exception of rarely powerful minds, for whom, as exceptional cases, no legislation need provide—the mass of students, after a good preliminary education, cannot possibly acquire a sufficient amount of professional and scientific information, for the decent performance of the duties now required of them, under the age of twenty-three years.

It is wholly unjustifiable to let loose upon the community medical tyros, who have only just attained their legal majority. Undoubtedly, for some time longer, they might be much more advantageously employed, as regards both themselves and the public, than in the irresponsible and uncontrolled exercise of their ingenuity upon "cases" which fortune or misfortune may throw in their way.

Yet the English College of Surgeons, after requiring* the attainment of twenty-two years for their diploma, actually lowered the minimum age for membership to twenty-one years, within a comparatively recent period.

The Scotch Universities do worse. They grant their highest honour, the M.D. degree, at twenty-one years! One knows not how to deal with bodies, any more than with persons, who glory in a ridiculous singularity.

§ 19. The exceptional regulations of universities, however, no less than the peculiar bye-laws of medical colleges, ought to be

* Regulations, Oct. 1829.

matters of secondary and subsequent consideration, if considered at all, in medical legislation.

If the State standard of medical qualification were determined on correct principles, and fully adequate to the public requirements, there can be no doubt that those institutions would soon conform. And, in that case, universities might possibly accept the State licence, by way of an *ad eundem*, as a sufficient guarantee of fitness for their primary medical degree. Reciprocally also (and this is most important) the central council might confer its licence, if applied for, on graduates of any British or Irish University, adopting a *curriculum* of education and a *minimum* age, not lower than that which, on the proposed scheme, would be required of all other medical students.

The late estimable Dr. Barlow, of Bath, who was the author of the first connected scheme of medical reform emanating from the provinces, proposed most wisely to identify the primary medical degree of the old universities—the Baccalaureate—with the uniform primary qualification to be demanded by the State.

§ 20. Some universities and colleges might deem it essential to their dignity to adopt a standard of qualification for their diplomas, more exclusive in its kind and more difficult of attainment. Why should their internal regulations be interfered with, in the event of the State providing independently and adequately for the public necessities?

So, with regard to the higher literary acquirements, and the lengthened period of study and probation, demanded by the older universities for their highest honours, and by colleges of physicians and surgeons[*] for their fellowships, such regulations might be left to their fate, if the State did its duty.

---

[*] The institution of the Fellowship in the London College of Surgeons, however reasonable in theory, however capable in original design of conferring a real benefit on the profession and the public, has been so miserably damaged in execution, that, with respect to the present generation of English surgeons, the mischief is irremediable. Successive attempts to redress the original grievance have only aggravated the confusion and injustice.

The primary mistake consisted in applying the distinction retrospectively. For

§ 21. With regard to the obstetric art, little need be said in this place.

It is clearly the duty of the State to ensure the thorough competency of those who practice midwifery.

The safety of mothers, the health and vigour of progeny, are matters deserving the highest consideration of a Government, for they concern most deeply the welfare of society.

If the proposed council, for the direction of medical education, contained one or more eminent authorities in obstetrics, we may rest assured that the best methods of training, for this branch of medicine, would be enforced.

In England, a certain proportion of physicians and the majority of surgeons practice midwifery. The art is not confined exclusively to the members of any particular college or grade of the profession. Nor should it be. It is therefore unreasonable to commit examinations in midwifery to single colleges, either of physicians or of surgeons.

All, who are to practise as accoucheurs, should be subject to the same *curriculum* of study and preparation in this department.

The amount of attendance at lying-in hospitals,—or, under the guidance and superintendence of experienced accoucheurs, among the poor in their dwellings,—would be determined by the proposed central committee; and the examinations would be very properly delegated to a separate section of a metropolitan examining board.

Arrangements ought certainly to be made for the due instruction and qualification of females in this branch of practice.

§ 22. The education and qualification of practitioners in phar-

---

this, the main pretext was the expediency of forming a constituency, from and by which the council might be elected. But this end might have been attained with equal security and more general satisfaction, by granting the elective franchise to all members of a certain standing—length of membership and mode of practice being both considered—and by restricting the new grade to those only, who chose to undergo the higher examination, and who, after obtaining the Fellowship, would have been entitled to participate with the senior members of the College in the election of the council.

macy is a more difficult matter for re-arrangement, in our anomalous condition.

By pharmacy, I now mean only the use and application of the "Materia Medica" recognised in the three metropolitan pharmacopœias, which will soon probably be combined in one national pharmacopœia.

For reasons already stated, and on other grounds, it seems that this branch of practice should be treated distinctly and separately.

A legal qualification in pharmacy should not be forced upon every holder of the State licence; although (as far as it can be taught) a knowledge of the action of all reputed medicinal agents upon the human frame, in sickness and in health, should be required of every one admitted to practise medicine.

So long as, and wherever, the mutual convenience of the public and the practitioner might be promoted by his combining with his other vocations the practice of pharmacy, suitable arrangements should be promoted for attaining this end; and it is very doubtful whether a simpler or more efficient machinery for testing the *pharmaceutical* knowledge of medical candidates could be devised, than that at present working in the examinations of the Societies of Apothecaries in London and Dublin, and the Edinburgh College of Surgeons. If not, why should their arrangements be disturbed further than to confine the special examinations of those Societies to pharmacy, and matters inseparable therefrom?

§ 23. But the public safety demands much more than a provision for the practice of pharmacy by *medical* men.

The greatest amount of pharmaceutical business in this kingdom is now conducted by chemists and druggists, who are not compelled to possess a legal certificate of competency.

Recent enactments, indeed, confer certain privileges on members of the Pharmaceutical Society, and on those who may choose to undergo an examination by that body; but there is no check upon, no control over, others who sell and prepare medicines without having passed that ordeal.

The public is, therefore, still unprotected against the very serious consequences of prevailing ignorance, error, and malpractice among this class.

With regard to improved regulations for the sale of medicines, this is not the occasion for details; and I would merely observe, that it is essential to any complete system of medical police, that every preparer and vendor of medicines should be duly examined, legally licensed, and placed under scientific inspection.

It is also expedient that such examinations should be conducted by a different board from that which tests the pharmaceutical knowledge of medical practitioners.

§ 24. It is scarcely necessary to point out to those who are at all conversant with the question of medical education, the wide difference between the principles of legislation which have now been submitted, and the views which appear to have guided the framers of measures recently laid before Parliament, or offered publicly for the opinion of the profession.

The measure most recently brought into the House of Commons, by Mr. Headlam, Mr. Brady, and Mr. Craufurd, alone demands notice, for it embodies many decided improvements upon previous schemes, and is a very fair attempt to reconcile rival claims and conflicting interests.

A complete analysis of the Bill would be quite out of place in this work.

It may suffice to mention that it provides for—

i. Examinations in general science and literature, to be considered equivalent to university degrees in arts, &c.; though, by some strange oversight, these examinations are not made, of necessity, preliminary to strictly professional studies:

ii. Some similarity in the *curricula* of medical study to be required by the several colleges:

iii. Control over the final examinations, so as to insure something like uniformity of qualification in the three divisions of the kingdom:

iv. A higher, though still insufficient, age on admission:

v. A general registration of medical practitioners: and

vi. A uniform national pharmacopœia.

Few will be disposed to deny that these are all desirable reforms, as far as they go. And it would be a profitless task to discuss the several details and minor points, in which the clauses differ from the general recommendations which I have now ventured to offer.

§ 25. But my principal reason for referring to this Bill, is to direct attention to the proposed method of constituting the "Council of Medicine;" which would be empowered merely to regulate the education, examination, and registration of medical practitioners. It would have no connexion with a central council of health. It would perform no duties of sanitary inquiry and deliberation.

Taking it, therefore, as analogous to the committee of medical education, suggested in these pages, I am tempted, in the first place, to ask whether the particular representative composition of the council, indicated by the Bill, is likely to satisfy the various collegiate and academical bodies and classes of practitioners, whose interests it attempts to reconcile, and whose favour it would fain conciliate.

The members of council are to be nineteen in number, eleven nominated by the several universities and colleges, and eight by the registered practitioners, after the first appointment by Government.

The reasons of the authors of this measure, for that precise apportionment of representation among the various professional bodies, may be hereafter explained to us. At present, we are without information on the point; but, if representation is to be based, in any degree, upon numbers, it will be difficult to show why, out of nineteen members, only eight are to be nominated in England, and five in Ireland, while six are to come from Scotland.

Setting England aside, it remains to be seen what Ireland will say to the offer of a minimum share of administrative power in the proposed governing body.

Surely, if a somewhat superior medical organization and polity, high collegiate reputation, and considerable parliamentary influence (all which mark the profession in Ireland), are to affect the ultimate distribution of seats in this council, the Green Isle ought to obtain a fairer proportion of representation, in the event of Parliament agreeing to any measure of the kind.

Whether it be desirable that the whole of the council should be representative is another question, requiring much thoughtful deliberation.

If the central controlling body, in the matter of education, were to constitute, as I have suggested, a medical committee of a central council of health; there would be less objection—probably none—to a purely elective constitution, because its proceedings would be liable to control and supervision by the superior body.

But if, as proposed in this Bill, there is to be no appeal from its decisions, the Legislature should pause before establishing it.

We have seen enough of the working of irresponsible medical boards, to prevent our expecting much benefit from the institution of another. Does not the late nomination of a Medical Council, for the purpose of advising the General Board of Health on preventive measures, point out the course that should be pursued in a medical reform bill? Why should we have *two* central *medical* councils, one for consultation in epidemic visitations, the other for medical organization, when these two subjects present so many points of mutual interest and interdependence?

§ 26. The conclusive and only unanswerable plea for legislative interference in the affairs of the medical profession, is that —THE SAFETY OF THE PEOPLE IS THE SUPREME LAW OF THE REALM.

It must prove an endless, as it has already proved a futile and thankless, labour, to devise a measure embodying a series of ingenious compromises between a host of rival professional bodies, to whom such an important power, as that of determining the number and qualification of those legally admitted to practise medicine, ought never to have been surrendered by the State.

§ 27. Strong grounds have been shown for the necessity of some system of control over licensed practitioners, in the exercise of their professional duties; but as this matter—although handled in recent medical-reform Bills—belongs to medical police rather than to medical education, it may be as well to suggest that matters of internal regulation would be most efficiently managed by Medical Faculties,* constituted in extensive districts, and presided over by a superintending officer of health.

In cases involving irreconcilable difference of opinion, an appeal to the central council should be authorized.

So again, if a general representation of the profession, in the proposed central council, be determined upon, it would, for obvious reasons, be more safely and beneficially conducted through a district organization.

§ 28. Most medical Bills, also, contain a clause empowering every practitioner to recover reasonable fees for attendance. Though not strictly belonging to our present subject, it may be remarked, in passing, that such a provision would confer a much greater advantage upon the public than upon the profession, provided no right were conceded to the general practitioner to recover, in addition to his proper fee for attendance, more than the actual value† of medicines and appliances furnished by him to the patient.

With regard, however, to the consulting classes of the profession, it may well be doubted whether any parties would be gainers by the substitution of a legal claim for the customary *honorarium*.‡

§ 29. Nothing remains to be said respecting recent projects of legislation, save on one point discussed in the commencement of

---

* See Essay V.

† Including a compensation for storing and compounding, &c.

‡ "I should be sorry to see the honorary character of fees of barristers and physicians done away with. Though it seems a shadowy distinction, I believe it to be beneficial in effect. It contributes to preserve the idea of a profession, of a class which belongs to the public, in the employment and remuneration of which no law interferes, but the citizen acts as he likes *in foro conscientiæ*."—Coleridge's *Table Talk*, p. 189.

this Essay, namely, penal clauses against unregistered practitioners and those who falsely pretend to be legally qualified. Here, I must risk unpopularity among my medical brethren, by protesting against the impolicy, to say the least, of attempting to enforce penalties against medical dissenters, until broad and comprehensive legislation shall have authorized all, without reference to their belonging to any particular medical sect, who may prove their competency to treat disease, and to promote health and longevity, by undergoing the discipline, completing the *curricula*, and passing the examinations (limited and regulated by a State council), which I have already presumed to recommend.

Then, indeed, penalties may be fairly enforced against those who attempt to practise without the State licence and registration. And then, also, it would be quite reasonable to deal more summarily with those, who, not having obtained the licence, assume the titles, and lay claim to the privileges, of legally qualified practitioners.

§ 30. I should have great confidence in an appeal to the calm and deliberate judgment of the entire profession on this subject. Anomalous and irregular as its condition may be, subject as its members have been to numerous influences calculated to disturb their equanimity, I believe in the elevating effect of Medicine, as a divine calling.*

Had there not been some internal correcting and renovating influence at work, the medical profession could never have so vigorously resisted the natural tendency of all institutions to deteriorate. The unconcern, the neglect, the careless repudiation of responsibility, in both its internal affairs and its relations to the State, which the constitutional government of England has ever evinced, have, indeed, depressed the social *status* of the

* Without assenting to the noted Dr. Parr's recorded opinion of the professions of law and divinity, I quote the passage, to show his view of the medical profession:—"The practice of the law spoils a man's moral sense and philosophic spirit; the church is too bigoted and stiff-starched; but the study and practice of physic are equally favourable to a man's moral sentiments and intellectual faculties."

medical body, cramped its usefulness, and suffered its want of regulation to injure the community; but they have not succeeded in crushing its vitality.

Coleridge said—" There have been three silent revolutions in England: first, when the professions fell off from the Church; secondly, when literature fell off from the professions; and thirdly, when the press fell off from literature."

Whether or not counter-revolutions may be expected with regard to the first and third movements, it is clear that a counter-revolution in medicine is now silently working as to the second. And, under a sound system of medical education, we may yet appeal to the truth of our motto—

"MEDICINA LITERIS."

ESSAY III.

ON SANITARY INQUIRY:

ITS METHODS AND DEFECTS IN ENGLAND—THE DIRECTIONS IN WHICH IT NEEDS EXTENSION UNDER STATE AUTHORITY.

THE State which founds its legislation on a knowledge of realities, which expects from the physical sciences information respecting human life collectively, considered in all its relations, has a right to demand from its physicians a general insight into the nature and causes of popular diseases."

HECKER's *Epidemics of the Middle Ages.* Preface to *Sweating Sickness.*—BABINGTON'S TRANSLATION.

ESSAY III.

CHAPTER FIRST.

Some of the Characteristics of Ancient and Modern Sanitary Inquiry.

§ 1. From the days of the Father of Medicine, different modes of life, personal habits, social customs, and places of residence, beside various circumstances of external nature—air and water, seasons and climate—have been noticed and recorded by celebrated public physicians, as tending to improve or to impair man's health, vigour, and activity; to lengthen or to shorten his existence; to render the greater portion of life beneficial to himself and to the general prosperity of the State, or to deteriorate and degrade both the individual and his race.

The observation of such influences upon persons and communities, constituted the earliest method of sanitary investigation; and the value of each observation depended upon the mental power of the inquirer to grasp a sufficient number of fairly selected instances, for the determination and expression of a general law.

The evidence, indeed, might be perfectly clear, even when the facts noticed were comparatively few; but, in such cases, positive conclusions were not to be relied on, unless made by persons of great discrimination and profound thought.

Statistical methods, so necessary for ordinary observers, and in modern times, were not in force among the few really great physicians of antiquity.

§ 2. Records of disease,—of its causes and treatment,—were,

however, preserved in the most ancient European hospitals, the temples or *Sanatoria* of Æsculapius and Hygieia; and it is said that the works of Hippocrates were, for the most part, composed after his study of these Registers at Cos,* although his conclusions are not presented to us in the form of induction.

It may be, as M. Littré and Dr. Adams have suggested respecting the treatise on *Air, Waters, and Places*, that the sanitary writings of the Coan physician were meant "as textbooks, on which were grounded his public prelections, wherein would no doubt be given all the necessary proofs and illustrations."†

We see, however, only the "grand results" of original observation and reflection. And we know not how far the laws of health, left to us by Hippocrates, may be due to his own extraordinary penetration and intuitive perception, rather than to deductions from recorded facts.

Some of his opinions with regard to the effects of locality and climate,—the influence of the site and aspect of cities upon the physical form, health, and constitution of their inhabitants,—seem often to have been founded simply on personal and cursory observations; while his statements as to the causation of particular maladies, under certain meteorological conditions, during the prevalence of certain winds, and at certain seasons, seem as if they resulted from more positive evidence; and indicate that the antecedent and concomitant circumstances of sickness had been carefully noted, and the relative importance of their respective shares in its origin and diffusion precisely weighed.

Subsequent ætiologists, for a thousand years, appear to have been scarcely more than commentators on Hippocrates.

* Φασὶ δ' Ἱπποκράτην μάλιστα ἐκ τῶν ἀνακειμένων ἐνταῦθα θεραπειῶν γυμνάσασθαι τὰ περὶ τῆς διαίτης.—Strabo. lib. xiv. p. 971.

Hippocrates, "cum fuisset mos, liberatos morbis scribere in templo ejus Dei, [*sc. Æsculapii*] quid auxiliatum esset, ut postea similitudo proficeret, *exscripsisse ea traditur.*"—Plin *Hist. Nat.* lib. xxix. s. 2.

† See note, p. 184, Adams's *Translation of the Genuine Works of Hippocrates*. 1849.

The precepts of health generally received and taught had more to do with the private life of the individual than with the polity of the State.

When and where public precautions were adopted, they were seldom, if ever, based upon a series of accurate inquiries. They rested on the authority of opinion.*

There has never been a second Hippocrates;† and if there were one now, we should not believe in him.

§ 3. Had Lord Bacon's principles of inquiry been carefully applied to the population of even a few States, numerous questions, upon which the vaguest opinions have since been formed, might have been almost definitively settled.

His remarkable *Historia Vitæ et Mortis* contains not only the substance of all previously recorded experience with regard to the influence of surrounding agencies and modes of life upon health and longevity, with many interesting and original observations of his own, but also some excellent rules for statistical inquiry, which have yet to be applied on a large scale.

(i.) He considered the body chemically as well as physiologically; the nature of its inanimate constituents, and the waste and repair of its vital organs.

(ii. and iii.) He advised that facts respecting the duration of life, and the causes of organic decay and nutrition, should be investigated; first, in the vegetable world; then, in the lower animals; and that the inquiry should thence ascend to the human race.

(iv.) As to man, he urged that the "inquisition" should be more exact in all particulars, and complete in all its parts, or confirmed by numerical calculations (*numeris suis absoluta*).

---

* Langius says—"Apud Herodianum invenio, miserabiliter urgenti in Italiâ peste, præsertim in urbe ob advenas undique sine discrimine eò advenientes, *ex consilio medicorum*, Laurentum secessisse, quod aëris frigidioris afflatû et odore lauri ejus regionis periculum evitarent."

This was at Rome in the second century. Laurentum is the modern St. Lorenzo.

† I need hardly explain that this remark applies to the man, and not to his name. He himself was the second Hippocrates, and there were several other physicians of the same name, in his own family.

(v.) Concerning longevity and brevity of life, said he, you must inquire with reference to historical epochs, regions, and climates of the world, places of nativity, and residence;

(vi.) About race and ancestry, for the causes may be hereditary; also about constitutions, temperaments, and habits of body; stature, manner and periods of growth; conformation and structure of limbs;

(vii.) About the times of birth,* admitting only common and manifest facts as to births in the seventh, eighth, ninth, and tenth months; also whether they occurred by night or day, and in what month of the year;

(viii.) About food, diet, exercises, and the like;†

(ix.) About occupations and modes of life, passions of the soul, and various accidental circumstances;

(xi.) About the signs and prognostics of a long or short life—not those which denote approaching death, for such belong to medical records—but those which are apparent in health, whether physiognomical or other.

Bacon wished further to extend the inquiry to the action of medicines,(x.) and other matters which were intended either (xii.) to preserve the human frame from decay, or (xiii.) to promote its alimentation and reparation, or (xiv.) to favour the removal or absorption of what was effete and useless.

He also recommended "inquisition" as to the manner in which life becomes extinct (xv.) through privation, defect of assimilation, and senile atrophy.

And lastly (xvi.), he directed diligent inquiry into the exact nature of the changes which take place in the progress from youth to age,—into the differences of condition and of the various faculties of the two periods of life.‡

---

* He added, "Ita inquirito ut astrologica et schemata cœli in presentia omittas."

† He understood the atmosphere, in which men dwelt, to be included under the former head—*places* of residence.

‡ Not having an opportunity of referring to a translation of Lord Bacon's *Historia Vitæ et Mortis*, I have given what I suppose to be the meaning of the greater part of his *Topica Particularia*, pp. 114—118, vol. x. *Opera Latina minora*, Montagu's Ed. 1828.

Although in that treatise he excluded the notice of facts relating to disease generally and to epidemics in particular, as belonging to "medical history," which, he elsewhere remarked,* " considereth *causes of diseases, with the occasions or impulsions*, the diseases themselves with the accidents, and the cures with the preservations ;" he no less strongly urged greater attention to medical records, which he found to be very deficient, " neither so infinite as to extend to every common case, nor so reserved as to admit none but wonders."

He also complained of the " discontinuance of the ancient and serious diligence of Hippocrates."

One cannot examine Bacon's principles and scheme of inquiry, without being struck with their singularly comprehensive character, their superiority to the state of science in the early part of the seventeenth century, and their obvious connexion with present subjects and methods of research.

The defects of his chemistry and physiology were those of his times. But his programme is minute enough for any modern statistical congress.

§ 4. In our own age,—since the numerical form of inductive proof has been generally applied to sanitary science and political medicine,—it has been too often discredited by a sad want of care and precision in the selection of instances, or rather in their classification for the purposes of deduction.

It has been well said that " the only facts which can ever become useful as grounds of physical inquiry, are those which happen uniformly and invariably under the same circumstances."†
Now the precise conditions of each of the several cases included

---

* *Advancement of Learning*, Book II. Chap. x. § § 2, 3,

† Herschel's *Natural Philosophy*, 1830, p. 119. He proceeds :—" If one and the same result does not constantly happen under a given combination of circumstances, apparently the same, one of two things must be supposed,—caprice (*i. e.*, the arbitrary intervention of mental agency), or differences in the circumstances themselves, really existing, but unobserved by us. In either case, though we may record such facts as curiosities, or as awaiting explanation when the difference of circumstances shall be understood, we can make no use of them in scientific inquiry."

in a single observation, have been very frequently neglected in sanitary inquiries. A series of instances which required careful analysis, and perhaps division into twenty or thirty groups, has been roughly treated as one. And a conclusion, wholly fallacious, has thus been hastily drawn, and laid down as a medical or sanitary law.

Results have been also deduced from too limited a number of cases,—selected, moreover, according to the opinion or prejudgment of the inquirer.

Examples of both those results of ill-conducted statistical research, of very recent occurrence, might be cited; verifying the proverb that "you may prove anything by figures."

§ 5. A curious instance of statistical blundering occurred not twenty years ago.

There was a great stir about workhouse dietaries. It was important to ascertain their effects upon health and life. The secretary of the Poor Law Commissioners, it is said, thought fit to examine the experience of Prisons on this subject. He therefore took sixty gaols, dividing them, according to their dietary tables, into three classes:—full, intermediate, and low diet. He noted the number of offenders committed, the number of those who fell sick, and the number who died in each class of prisons.

And he found this tabular result:*

	Daily Cost of Food.	Sick per cent.	Deaths.
Twenty *low* diet	$3\frac{1}{4}d.$	$3\frac{3}{4}$	1 in 622
Twenty *full* diet	$5\frac{1}{2}d.$	$23\frac{1}{2}$	1 in 266

By raising the expense of maintenance of each prisoner to $5\frac{1}{2}$d. per diem, he inferred that the sickness was increased six-fold, and the mortality more than doubled!

A closer examination of the facts soon exposed the following errors in that extraordinary assumption :—

(1) The number of persons committed had been reckoned, instead of the average population of each prison :

* The "intermediate diet" class is omitted as not affecting the question.

(2) No notice had been taken of the fact,—that "cases of sickness" were very differently registered in different prisons. In those classed under "full diet," every complaint, however slight, seems to have been recorded; while only severe cases, sent to the infirmary wards, had been entered in gaols where the prisoners were more hardly treated:

(3) The difference in the term of detention in the two extremes of prison classification, was also omitted; and it proved that in what were called "full dietary" prisons, the average term of detention was 84 days; while in the "low dietary" prisons, it was only 34 days, a period too short for the development of the injurious effects of residence in the insalubrious condition of imprisonment:

(4) The ages, sexes, and previous sanitary state of the prisoners, in the respective classes, were also omitted.

The result of a more accurate investigation showed that a slightly higher rate of mortality prevailed under low dietaries, notwithstanding the short term of imprisonment; and that in the full dietary prisons, only 15 cases in 1000 ended fatally; while in the others, no less than 40 deaths occurred in 1000 cases. The practical conclusions of the economist were therefore reversed.*

§ 6. Another instance may be cited as still more clearly illustrating the nature of those defects in sanitary inquiry, to which I have called attention. The average age at death of different classes of the community, was assumed, a few years ago, by some ardent sanitary reformers,† to be a test of the salubrity of the circumstances under which those classes respectively lived. And it was thus made to appear that the gentry are longer lived than tradesmen, and tradesmen than artisans or labourers.

But (1) it was not shown how many of those who *died* in

* See an able statistical review of Mr. C.'s paper in the *Lancet*, 1838, p. 779.

† The error arose from the incautious use made of certain returns in the General Sanitary Report and its Supplement, of 1842 and 1843; and the results were still more boldly misapplied by the Metropolitan Sanitary Association.

The question was treated at considerable length, and the fallacies fully exposed, in a celebrated article in the *Brit. and For. Med.-Chir. Review*, Jan. 1848.

advanced age as gentry, had lived during the active period of existence as labourers, farmers, or tradesmen, and had laid the foundation of their longevity in those "inferior" circumstances:

Nor (2) was the great proportion of the labouring classes who died at advanced ages in workhouses, taken into account:

Nor (3) were the deaths of a numerous "undescribed" class analysed:

While (4) the greatest source of fallacy in this assumption, consisted in omitting to estimate the average age of the living (a fact which I know to be extremely difficult to ascertain in any district, under existing public arrangements) in each of those classes, for which the age at death was recorded.

Subsequent inquiries on a larger scale tend to the conclusion—though the proof is not complete—that the working classes, in places where there are no gin-palaces, notwithstanding their miserable dwellings and exposure to casualties, are longer lived than the affluent and luxurious.

§ 7. But beside want of accuracy in the statistical method, other peculiarities were to be noticed in the principal inquiries which immediately preceded recent legislation on the public health.

Here, I must premise that these inquiries established certain conclusions, which it may be as well at once briefly to detail, for the purpose of showing the scope and direction of the late "Health of Towns" movement in this country.

i. Public arrangements for town sewerage and drainage and for cleansing the surface of streets and pavements were proved, generally, to be most defective.

ii. Sewers were extremely rare in comparison with the streets and places which required them, and were generally constructed on erroneous principles, forming "elongated cesspools," and generating mephitic exhalations.

iii. Domestic arrangements for the reception of refuse, in an immense majority of instances, had no communication with the public sewers, even where these existed.

In the absence of house-drains, the subsoil of towns was generally found to be studded with sinks and cesspools; the surface of courts, alleys, and bye-places, covered with middens and heaps of refuse, and the atmosphere laden with impurity and charged with deadly gaseous emanations.

iv. The drainage of *lands*, and the consequent removal of stagnant moisture in and around populous districts, where adopted, had apparently produced great improvement in the climate and in public health; but these places were found to be few compared with others in which nothing of the sort had been attempted, and which accordingly suffered from malaria.

v. Water, the second great necessary of life, was very insufficiently supplied to the inhabitants of towns. Its quality, generally inferior, was found to be further deteriorated by the methods of its distribution, supply, and detention in houses and premises; and thus a main source of comfort and cleanliness was rendered a probable cause of preventible disease and mortality.

vi. Suburban districts were stated to be frequently intersected by open ditches and foul water-courses, laden with the decomposing impurities of the towns. Offensive occupations and deposits were often found to exist in greater numbers, and with fewer attempts at palliation, in the outskirts, than in the streets and courts of towns.

vii. Owing to the last-mentioned evils, and the absence of public walks, parks, and gardens, for the poorer classes of towns, opportunities for breathing pure air and for healthy exercise were found to be everywhere sadly deficient.

viii. Grievous abuses and mismanagement were discovered in the internal economy of factories and places of work. Want of ventilation was almost universal.

ix. The defective structural arrangements, and the damp and filthy state of lodging-houses, cottages, and the closely-packed dwellings of the poor in towns, the condition of their sleeping apartments in particular, were shown to be generally detrimental to health and life, degrading to their moral and physical constitutions, producing a disastrous amount of intemperance and immorality, successfully opposing the progress of education and the influence of religious teaching, disgusting to all who were not inured to an atmosphere of impurity; promoting and intensifying attacks of epidemic disease, and deeply injurious to the welfare of society at large.

x. The practice of intramural burial of the dead was shown to lower the public standard of health, virtue, and decency. All inquiries confirmed Mr. Walker's* original statements as to the disgraceful condition of grave-yards in the metropolis and other populous places; the prevalent disrespect to the remains of the departed, occasionally even their horrible mutilation and indecent exposure. The destructive effects of mephitic gas, from bursting coffins and prematurely opened graves, were stated on credible evidence. Instances were adduced of the communication of disease from human remains. Solid objections were urged against all endeavours to preserve bodies from their natural return to dust, *i. e.*, to inorganic matter fit for re-admission into living combinations.

xi. The needless expense of interments, the sordid practice of undertakers, and the shocking haste and irreverence common to the burial of the poor in crowded localities, were justly exposed.

Frightful abuses were proved to exist in burial societies among the working classes; the temptation of realizing small insurances even leading in some instances to murder.

xii. Social evils of great magnitude were fairly traced to the undue retention of the dead in crowded apartments, and in horrible familiarity with their miserable living inmates.

xiii. The advantages of scientific expedients and precautions as to modes and places of burial, and for the protection of

* Mr. Walker's arduous and unpaid labours in this cause were never even alluded to in the *Report on Interment in Towns*, 1843. This is an instance of the unfairness which characterizes too many of Mr. Chadwick's sanitary writings.

survivors, and the superiority of the German system of sanitary police in the regulation of interments, were well shown.

xiv. Heavy expenses and pecuniary losses, far exceeding the cost of most comprehensive measures of purification, regulation, and prevention, were estimated for families and communities.

xv. Existing laws were shown to be wholly inoperative for public protection against local nuisances, and wholly inadequate to enforce the required reforms in unhealthy places.

xvi. A heterogeneous and perplexing medley of petty and inefficient local jurisdictions was proved to exist, especially in the metropolis, checking spontaneous efforts at amendment, and hopelessly impeding the execution of sanitary measures.

§ 8. To prove the injurious effects of all these *gravamina et lædentia*, medical evidence was called by each successive Commission.

Indeed, the originators of the several Government inquiries, and the real workers in them, were, with very few exceptions, physicians and surgeons.

Medical reports of high literary and scientific merit were gratuitously placed at the disposal of well-paid legal and engineering functionaries.

But it is perhaps needless to add, that the whole body of evidence, however trustworthy in itself, however valuable as indicating subjects and fields for future inquiry, was necessarily based on limited researches. The principal witnesses and sources of evidence were, moreover, arbitrarily selected.

In this respect, the older methods of sanitary investigation and report in our fleets and armies were superior; for in those services, the whole body of medical officers employed in the entire field of observation contributed their quota, and thus exceptional facts and opinions met with their compensations.

Further, the materials for arriving at positive conclusions were extremely defective, as will be presently shown. The mortality records of the Registrar-General were the only incontrovertible documents cited in proof, and these, without collateral information, might lead, as they have done, to mistaken inferences.

Again, while many important and interesting particulars were accumulated and published, the Sanitary Reports were the less available for practical use and reference, owing to their diffuseness and their want of methodical arrangement.

Scientific, technical, statistical, economical, and administrative facts and suggestions, with historical and continental illustrations, were heaped together in "most admired disorder," through many hundred pages of Blue-Book. The whole mass of reports needed almost another Record Commission to arrange, digest, and condense them.

§ 9. Once more, I would call attention to a distinctive feature of recent official inquiries. They related mainly to towns and dwellings, to isolated communities, to one condition of human society, to one set of influences upon human life; and nothing was more clearly proved by these most valuable documents than the necessity (1) for instituting an organized corps of observers throughout the land; (2) for a division of labour in the central department; and (3) for the delegation of particular subjects to distinct and specially qualified committees of one council of health.

If, as may be safely admitted, the first General Sanitary Report and its Supplement, contained the largest amount of original matter, and manifested the greatest extent of design, the Reports of the Health of Towns' Commissioners in 1844, were generally understood to furnish more minute and accurate information upon the special matters for which they were appointed,— namely, "the drainage of land, the erection, drainage, and ventilation of buildings, and the supply of water, whether for purposes of health, or for the better protection of property from fire."

These volumes had also the advantage of embodying original observations and opinions in the respective departments of scientific inquiry, for which the eminent reporters, who constituted that commission, were severally distinguished.

The Metropolitan Sanitary Commission, afterwards appointed,

although exceeding the objects of its appointment by entering upon the cholera question, and discussing ætiological theorems connected with epidemic disease (which would have been more fitly committed to a medical council), nevertheless progressed a step in the direction of the preceding reports, with more particular reference to the advancing state of art in the skilful construction of sewers and drains.

§ 10. With reference to more recent *local* inquiries, some of which have been made here and there by philanthropic and intelligent medical volunteers, others by the engineering inspectors of the Board of Health, and a few of the best and latest by the new medical officers of health; the first class could not be expected to exhibit uniformity of design or similarity of material; the second class was unavoidably defective in the most necessary element of sanitary investigation; while scarcely any of these reports on physical topography and vital statistics, by whomsoever prepared, do more than indicate the particular impressions of earnest inquirers, at particular times, with regard to facts selected by themselves and occurring within their own limited fields of inspection.

Such efforts, however creditable to their authors, could form no consistent or regulated elements of a permanent national system of inquiry, although many of them will always possess a kind of historical value.

§ 11. Looking generally upon the mass of these printed statements, official and private, and at what has been actually gained by them; looking also at the confined range of matters under investigation, at the brief periods of observation, at the avowed motives and preconceived views of the reporters, some of whom have written in an arrogant and polemical tone; it is hardly possible to avoid the conclusion, that, as a nation, we are yet stumbling at the threshold of the temple of Hygieia, not seeing our way clearly to enter it, as sincere and humble votaries, in the true spirit of philosophical inquiry.

The most vivid and faithful of these irregular and occasional revelations of sanitary truth, are but as bright spots opening in a cloudy sky, and soon obscured by the next shifting stratum of mist. A thousand circumstances may arise, in seemingly capricious succession, to modify, perhaps wholly to invalidate, the conclusions of isolated and ephemeral observers.

The relative value of the several ascertained causes of sickness and mortality, debility and deterioration of race, is still undetermined; many causes are yet, probably, undiscovered; all, whether remote or proximate, are too complex, in their various combinations and correlations, to be fairly dealt with by any number of temporary commissions called into action on sudden emergencies and alarms.

Legislation based upon such inconclusive evidence must, of necessity, prove defective and unsatisfactory.

CHAPTER SECOND.

Subjects on which Public Sanitary Inquiry needs Extension and Permanence in England.

§ 1. It is a striking fact, that Great Britain stands almost alone, among the most civilized nations, in leaving to private and voluntary effort, the record, collection, and publication of many classes of events and circumstances, a careful study of which is essential to any correct inferences as to the causation and prevention of disease.

Any attempt to elevate the physical and social condition of the people, without such knowledge, is mere sanitary empiricism.

The employment of a scientific agency by national governments, for the general record of statistics, bearing in any degree upon the public safety, is by no means a visionary or untried scheme.

But, in most districts of the United Kingdom, numerous valuable materials remain unemployed; a multitude of important facts are unnoticed, or if casually and partially registered, their records are inaccessible and therefore practically useless to the many, who, in this country, rule the Government.

§ 2. The only marked and general exception to this characteristic imperfection of our Civil Service, I believe, is to be found in the department of the Registrar-General of Births, Deaths, and Marriages.

The State and the public are supplied by him with annual reports and quarterly returns of the principal facts of mortality and reproduction in every part of the kingdom, and with weekly health-bills for the metropolis.

Invaluable records of epidemic visitations (as the Reports on Influenza and Cholera,) are compiled by his medical coadjutor; and a decennial census of the population, remarkable for the variety and extent of its information on vital and social statistics, is now made under his authority.

Thus, in effect and in public estimation, the General Register Office constitutes the only authentic source of information, if not the ultimate court of appeal, in all occurrences seriously affecting the public health.

The regular periodicity, the universality, and the calm freedom from controversy, which characterize the documents emanating from this office, place them in striking contrast with the earlier publications of the General Board of Health.

§ 3. Nevertheless, it must be recollected that the returns of mortality relate only to those deviations from health which terminate fatally; and that the annual sum of DEATHS in any locality is the only datum at hand for an estimate—which must be merely approximate and theoretical—of the comparative vigour and physical soundness of its inhabitants.

The ages at death, and the ages of the living, in any parish or district, which go far to correct such an estimate, can be ascertained only by much personal sacrifice of time and labour. In the absence of a local machinery for abstract, these facts cannot be generally employed for the public advantage.

It must also be confessed that the certification of the causes of death, although steadily improving, is still defective in completeness and accuracy.

Some official information, not unimportant, on this point, has very recently come into my possession.

In a correspondence with the medical officers of health, lately appointed in a few towns of England and Wales (of which I shall have occasion to make extensive use in a subsequent Essay), only two, out of nine who replied on this subject, considered the certified statements of the causes of death to be "full and satisfactory."

CAUSES OF DEATH. 103

These two reside in the county of Durham, while the returns of seven others, in different parts of the kingdom, are as follows:—

No. 3. "Incomplete."
No. 4. "Often defective," with some curious instances in proof.
Nos. 5 and 6. "By no means satisfactory."
No. 7. "Not as it ought to be. The registrars take certificates from all kinds of illegal practitioners. Some time ago I took off from one file *nineteen* certificates given by a druggist. Government ought to prevent this, as it defeats the intention for which the registry of deaths was ordered."
No. 8. "Not full or satisfactory."
No 9. could only say they were "tolerable."

§ 4. Now, it must not be forgotten that the certification of the causes of deaths, is the result of an appeal to the public spirit and good feeling of the medical profession; that the entire mass of information thus afforded to the community is gratuitous; and that the Registrar-General has done his utmost to insure a careful and trustworthy record of the alleged causes of mortality.

Granting all this, as well as the progressive amendment in the certificates, it cannot be doubted that the unsatisfactory, incomplete, and inaccurate statements to which the officers of health bear testimony, are not infrequent in most large towns, and that the system is capable of a much nearer approach to perfection.*

In crowded and neglected localities, where life is at a low value, the consequence of the non-requirement of medical certificates may be readily imagined. Yet, in such places, many deaths do occur, especially among children, without the cognizance or

---

* In my Report (1848) to the Registrar-General, on the mortality of Gloucester, it was shown that, excluding the deaths in public institutions, and those on which coroner's inquests had been held, "no fewer than 39 per cent. of the other deaths were registered without medical certificate, on the mere authority of survivors, or nurses! Hence deaths were reported to be from 'strictures in the wind-pipe,' and 'rheumatism in the bowels'!

"The extreme importance of not depending on the unauthorized statements of parties who may have an object in concealing or mis-stating facts, was urged by one of the Registrars, who told me that he had discovered in the year, two in-visit of a legally qualified practitioner.* In a still greater number of cases, some medical man is asked to see the dying person barely in time to warrant an application to him for the certificate.

What reliance can be placed on a casual opinion respecting the cause of death obtained under such circumstances?

Here, the remedy would be to enforce, by law, medical inspection and report, in every instance. If the death occurred before the medical visit, a post-mortem examination should be imperatively required.

It must indeed be a rare case, even under the present non-compulsory system, in which the practitioner, who has attended, declines to grant a certificate; yet, absence from home or some accidental occurrence must often prevent his compliance with the first request of the registrar or the survivors; and all the parties concerned are naturally disposed to save themselves trouble.†

Thus, from one circumstance or another, proper certification is very frequently omitted, or imperfectly performed, especially in dense populations.

And it is plain, that, until medical certificates, based on accurate investigations, are peremptorily required by legal enactment in all cases, from duly qualified practitioners, the community can possess no adequate security against secret crime.

Nor can this department of public inquiry be considered com-

---

stances in which the deaths of infants *born alive*, were represented to him as *still-births*."

In most places, doubtless, a marked improvement has taken place in the certification of deaths. The following figures, for which I am indebted to Dr. Greenhill, afford an instance in proof:—

HASTINGS DISTRICT.

Per-centage of not *certified Deaths.*

Year.	Per cent.	Year.	Per cent.	Year.	Per cent.
1846 }		1849 }		1852 }	
1847 }	. . . 33·71	1850 }	. . . 28·16	1853 }	. . . 16·85
1848 }		1851 }		1854 }	

* See Registrars' Notes at the end of several "Quarterly Returns."
† See instances in *Medical Times and Gaz.*, March 24, 1855.

plete, until the registration of births be made compulsory, and a separate record be kept of still-births.

§ 5. But if our only thoroughly organized system of civil sanitary record be thus open to criticism, what can be said for the department of medical statistics?

The truth is, that no complete, authentic, and generally available returns are made and published in this country, with regard to the sickness, accidents, and infirmity, which occur,—either among bodies of work-people under legal protection and in public employ,—or among inmates of our civil institutions, whether penal, reformatory, or eleemosynary,—or among the masses, whose maladies are relieved partly by the medical officers of unions, and partly by means of hospitals and dispensaries, but who are too often abandoned to a miserable self-provision—to private professional charity, or to utter neglect.

§ 6. Lists of cases are indeed prepared weekly by the Union medical officers, in order that Boards of Guardians may review, from time to time, the progress and extent of local pauperism, and may determine the amount or confirm the grant of other relief; but these returns, being intended merely for economic uses, are unavoidably defective in a scientific or sanitary point of view.

Even the occasional reports, which the medical officers are directed by the Central Board to make, on the advent of epidemics, or on the existence of nuisances and local causes of disease, lose almost all their possible value from being made unsystematically—on the spur of exigency—and presented to bodies notoriously indisposed to incur expense, by acting upon the information thus obtained.

So likewise, from what has transpired respecting the quarterly abstracts of medical relief,* kept by the Poor-Law Board, I infer that they are of little avail, even for the purpose of ascertaining the actual amount of sickness; still less do they show the

---

* Vide Appendix (A) *Health and Sickness of Town Populations,* p. 77.

nature and causes, the personal conditions, the duration and results, of the cases which come under the care of the parochial surgeons.

The annual reports of the Poor-Law Board contain no information whatever, respecting either the sickness of the poor or the medical attendance provided, except its total cost in every Union!

§ 7. Nevertheless, in Ireland, where a medical commissioner and medical inspectors are appointed, the amount of sickness, publicly attended, is far more correctly returned; and the finance and general administration of the system are clearly revealed. Yet, it is said, by persons well qualified to form an opinion, that the medical returns from the dispensaries in Ireland are but of little value to science.

But in England, even the Irish amount of order, accuracy, and completeness, is, and must be, impossible; for, in the large towns especially, the greater portion of sickness among the poor is not even seen by the Union medical officer.*

On the other hand, the medical charities, the sick-clubs, and other voluntary contrivances, for administering that aid, which the State does not provide for the poor, are under no obligation to report their proceedings.

§ 8. Again; the records of the excellent hospitals and dispensaries of this country, relate, for the most part, merely to curative medicine.

Rich stores of information concerning the ætiology of disease and the vital statistics of their respective localities, which they might open to the physician and the statesman, lie almost untouched.

Even their registration of cases exhibits no uniformity of system, and therefore affords no accurate means of comparing results.

Facts of great moment to society, which are, or might be, noted by their medical staffs, are, at all events, unpublished.

---

* See *Report on Medical Poor Relief*, Parliamentary Committee,—1844, cited in Appendix A to *Health and Sickness of Town Populations*, pp. 78—89.

Individual, local, and temporary exceptions to this statement, may, of course, be brought forward, but these serve only to establish the rule,* and Dr. Clifton's "Proposal for the Hospitals," a century and a quarter old, still remains to be carried generally into execution.

"First of all," said he, "three or four persons of proper qualifications should be employed in the *Hospitals* (and that without any ways interfering with the gentlemen now concerned) to set down the cases of the patients there, from day to day, *candidly* and *judiciously*, without any regard to private opinions, or public systems, and at the year's end publish these facts just as they are, leaving every one to make the best use of them he can for himself. Would not some such method as this let us more into the *nature* of diseases in a few years than all the books of *theories*, or even the books of *observations* hitherto published? Certainly it would: and yet, if proper encouragement was given, 'tis not at all unlikely but that persons enow wou'd soon be found every way qualified for such an undertaking. And even if good salaries were allow'd 'em, and everything made as easy and agreeable to 'em as they cou'd desire, the benefit the publick wou'd receive from 'em wou'd vastly more than balance the expence. . . . Private men may labour and tug at it as much as they will, but they can never bring it to a bearing like the publick."†

Legal and constitutional objections might be fairly urged against requiring hospitals, infirmaries, and dispensaries—supported by private endowments and subscriptions—to furnish gratuitously such information as a council of State Medicine might deem desirable. But, provided a reasonable remuneration were secured to the secretaries or resident officers for making returns, it would be quite justifiable and practicable to place recusant in-

---

* It is especially due to the staff of St. George's Hospital, London, to mention their appointment of medical and surgical registrars, and their publication of the general results of treatment in certain kinds of disease and injury.—*Medical Times and Gaz.*, Nov. 1853.

Other hospitals, as the Canterbury Infirmary, may have done the same. The Report of the "Consumption" Hospital at Brompton is a proof of the value of medical statistics, when applied on a large scale, to particular diseases.

† *Clifton's State of Physick*, 1732, pp. 171-2.

stitutions in the predicament of being neither legally recognised for the education of medical students, nor entitled to their present privilege of freedom from general and local taxation.

§ 9. "A miserable self-provision" of medical aid by the poor has been mentioned; and in this phrase, I would comprise not only their constant resort to ignorant druggists and mischievous quacks; but, also those contracts, which are made by "sick-clubs" with medical practitioners, for attendance and medicines to their ailing members; and lastly, societies instituted solely for the *medical* relief of labouring families, and called " Medical Clubs."

It may be observed, by the way, that these arrangements are removed from the wholesome influence of public supervision; and, as they will come under consideration in the following Essay, I allude to them now, only for the sake of calling attention to the fact, that they have to some extent obstructed and vitiated the results of statistical inquiries into the actual sanitary state of the people. A public registration of the nature, causes, and amount of sickness in every locality, would lead to very desirable changes in these ill-regulated compacts.

§ 10. The preceding remarks on the statistics of medical relief apply almost entirely to the diseases and infirmities of an *undefined class*, the number of which, in any place, it would be extremely difficult to ascertain; although on the average it may be safely estimated to amount to half the population.

How great would be the benefit to the country, if correct information were periodically and generally supplied respecting the sickness and non-effectiveness of even a moiety of its inhabitants!

§ 11. There are, however, in England, other portions of the population, definable in number and condition, in which the ratio of sickness to health could be determined with tolerable accuracy, if the requisite machinery were provided by the State.

Thus, Friendly or Provident Societies, established on correct principles of insurance, and under legal protection, might contribute very valuable materials towards sanitary conclusions.

Their "Quinquennial Returns" have already been employed in this way, with good effect, by some of our leading actuaries.*

But the periods during which numbers of these societies receive "pay," are far from always corresponding with the duration of illness and incapacity; and the returns, as now made, afford no sufficiently distinct evidence of the influence of site, residence, occupation, and habits of living upon the physical condition of the labouring classes. These registers and returns require, therefore, material improvement in form, more careful compilation, and annual abstract and circulation, before they can be enlisted, with their utmost utility, in this cause.

§ 12. So, with regard to large classes of persons employed in public works, in the Police and Revenue departments, and in our great factories, mines, and railways, worked by private enterprise, though subject to legal supervision, the sanitary statistics of these immense bodies are to be ascertained only by referring to ponderous Blue-Books, or to the archives of separate public offices. Here, again, we need the same periodical abstract and publication of results.

§ 13. Passing on to a larger department of inquiry, not un-

---

* "Friendly Societies in general make these returns very reluctantly, and are careless as to their correctness or completeness. A very large proportion of the total returns from these societies has been rejected by Mr. Neison and Mr. Finlayson as unavailable through obvious defects arising from negligence, wilful or otherwise."

The above is taken from a valuable series of papers on the *Laws of Mortality and Sickness of the Labouring Classes of England*, by the eminent actuary, Mr. T. R. Edmonds. We have no higher authority on this subject.—See *Lancet*, vol. ii. 1854, pp. 329, 453.

Another paper, full of useful information upon the proportion of sickness to health, among members of Friendly Societies, was read by Mr. H. Tompkins, at the Institute of Actuaries, in 1854.

His facts, based on parliamentary returns, show the influence of age upon sickness in rather a new light.

Some of his theories will astonish the medical reader.

"Locality had very little to do with the ratio of sickness."

"The duration of sickness is in direct proportion to the vital power."

If such conclusions as the above are hitherto unsupported, the following coincides with medical observation:

"Light labour in the open air" is the most healthy condition of human existence.—See Abstract of Paper in *Med. Times and Gaz.*, July 15, 1854.

connected with the two latter groups of facts, it appears that the United Kingdom, in common with most continental nations, is, at the present time without the means of determining the comparative influence of various trades and occupations upon health and longevity.* Yet nowhere do correct observations on this subject seem to be more urgently called for, or more likely to be beneficial, than in a country so unrivalled for the variety and extent of its manufacturing industry as England.

To be really satisfactory, this investigation should apply to every portion of the population, which depends for subsistence on labour, or employment of any kind. It should note the occurrence of particular maladies and injuries in special occupations; the ulterior results of such ailments, with respect not only to the primary sufferers, but also to their families and posterity; and the effects upon the inhabitants of their respective neighbourhoods, as far as can be ascertained, of certain processes from which mephitic vapours or gaseous emanations arise. It should record all the known circumstances and precautionary expedients, which have been found to lessen the hazard of insalubrious employments.

§ 14. In this department of sanitary inquiry, a regular and periodical repetition of observations is most essential.

For not only are the remarks of the earliest systematic writer on this subject, the learned and accurate Ramazzini, now generally inapplicable to English industry; but, even since the modern researches of Patissier and Thackrah, several occupations on which they treated have been wholly superseded by the advance of civilization, while other processes have been so modified as to diminish, if not to remove, their injurious re-actions and effects.

Moreover, the ever-changing demands of a rapid social progress are continually developing new employments and new arts, some of which, if we may trust recent accounts, are still more

---

* The French Government has promoted inquiries, and preserved annual returns on the subject, for some years.

deleterious to the operatives than those which have become obsolete, or have been rendered comparatively harmless.

A permanent machinery for record and comparison is therefore the more needed, in proportion to the variety and rapidity of the changes made.

Possibly, at the present time, a greater number of working people suffer loss of health, bodily injury, and reduction in the natural term of life, from the want of legal regulation and sanitary precaution, than at any former period.

Thus, from age to age, does man travail mortally with the offspring of his brain and the work of his hands; while few indeed of those, who enjoy the fruits of this labour, stay to reflect how they might derive equal gratification of a higher kind from a less lavish expenditure of vital force, health, and happiness.

Still more slowly does the Government of a State perceive that, as guardian of the people, its truest policy is to watch, and sometimes to control, inventive and productive energy; that the weaker and poorer classes need protection against the unrestricted influence of capital upon labour; and that the real prosperity of a community depends more on the prolongation of its effective lifetime, and on the preservation of its moral and physical integrity, than on the amount of its exports and imports.

§ 15. With the laudable intention of assisting to determine, by strict statistical method, the effects of certain kinds of labour upon human life and health, Dr. Guy and Mr. Neison have each contributed, within a comparatively recent period, some valuable essays; the former taking his facts from mortuary registers and the case-books of his hospital; and the latter, on a most extensive scale, from the quinquennial returns of Friendly Societies; but, their materials being either limited or defective, their deductions, however carefully made, are confessedly inconclusive.

No one, then, need be surprised to hear of another spontaneous effort, promising, for the time, more precise results. I allude to the appointment of a committee by the Society of Arts, to investigate what they aptly term the "industrial pathology" of the kingdom.

The names* of the gentlemen, who have undertaken this task, are guarantees for a vigorous and minute research, as well as for a scientific and truthful report; but, since they are armed with no official authority, they must depend on their own tact and personal influence in obtaining evidence; and they must expect to encounter peculiar obstructions and difficulties, for master-manufacturers and employers are known to be generally averse to such inquiries. It would, in fact, be unsafe for the legislature, or for a council of health, to act upon conclusions derived from voluntary and partial information.

Nor will much be gained by appointing temporary commissions to meet temporary popular demands. Scientific gentlemen, who feel the burden of leisure, are always ready to press on the Government the vast advantage of such appointments. A private job is thus created out of a public grievance, and a plausible excuse afforded for delaying a permanent national organization for the more complete attainment of the object.

It seems obvious that, under the direction of a committee of the proposed council of health, the necessary inquiries should be instituted in every district and at regular intervals, and that the duty of abstracting and analysing the returns should be committed to public functionaries, removed as far as possible from all personal predilections and local influences.

§ 16. Although recent sanitary inquiries have been mainly limited to the circumstances of populous districts, there are still some characteristics of our "great-town system" which require more thorough investigation.

One ought to know the specific density of the population in its smallest practicable divisions. One ought also to be able to compare this density with the physical features of the site, with

---

* Dr. T. K. Chambers, John Simon, T. Twining, Junr. An elaborate report of those trades which affect the eyes, has been recently issued by this committee; and reports on other departments are contemplated. (1855.)

meteorological records, and periodical returns of the vital, sanitary, and social state of each subdivision.

The average extent of surface (breathing space) allotted to each resident upon every acre of crowded districts, should be annually reported. The nature of the localities, as to site and soil, selected for the aggregated abodes of human beings, and the methods in which their dwellings are constructed, should be everywhere carefully examined and noted.

It is no less important to register the number of inhabitants, floors, and rooms, and the cubic space, of every dwelling-house.* And this should be done more frequently in places where the rates of sickness and mortality are high, or where other insalubrious conditions are manifestly present.

Such investigation would, in a short time, decide a question often mooted of late, and bearing directly upon all enactments for regulating the construction of houses.

Some philanthropic and public-spirited persons have tried the experiment of introducing into London and other large towns, the continental and Scotch practice of accommodating entire families on separate " flats," or horizontal sections of large and lofty houses; but they have not yet proved that, by this additional means of condensing the population, the general health and social welfare of the residents, and of the neighbourhood, are promoted more effectually than by enabling each family to occupy its perpendicular section of a lower range, on a laiger area, as is generally the case in England, where every householder prefers to claim his right† *a solo usque ad cœlum*.

Of course, no comparison could be fairly instituted where both descriptions of houses were not in other respects equal as to their sanitary condition.

Unless very unexpected advantages were proved to attend the

* Introductory Essay, p. 10 (I. A. 5.)

† There is an interesting extract in the *Report on the Census*, 1851 (8vo, 1854, p. 7), from *The King of Saxony's Journey through England and Scotland in* 1844, by Dr. C. G. Carus, with remarks by the Registrar-General and his coadjutors on the two systems of house accommodation.

new system, it would surely be undesirable to disturb notions and habits of independent reserve, so characteristic of the English, and so plainly connected with their structural and domestic arrangements.

§ 17. A public system of inquiry is not less urgently called for, respecting the different kinds of aliment consumed by the working population, in different places.

This question is one of deep interest to statesmen, to the managers of public institutions, and to all who are entrusted, medically or otherwise, with the care and supervision of poor-houses, prisons, ships, asylums, and hospitals; while to the officers of our land and sea forces it is of paramount importance.

With regard to bodies of persons assembled under authority, observations might be readily made and compared; and much has already been done, and is doing, in this way: but, as concerns the poorer classes at large, the inquiry has been wholly neglected.

Yet, believing that extensive and continued investigations would lead to very beneficial results, I would suggest that in all cases of sickness and injury attended at the public charge, whether at the homes of the poor or in charitable establishments, the medical officers should be directed to ascertain and record,—

(*a*) the nature, quality, and quantity of the ordinary diet, not only of the patients, but of the families to which they belong;

(*b*) their methods of preparing, cooking, and preserving victuals;

(*c*) their liability to vitiated and deteriorated articles of food;

(*d*) and specially the amount and nature of the fermented and alcoholic drinks which they consume.

By this means, a very large body of facts would be collected, from which it would be no difficult task to determine the comparative advantages of various kinds of nutriment and beverage, under differing circumstances; or to show what, on the whole, conduces most to the bodily soundness and efficiency of the labouring classes. I am satisfied that no order of men could obtain more correct information on this subject than their medical attendants, with whom they are ready at all times, especially when ill, to communicate unreservedly: and whose advice, on this and other matters, they are disposed thankfully to receive and adopt.

The extreme ignorance of the poor, and the practical blunders of their daily life, with regard to the choice and preparation of food, are too well known to call for accumulated evidence.*

§ 18. Many important facts in physical science and in political economy, directly bearing on the public health, have been at times noticed in this country, partly by collectors of *agricultural statistics* (a general and constant registration of which, under Government authority, is now an acknowledged necessity of the State), partly by writers on medical topography and amateur meteorologists, and to a very limited extent by inspectors or commissioners employed for special and temporary objects by the Government.

But these spontaneous or casual reports are on no systematic plan; they relate only to separate localities, during occasional periods, and are therefore quite insufficient for the purposes of safe induction, and unavailable for the permanent objects of sanitary administration.

Yet all the essential matters to which they relate might be registered periodically in every district by the same official agency which is required for a perfect system of statistical record, local inspection, and care of the public health.†

There are both theoretical and practical reasons for combining these researches with the higher department of agricultural statistics,‡ and committing the returns, for classification and

---

* "At our national schools . . . we have classes for reading, writing, arithmetic, &c., but where is the cooking class?—in other words, teaching how to economize the *vivres* of the country;—to live well upon small means;—to prepare food in the best form, by giving it bulk and flavour; and when coarse, to make it palatable and nutritious;—to put everything to its proper use;—to waste nothing, and save every thing."—*Notes and Recollections,* by the late Dr. Ferguson, Inspector-General of Hospitals, pp. 78, 79.

† Introd. Essay, pp. 10, 11, 12 (I. A. 6 and 7. I. B.)

‡ More minute details are probably required by the practical agriculturist. The

report (quarterly, and more frequently in emergencies), to properly qualified officers connected with the proposed district courts of health.*

It is scarcely necessary to remark, that—although blights and other diseases of the vegetable kingdom (epiphytics), unusual phenomena of insect life, and especially murrains and contagious diseases among horses, herds, and flocks (epizoötics), have been observed, in all ages, to connect themselves more or less closely with epidemic visitations, and to affect generally the vitality, health, and welfare of the human race,—no measures have hitherto been adopted by the Government to determine accurately their degrees of morbific influence.

§ 19. Among the most ancient topics of sanitary observation were climate and meteorology.

Unreflective persons are too apt to overlook the ordinary successions of day and night, seasons and years, with their alternations of heat and cold, wind and calm, rain and sunshine, mist and dew, because they are "common things;" not fully recognising their agency for good or harm upon human life and vigour, according as they are used or encountered.

Wiser men, however, have thought differently. And when they noted the frequent connexion, as to time and place, between some less common atmospheric changes and the advent or decline of different diseases; especially when extraordinary meteorological phenomena and cosmical movements were observed in certain relations with destructive and appalling bursts of pestilence,† the subject became a science.

village schoolmaster, or the sub-district registrar, might be here available. The plan suggested in the *Journal of the Statistical Society*, June, 1854, seems feasible.

At all events, a *sanitary* registration of agricultural statistics is far more likely to elicit truthful information than the Poor-Law machinery now employed upon, and interfering with these inquiries.

* Introd. Essay, p. 51. (iii. B. 4. (*d*) to (*g*).)

† Noah Webster's *History of Epidemics* is full of these marvellous coincidences. See also Hecker's unrivalled description of the telluric commotions and psychical perversions which accompanied the "Black Death" in the fourteenth century.

It may not be out of place to recall to the mind of the reader some of those natural phenomena to which we attribute the simplest of these effects.

Think of the regularly recurring changes produced in the atmosphere by the diurnal and annual revolutions of the earth and the monthly circuit of its satellite. Then recollect the successive modifications of solar and lunar influence upon different parts of the earth's surface—upon the abrupt or undulating elevations and depressions of its solid face—upon the far wider domain of its watery level, and upon the rapidly changing masses of vapour, seen and unseen, in the air. Think of differences of climate, as resulting—mainly from our planet's particular course and position in the solar system,—partly from the singular discrepancy between its circles of latitude and its isothermal zones, —and incidentally from ocean currents, from atmospheric movements, and from the peculiar conformation and physical features of certain localities. Think of the continuous, yet wonderfully varying, action of the imponderable physical forces, light and heat, electricity and magnetism, all inscrutably connected with that MOTION which marks these successions. Consider the chemical processes ever silently at work under the same influences; for example, the actinism of the sun's rays, and the ozone produced in the oxygen of the air by electric disturbance. Think, again, of the operation of mysterious subterranean agencies, some directly affecting the air through volcanoes and cracks in the earth's crust, all indirectly through the soil. Recollect that all these changes are developing in varied and ever new combinations, most of which are yet unexplained.

And, to bring such considerations nearer home, observe how all these physical phenomena and climatic circumstances influence the structure and life, not only of the fauna and flora inhabiting and characterizing different regions of the world, but of man himself.

Can any one thus reflecting stop short of the conclusion that this group of "causes,"—not to mention the reaction upon the atmosphere of the organic forms which it maintains, or the effect upon climate of human labour and civilization,—has a more important bearing upon the health of the human race than any other class of external circumstances?

And since the Great First Cause, the Creator and Regulator of these influences, has endowed man with the understanding which enables him, by a study of the "laws of nature," to adapt himself to these various conditions, to avail himself of their beneficial agencies, to avert or to protect himself from their dangerous or injurious effects; can one doubt that this department of knowledge is essentially and inseparably connected with the art of preventing disease and prolonging life?

§ 20. A more intimate and comprehensive acquaintance with these conditions and changes in relation to disease, is now indeed generally admitted to be of paramount necessity. Hence, we see scientific societies* instituted, specially or partially, for the promotion of such studies. Hence, also, minor voluntary arrangements among groups of diligent and intelligent observers.

Hence, again, the Registrar-General, fully alive to the importance of the subject, adds to his most useful "Quarterly Returns," full reports of the weather from the Royal Observatory, accompanied by trustworthy meteorological contributions from men of science in different parts of the country.†

How long, then, is a department of registration, so necessary for the public welfare, and thus sanctioned by official authority, to be limited to a few localities, casually favoured by the residence of zealous scientific volunteers?

---

* The British Meteorological Society and its labours deserve special notice.

† A recent contribution on *Medical Meteorology*, by Drs. Moffatt and Richardson, to the Epidemiological Society, suggests that these observations ought to be conducted at various points of the earth's surface, including areas of not more than twenty miles (square?); and that the results thus obtained should be regularly forwarded to a central office.—See *Rep. of Epid. Soc.* March, 1854.

Oxford was the first provincial city to publish periodical reports, combining meteorological notices, with returns of the births and deaths, and general remarks on the state of the public health. These were compiled with great care, and issued, monthly and quarterly, by Dr. Greenhill and Mr. Allen, for two years.—See *Report on the Mortality and Public Health of Oxford, during the Years* 1849, 1850, recently published by the Ashmolean Society.

§ 21. In order to carry public sympathy and approval along with a national organization for the purposes of sanitary inquiry,—in order to bring home a sense of the personal importance of the subject to every family,—the information collected must be made use of in each locality.

The facts and events observed in every district should not only be reported to official authorities, but should be compiled on the spot, in a form easily available for reference to the inhabitants. For as these become better informed on the various circumstances which affect their physical well-being, prejudices will subside, opposition to improvements will cease, and local councils will become more useful and effective.

The regular publication of such complete sanitary records in the several localities, would also lead to a very beneficial competition between adjacent districts in the race of sanitary improvement.

Under present disadvantages, any zealous inquirer into medical and topographical statistics must either depend on the good-nature of central and local officials,—and this species of civility ought not to be recklessly taxed,—or he must pay for the information he requires.

Registrars, clerks, secretaries of local institutions, and parochial officers cannot be asked to devote their time gratuitously to the preparation of returns, which are no part of their official duty.

On the other hand, it is extremely hard upon those few who may be willing to bestow time and labour upon public objects, that they should be compelled to purchase the materials which they are ready to employ for the general good.

And in fact, reports thus prepared, ought not to be relied on in public administration.

Objections are made by certain parties to minute investigations on some of the points suggested. Short-sighted persons suppose that the value of property and the success of trade, in their respective neighbourhoods, depend on the concealment of such facts. They hastily assume that local interests may be injured by unwelcome disclosures; forgetting that sound measures of police, based on impartial inquiry, are particularly calculated to improve every legitimate source of income, and to promote all just and right investments of capital. But let us hope that the objectors are in a miserable minority. It is said that Englishmen generally are proud of stating, and desirous of hearing, the whole truth. Public and personal veracity, we are told, is a national characteristic; and certainly these are not the times for concealment of abuses in general or local administration. Happily, the moralist, the philanthropist, and the political economist are agreed, that the permanent prosperity, collective and individual, of any community, depends on an open and fearless exposure of whatever circumstances tend to deteriorate the physical condition, and to impair the vital force of those who compose it.

§ 22. On the other hand, an unreserved publication of local facts and circumstances, would serve in time to dispel an unphilosophical notion which the recent current of sanitary reform has led many benevolent persons to adopt; namely, that FILTH,—in some form or other, aërial, fluid, or solid, is the sole cause of preventible disease; and that public cleansing and the care of the public health are convertible terms.

Far be it from me to discourage by a single word, if that were possible, the very reasonable and obviously necessary efforts which are now being made in many towns, and with much apparent benefit, to insure the removal and abolition of whatever is offensive or incommodious to persons of civilized habits; whatever is incompatible with the social comfort, intellectual progress, and moral welfare of the people. Eccentricity is the mildest term one can apply to those who deny or doubt that all such reforms are truly "sanitary."

But the best cause often suffers from the heat and prejudice of its advocates: and in this great question of the day, it must be confessed that some promoters of the Public Health Act have laid themselves open to the imputation of having either denied or ignored or underrated the influence of all causes of sickness and premature mortality, except those which they were so resolutely and (it must be owned) so laudably bent on removing. Fully admitting that it was satisfactorily ascertained, by reports of self-sacrificing medical inquirers, that in certain towns and neighbourhoods, excessive rates of mortality and a greater prevalence of epidemic disease co-existed with a remarkable degree of social degradation, with grievous neglect and mismanagement in civic and domestic arrangements for cleansing, ventilation, drainage, and water-supply, and with gross abuses in mortuary interments; admitting all this—the philosophical inquirer may nevertheless hesitate to join in the loud *eurekas* with which these discoveries were announced. Still less could he agree with those who boldly scoffed at the notion of other less obvious, but not less real, predisposing and exciting causes of preventible disease.

One cannot doubt that the fallacy of any conclusions, and the limited success of any measures, which may have been founded on predetermined views and partial investigations, will become manifest at no distant period.

But we need not speculate on the turn which events may take upon the discovery of such fallacies and failures by a disappointed people.

It may suffice to have shown that the institution of a comprehensive system of inquiry, such as I have now suggested, by an organized body of specially trained, experienced, and unbiassed observers, was not treated as indispensable to the formation of a code of public hygiéne by those who devised, and who were afterwards appointed to carry into effect, the Public Health Act.

CHAPTER THIRD.

INVESTIGATION OF EPIDEMICS.

§ 1. In no department of sanitary inquiry is an accurate, permanent, and general record of facts more urgently demanded, than with regard to the origin and extension of zymotic diseases.

Our knowledge of the more recondite sources of endemics, in different regions and climates, is extremely limited. We talk indeed of *malaria* and *miasmata*, but we know scarcely anything about them.

Equally at a loss are we to assign reasons for the continual outbreak of epidemics of different kinds, whether indigenous or naturalized to this country.

More uncertain, if possible, are we as to the importation of those malignant foreign epidemics, which we call pestilences.

Then, as to the various modes in which all diseases of these three divisions of the zymotic class are diffused—why, under certain circumstances, and at different periods of its prevalence, the same epidemic should assume an altered character, as regards its communicability; whence comes the specific *materies morbi* which probably belongs to each of these diseases; how it is propagated; how received by those who suffer from it; why others escape it; where it goes, and what it is about until the next outbreak: these are all questions on which we are much in the dark.

§ 2. Again, in no kind of medico-political inquiry is it more essential that those who are charged with the duty of collecting facts and reporting upon evidence, should be men of acknowledged reputation, well esteemed in and out of their profession, reflective, acute, and honest; and, above all, rendered independent of any set of official authorities, which may be pledged to particular opinions, or interested in the establishment of certain views.

I am aware that the bare supposition that there are epidemic and pestilential diseases, which, under favouring circumstances, spread by human intercourse, and which may be thus imported into a country or introduced into a district, renders one liable to misconception or misrepresentation.

But while prepared to defend the use of expressions obnoxious to an extreme party, it is, perhaps, as well to endeavour to allay prejudice by avowing, *in limine*, that I am not a "contagionist," in the ultra or exclusive meaning of that term, and that I believe in the superior efficacy, in general, of internal precautions—civic, domestic, and personal—as compared with external defences and prohibitions of communication.

I may also be excused for adding, that I am in no way personally affected by the attacks made or promoted by the first members of the (so-called) General Board of Health upon distinguished officers of the War and Quarantine departments, who had been led to believe that certain malignant diseases might be conveyed from country to country, might be communicated from person to person; and who had, therefore, proposed or defended measures of separation and isolation.

§ 3. But my readers need not be reminded that no body of men have contributed more largely to our knowledge of preventive medicine, none have had more extensive opportunities of observation, and none stand personally or professionally higher, than the medical officers of our navy and army.

On the other hand, of all public departments, the Board of Sanitary Works was surely the least entitled to accuse another of unfairly pressing professional testimony in favour of its peculiar views. Its members, however, dealt pretty freely in such aspersions. For instance, in referring to the medical departments of the army and navy, they said:—"The discipline

". . . . predisposes the subordinate officer to adopt the views and support the opinions, which are understood to be most acceptable to the head of the department, upon whom his future professional prospects may depend."*

This was not a very safe or wise method of argument, considering the controversial position assumed by that Board. However it might have lacked the confidence of the public and the medical profession, it likewise had not only its "subordinate officers," but its expectant *employés*, whom no one should be tempted, by a *tu quoque*, to accuse of interested motives, for the singular agreement of their strongly-expressed sentiments on this subject.

That a Quarantine Board and its officers should manifest a bias towards the doctrine of Contagion, and the employment of *cordons* and pest-hospitals, is not more remarkable than that a Board of Works and its adherents should display a zealous preference for the doctrine of Filth, and the formation of drains and aqueducts.

And that the medical profession has declined to commit itself unreservedly to either party, redounds, I think, to its credit.

But to treat adequately, however briefly, of the matters involved in this discussion, would lead me to consider in what degree those, who constituted a Board, which originally professed to be merely one of Sanitary Works, were especially qualified to control certain measures of precaution, or to attempt to settle some vexed questions relating to epidemic disease, which were so strangely committed to them.

It would also compel me to review a large portion of their proceedings; to point out the sources whence, without acknowledgment, they derived their most successful measures; and to criticize the course which they thought fit to adopt—in various publications—by way either of supporting their own opinions, or of invalidating those of medical bodies, and of other administrative departments, from which they differed.

---

* *Second Report on Quarantine of General Board of Health*, p. 130.

The necessity, however, for so comprehensive a review of their proceedings, is now almost at an end; although some of these matters may have to be noticed incidentally as we proceed.

§ 4. Some have thought that the earliest advent of pestilential cholera into this country was connected, not remotely, with the origin of the present sanitary movement.* And certainly, the second and third invasions of the same tremendous epidemic have been attended with, at least, one good result. They have given a stimulus to more rational, vigorous, and honest methods of research into the causes of its outbreaks, its course, and its diffusion.

If the State, the municipalities, and the people have been impelled by these awful warnings to adopt, not too hastily, some empirical, though useful, preventive expedients,—the medical profession has been taught to investigate more reasonably, to assert less rashly, and to conclude more cautiously.

§ 5. The choleraic pestilence of 1848-9 was the subject of no less than three official inquiries and reports, each of which may possess its peculiar merits.

That which issued from the Board of Sanitary Works had, however, the disadvantage, before alluded to, of mingling unmethodically scientific researches and arguments, pathological and ætiological facts, statistical returns and topographical descriptions, with details of administrative mismanagement and the suggestion of palliative and preventive measures.

* "All analogy," says Dr. Farr, "proves that no extensive or permanent degeneration of a race can be accomplished in less than two or three generations. The great change is as slow and insidious as it is certain. It is rarely perceived by its victims, who remain rooted and benumbed on the spot, unless they and the community are aroused by sudden and terrible catastrophes. That angel which, it would seem, it has pleased the Almighty Creator and Preserver of Mankind to charge with this dread mission, is the Pestilence. Wherever the human race, yielding to ignorance, indolence, or accident, is in such a situation as to be liable to lose its strength, courage, liberty, wisdom, lofty emotions—the plague, fever, or cholera comes, not committing havoc perpetually, but turning men to destruction, and then suddenly ceasing, that they may consider. As the lost father speaks to the family, and the slight epidemic to the city, so the pestilence speaks to nations, in order that greater calamities than the untimely death of the population may be averted."—*Report to Registrar-General*, p. xcvii. 1852.

The attention of the Board was thus partially withdrawn from their appropriate duties, to treat of several specialities, requiring separate study by scientific reporters.

Their cholera Report contained a minute and interesting account, founded upon Government documents, of the progress of the epidemic from the East; and these facts, viewed in connexion with others noticed by individual observers here and on its route, lead inevitably to the inference that the cholera generally follows great lines of human communication, especially those of navigation, inland and by sea. A mode of diffusion, to which the opinions of that Report are diametrically opposed, is shown, by it alone, to be quite possible.

With the exception of important official particulars, such as are to be procured and circulated only by a central department of the State—all the really valuable matter of that document is derived from the excellent tributary Reports of Dr. Sutherland and Mr. Grainger.

§ 6. The second and third inquiries might perhaps have been suggested by the obvious imperfections of the first.

Dr. Farr's Report to the Registrar-General has already taken its place among our best English classics, as a remarkable application of facts in physical geography and of events in the history of civilization, to illustrate and explain the ravages of a pestilence.

While marshalling his vast array of figures with all the dexterity of a practised mathematician, he tempts his readers from the exact and dry domain of statistics, in the impressive language of a genuine poet, to realize momentous truths in the wider fields of social science and public duty; truths, which, however plain to the awakened mental vision, need the magnifying power of a destructive plague to arrest and fix the attention of the thoughtless, the sordid, and the slothful.

He is not, however, led away by mysterious and transcendental analogies, such as Hecker delights in when describing those strange moral and cosmical phenomena which accompanied the epidemics of the middle ages.

Dr. Farr's great point is the connexion between certain natural features of inhabited spots and their liability to epidemic visitations.

He directs attention to a question almost wholly neglected by modern governments—the sites of cities;* bringing historical and topographical illustrations to show how various degrees of elevation of land-surface affect the condition of the human and animal races which subsist upon it. And, with especial reference to mortality from cholera, he demonstrates that in the metropolis the number of deaths varies inversely, in definite progression, with the altitude of the localities in which they occur.

So far as we know at present, it is extremely doubtful whether the specific leaven of other diseases † of the class, which he has so appropriately named *zymotic,* takes effect in obedience to the same law; but the experience of both the last visitations of cholera in London supports generally the principle, which he may almost be said to have established.

§ 7. The third inquiry, touching principally on the medical history of this epidemic, fills up a blank left by both the former reports, and (may I be permitted to add) does infinite credit both to the College of Physicians from which it emanated, and to the learned and candid Fellows of that College to whom was committed the task of reporting.

Dr. Baly's branch of this inquiry specially concerns our subject.

Not the least valuable feature of this Report is its presentation of facts and opinions, collected from a number of intelligent and trustworthy medical observers, respecting the origin and diffusion, the severity and duration of the epidemic in different

* No one of the present day has devoted more sedulous and successful attention to this subject than Mr. J. R. Martin, formerly of high rank in the medical department of the Indian army, the promoter of most important sanitary reforms in Calcutta, and lately one of the Health of Towns' Commissioners.

† The effects of elevation upon tropical fever have been noticed by the late Dr. Ferguson. He gives a very remarkable instance at St. Domingo, of the diminishing effect of fever in proportion to altitude; and of another at Trinidad, which, at first sight, makes against the theory.— Ferguson's *Notes and Recollections,* pp. 152, 192.

towns and places, with information as to their "character of site," local circumstances, and sanitary provisions.

All the returns appear to be treated with perfect fairness, and equal prominence allowed to opinions and circumstances tending to favour contrary theories.

Thus, doubts are multiplied rather than certainties determined. But then, as Bacon said, "The registering of doubts hath two excellent uses; the one, that it saveth philosophy from errors and falsehoods; when that which is not fully appearing is not collected into assertion, whereby error might draw error, but reserved in doubt: the other, that the entry of doubts are as so many suckers or sponges to draw use of knowledge; insomuch as that which, if doubts had not preceded, a man should never have advised, but passed it over without note, by the suggestion and solicitation of doubts, is made to be attended and applied."*

Dr. Baly analyses with great precision the materials already furnished by the Registrar-General, and employs them to elucidate, as far as possible, different properties of the epidemic.

§ 8. One of these properties—namely, its relation to density of population—has been lately controverted, and therefore I wish to recall attention to Dr. Baly's important inference on the point.

He found that in the 134 more thickly inhabited registration districts of England, where the higher rate of cholera mortality occurred, the population being 915 to the square mile, the deaths averaged 65 to 10,000 living. In the 404 districts of lower cholera mortality, there were on the whole 235 inhabitants to the square mile, and the deaths averaged only 7 in the 10,000. While there were *no* deaths from cholera in the remaining 85 districts, where only 122 persons, on the average, resided on a square mile.

This is a remarkable numerical confirmation of records, made at all times and in all places, of the co-existence of epidemic ravages with closely packed assemblages of living beings.

Nor is the received opinion invalidated by the metropolitan records of the epidemic in 1854.

---

* Bacon's *Advancement of Learning*. Book II. chap. viii. § 9.

The " Scientific Committee" of the late Medical Council show, indeed, that, in this instance, and upon an area of 78,000 acres, the mortality from cholera, in the several sub-divisions, was not materially influenced by their respective densities of population.

But, as they candidly remark, the *materies morbi* of cholera was evidently diffused over every sub-district of London ; and we may infer that the aggravating effect of the crowd told throughout the metropolis ; and rather contributed to its total excess of mortality, than acted solely upon those smaller sub-divisions in which the crowd was closer. Besides, in some of these districts, there might be other modifying influences, temporary or permanent.

That the apparently slight effect of aggregation was on this occasion accidental and exceptional, becomes more probable from the circumstance that some of the most confessedly healthy parts of the metropolis—*e. g.*, Hampstead—exhibited at the same time a disproportionate amount of mortality,—telling as much against a law of altitude as against a law of aggregation.

This circumstance affords an illustration of the insufficiency of limited and temporary observations. It shows the caution necessary in making use of them.

Among Hecker's admirable remarks on State inquiry, occur the following, which are quite pertinent to this matter :—

" Such an insight into the nature and cause of popular diseases as is worthy the dignity of a science cannot be obtained by the observation of isolated epidemics, because nature never, in any one of them, displays herself in all her bearings, nor brings into action, at one time, more than a few of the laws of general disease. . . . . The experience of all ages is the source whence we must in this case draw, and medical investigation is the only road which leads to this source, unless, indeed, we would be unprepared to meet new epidemics, and would maintain the unfounded opinion that medical science, as it now exists, is the full result of all preceding efforts."*

§ 9. It is to be inferred, though it is not stated in so many words, that a decided majority of the respondents to the inquiries

* *Epidemics of Middle Ages*—Syd. Soc. p. 178.

circulated by the College of Physicians, either assert that disease is communicable from person to person; or manifestly le to that theory, without excluding other modes of its diffusion; cite instances which can be explained on no other hypothesis but that of human communication, without expressing an opinion about them.*

This apparent decision of a probable majority of the profession in England, is corroborated by the recorded experience of the Dispensary Commissioners in Ireland, and by the majority, I believe, of the ablest foreign writers on the subject.

I am not now arguing a disputed question, as to the outbreak and extension of cholera in localities, or I might adduce additional facts which seem to admit of no other solution than the above. But it is to my purpose to notice that, while Dr. Baly is opposed to the exclusive theory of its spread by personal infection—that is, by a material emanation from the bodies of the sick—he states that "a large body of evidence renders it certain that human intercourse has, at least, a share in the propagation of the disease, and that it, under some circumstances, is the most important, if not the sole means of effecting its diffusion." The probability of its being conveyed in this way by ships,† by importation,‡ and along main lines of military march or commercial traffic‖ on land, is almost converted into a certainty, by the facts which he brings to bear upon the discussion.

§ 10. The College reporter leaves, and wisely leaves, several important points undetermined, for future investigation. Had the official machinery for collecting facts been universal, and their registration compulsory and systematic, conclusions on one or more of these points might have been irresistible.

At all events, enough has been done thoroughly to explode and demolish the unphilosophical arguments and the dogmatical assertion of the first General Board of Health,—namely, that diseases, so specifically and essentially different, as the typhus of

---

* See Dr. Baly's *Summary of* 84 *Medical Communications,* pp. 3, 4.
† Page 128. ‡ Page 131. ‖ Page 135.

estern Europe, the carbuncular or glandular plague of the East, the hæmagastric pestilence of the Tropics, and the cholera of the whole world,—each and all arise from the same cause or set of causes.

It is marvellous that a Board, which, through its favourite organ of periodical criticism,* presumed to accuse learned and painstaking medical writers of "ignorance of the most obvious rules of evidence"—" want of inclination or ability to analyse testimony," and "unreasoning credulity"†—should itself have ventured upon statements and conclusions so rash, so illogical, and (it must be added, when one considers the character and qualifications of the persons attacked) so dangerous to its own reputation.

§ 11. Doubtless, some advantages resulted from the independent and often differing views and conclusions of the three official reports on the second invasion of cholera. The plurality of reports afforded greater scope for originality of design and expression. Distinct lines of investigation were perhaps more boldly followed out.

But it was probably to avoid the repetition of a comparison so disadvantageous to the Board of Sanitary Works, that the acute and energetic baronet, who recently presided at that Board, determined upon comprehending within his own department the labours of the same statistical and medical authorities who had given the literary *coup-de-grace* to his predecessors.

His Medical Council accordingly contained the very authors of the two ætiological reports last mentioned, And the result of his arrangement proves that the State is no loser by enlisting the co-operation of science, or by confiding sanitary inquiries to those whose special education and pursuits entitle them to be thus trusted.

It is, however, no less to the honour of medicine than to the discredit of the Government, that this medical council was unsa-

* *Edinburgh Review*, Oct. 1842, "Quarantine," &c.
† What would the venerable author of *Medical Logick* have said to such impertinence ?

laried; that the whole body of local evidence from medical practitioners was supplied and collected by voluntary effort; and that the labours of the three committees* were rewarded only by the gratitude and approbation of those who were capable of appreciating them.

It is also painful to add that the council seems to have been dismissed without an assurance on the part of Government that some comprehensive measure of public health should be forthcoming, which would recognise the medical profession as a main and independent constituent of the central and local organization requisite for sanitary inquiry and administration.

This is the more surprising, as the same council forcibly pointed out the necessity of an uninterrupted continuance of scientific inquiries during seasons of comparative immunity from epidemic disease, and the disadvantage under which they themselves laboured from not being called into existence until the pestilence had already passed its culminating point. Whether referring to former official reports, or by way of suggestion for future arrangements, they went on to remark, very truly,† "The way had not been sufficiently cleared by preliminary inquiries, and the prospective path of investigation had not been traced or enlightened by any scientific pioneers."

§ 12. The report of the 'Scientific' Committee at once declares, what I have already laboured to prove, that no correct idea of public disease in its relations to public health can be formed until the State establishes a registration of sickness.

"The list of the killed is complete; what was the number of the wounded?"‡

More than three hundred medical men afforded information as to the attacks attended by themselves; and the committee draw

---

* (1) The Committee for Scientific Inquiries, (on the history, statistics, ætiology and pathology of this cholera visitation); (2) the Treatment Committee; (3) the Committee for Foreign Correspondence.

The Administrative Reports were committed to Drs. Sutherland and Milroy.

† *Gen. Rep. Medical Council*, p. 4.   ‡ *Rep. Scientific Committee*, p. 9.

certain inferences from those returns as to the number attended by other practitioners. How different might be the result, how much more reliable the conclusion, how beneficial to the sufferers from disease, and how useful to the public, if the State possessed a competent machinery for discovering, inspecting, and recording disease in every district and institution of the land!

In a scientific aspect, perhaps the most interesting feature of this inquiry is Mr. Glaisher's Report on the relations possibly subsisting between the outbreaks of cholera and certain meteorological conditions.

These observations, confined to the metropolis, seem to throw some light upon Dr. Farr's law of greater mortality at lower altitudes.* But on this point also no satisfactory conclusions can be drawn, until meteorological records and other physical researches are made compulsory everywhere.

§ 13. In this department of medical investigation, as in many others, voluntary association has attempted much, and indeed has performed more than can be permanently expected from it.

The foundation and progress of the Epidemiological Society are facts most suggestive to all who are interested, officially or as amateurs, in the improvement of the public health.

Its objects were high and noble:—"To institute a rigid examination into the causes and conditions which influence the origin, propagation, mitigation, prevention, and treatment of epidemic diseases; to collect and promulgate, with relation to these subjects, such facts as appear to be established on sound and sufficient evidence; and to point out those methods of investigation by which the misleading influence of false or deficient evidence may be best avoided."

The Society further proposed "to institute in this spirit of careful inquiry" original and comprehensive researches into the

---

* "Mr. Glaisher has clearly shown, that in the low-lying districts, wherein the epidemic assumed its highest malignity, the air was stagnant, and moisture, impregnated with impurities, was especially induced to hover."—*General Report of the Medical Council.*

nature and laws of diseases connected with soil and climate,—of fever in its various forms and *habitats,*—of cholera and other pestilences,—and of eruptive fevers. It proposed to include in its inquiries all those matters relating to towns and buildings—to overcrowding and filth, which have been already so carefully investigated under Government authority;—also, some of the collateral topics which have been suggested in this Essay, as epizoötic and epiphytic diseases.

But it aspired to yet more vigorous efforts, to extensive practical operations:—" Immediately on the outbreak of an epidemic in any place, the Society will consider it *its special province* to institute a searching inquiry, tracing with scrupulous minuteness the history of the first cases . . . up to their causes; to examine such causes thoroughly; to ascertain whether they admit of prevention and by what means;" and "particularly" to investigate "the influence of isolation and of unrestrained intercourse" in the spread of epidemics.

Their inquiries were to be conducted not only by committees and individual members, but by "paid agents;" and "apparatus" was to be supplied "for scientific and experimental researches into chemical, meteorological, and other influences."

One step further towards the exercise of administrative power. "It will be a part of the Society's province to ascertain the operation of existing legal enactments," and to "point out such alterations as may be necessary for the protection of the public health."

Lastly. "The Society propose to communicate with the Government and Legislature in matters connected with the prevention of epidemic diseases."

§ 14. Now, it may be asked—If a private society could really carry into effect the whole of this investigatory and administrative project—obviously appertaining to a central and local State organization—what necessity is there for any interference of the Government in this department of public health?

The answer is to be read in the recent confessions of this society.

Whilst a few active and zealous members of the medical profession (all honour to them!) contribute admirable papers, diligently discuss controverted points at their meetings, correspond with scientific *confrères* at home and abroad, and endeavour to work upon the Government by deputations and reports,—the vast majority of the profession stands aloof; local inquiries cannot be conducted for want of funds; the Government declines to aid (we may hope from a perception that the whole matter belongs to itself); and one of the most aspiring societies ever formed must prepare for gradual extinction.

Happy for the country will it be if that event be caused by the institution of an efficient machinery by the State for scientific, unprejudiced, and continuous inquiry, in every part of the kingdom.

If the inquiries promoted by the Epidemiological Society have been necessarily incomplete, owing to the inherent defectiveness of the voluntary principle—its want of power and permanence; if some of the plans and recommendations of this Society manifest a limited acquaintance with practical difficulties, and undue dependence on theory; if in design and operation it may have sometimes overstepped the boundary line of investigation and discussion to which its correspondence and meetings might have been more usefully confined; no fair and competent observer can deny that it has done essential service to the cause of science and the public health.

§ 15. A more recent, and in some respects a more interesting, example of spontaneous and associated effort in this good cause, is afforded by the International Statistical Congress at Paris.

Its committee on epidemics (containing a large proportion of our own countrymen), and the able reporter, Dr. Tholozan, have sketched a very excellent programme of the facts and circumstances, which they invite competent observers in all civilized countries to register, and which they believe may be collected in "nations even the least advanced in statistical organization."

It is needless here to specify the details of their scheme. It includes all the leading particulars which have been demanded by public bodies or private societies in this country. The authors might, perhaps, have specified more distinctly the precise density of population and altitude of surface, as facts to be observed in connexion with the number of attacks and deaths in every district. But the section very judiciously pleads as an excuse for the omission of several articles, that a more comprehensive and minute scheme was inapplicable to some states, " on account of the want of observers in a position to execute all the conditions of a vast and difficult programme."*

This remark applies especially to the present state of organization for scientific inquiry in England.

§ 16. Success in this, as in every other department of sanitary inquiry, depends mainly upon the VERIFICATION of original facts.

No considerations of cheapness should prevent the constitution of an efficient machinery. In the notation of facts of so great importance to society, I would especially deprecate the employment of any order of inferior and incompetent officials, simply because it happens to be already in existence.

It was Cullen, I think, who said that there were in physic more false facts than false theories.

If TRUTH be the object; if something better be intended than mere concession to temporary and importunate demands; the Legislature should promptly provide for the appointment of a superior staff of agents, to form the base of the pyramid of a State system.

§ 17. In England, at the present time, three kinds of local

---

* "As to the localities which are wanting in competent observers, or where there is an absence of statistical organization, or where there is a want of labourers for the registration and classification of the data of the statistics of epidemics, the section has considered that the most restricted programme would, for the most part, be still too extended in these circumstances, and that it ought not in any manner to subject statistical researches to a kind of mutilation, in which the wants of statistics, of medicine, of civilization, of governments, would be sacrificed on account of certain difficulties or impossibilities, which are fortunately almost everywhere of a very transitory and accidental nature."—Dr. Tholozan's *Report*.

agency are legally established, which, under improved organization and with the regulated assistance of other official machinery, might co-operate in the collection and registration of various particulars of information, relating to the vital statistics and sanitary circumstances of the people.

Each of the three is capable of being rendered vastly more available and efficient than it now is; not merely for taking its own share in such investigations, but for promoting, practically and energetically, the physical and mental improvement of the masses in every district.

These three official bodies are—

1. The medical attendants of the sick poor under the Poor Law;
2. The medical officers of health under the Public Health Act;
3. The local registrars of births and deaths.

The first and third may be said to exist in every locality; for the comparatively few parishes still exempted from the superintendence of the Poor Law Board, provide medical relief on much the same principle as the rest of England and Wales.

The second class—officers of health—are to be found only in a few places, of limited area. Their appointment, except in London, is merely optional with local boards. Their position and duties are not, as yet, settled on any definite principle.

§ 18. It will therefore be my object, in succeeding Essays, to treat of the condition of each of these departments of the civil service.

And I may conclude this Essay with Sir John Herschel's admirable summary of the functions of an organized system of public inquiry:—" First, to ask distinct and pertinent questions, admitting of short and definite answers; secondly, to call for exact numerical statements on all principal points; thirdly, to point out the attendant circumstances which ought to be observed; fourthly, to call for their transmission to a common centre."*

* *Discourse on the Study of Natural Philosophy*, p. 134.

ESSAY IV.

THE MEDICAL CARE OF THE POOR IN ENGLAND, WITH NOTICES RELATING TO IRELAND.

PART I.

HISTORICAL.

"Few questions are well considered till they are largely written about, and the minds and judgments of great functionaries transacting business *inter mœnia* labour under the deficiency of bold checks from oppugnant minds."

Taylor's *Statesman*. *Reform of the Executive.*

ESSAY IV.

PART I.

CHAPTER FIRST.

FROM THE REFORMATION UNTIL A.D. 1827.

§ 1. IN order to present a correct view of our national provision for the sick poor, in its relations to the public health, and to clear the ground for the adoption of certain principles essential to the successful administration of any such provision, it will be necessary to notice, as concisely as the importance of the subject permits, some particulars of its history in this country.

When a legal assessment for the relief of the poor was first established in England, the diseased and maimed among the common people had been for some years deprived even of that casual supply of medical care, which, until about the year 1536, had been made for them in most parts of the kingdom by the monasteries, hospitia, and lazar-houses of the middle ages.

It is true that the hospitals of those days corresponded but little with modern institutions bearing that name. Receptacles for the aged, the wayfarers, the lame and blind, the infirm and incurable, they rarely afforded anything more in the way of medical treatment than could be administered by those monks and lay brethren, who had studied medicine and were maintained on the charitable foundation purposely for such attendance.

Nurses seem also to have been appointed.* Baths—hot, cold,

---

* " Eadmer relates that Gundulf founded lazar-houses of wood at Canterbury, and erected a house of stone, handsome and spacious,—*lapideam domum decentem et amplam*,—with several small dwellings, and a spacious court. It was the nearest approach to modern hospitals that I have discovered. He divided it into two parts—one for men afflicted with different kinds of sickness, another for female and medicated—were provided. And some idea of the extent of aid and refuge thus bestowed on the poor, may be formed from the long list of these hospitals given in Dugdale's *Monasticon Anglicanum*.*

The philosophical historian of the medical profession in England, of whose valuable labours I now gladly avail myself, beautifully adds to his interesting notice of these institutions:—
" So it was ever: the humanity of the age promised infirmity a home, a christian grave, and heaven, when it could not provide healing."

Considering the state of the medical art at that time, we may safely assume that the poor inmates of the hospitium had but little cause, and probably no desire, to blame either the governing powers in general, or the founders in particular, for this defect. For to be treated by such a "Doctour of Physike" as Chaucer describes, had there been enough of them for the whole population, might perhaps have shortened the sufferings of the sick, but could scarcely have prolonged their lives: although by his "magike naturel" he might have foretold their release.

§ 2. The real and original wrong inflicted on the people,—an injury irreparable for centuries,—was perpetrated by the rulers of the mediæval church, who forbad the clergy to study and practise medicine, and under whose influence ecclesiastical endowments were restricted to "mere theologians."†

As the elegant writer, just quoted, says elsewhere‡—

" When the Church obtained its immense possessions, the clergy (*clerus*) embodied, like the priesthoods of Egypt and Asia, the learning

patients: he provided the inmates with clothing, daily food, servants, and nurses (*custodes*), to watch them, and to see that they wanted nothing."—Farr's "History of the Medical Profession in England," *Brit. Med. Ann.* 1839, p. 129.

* About one hundred were recorded by Dugdale himself; and nearly two hundred and fifty, of the order of St. Augustine, were added in the last edition.—Vol. vi. p. 2.

† Napoleon I. reversed the ecclesiastical decree, and authorized the clergy of France to devote themselves to the healing of diseases.—Frank. *Med. Poliz.* b. 6, s. 63.

‡ Ibid. p. 134.

of the nation; they were the students, professors, repositories, teachers of the Anglo-Saxon cyclopædia of science. The poetry, the history, the natural philosophy, the music, the architecture—all the arts—all the professions, were branches of that religious Catholicism. What works and what memorials did Alcuin, Bede, Dunstan, Aldhelm, Bacon, the scholastic writers, the body of the clergy, transmit to posterity? Sermons and homilies? Few of these. But innumerable scientific treatises; and the cathedrals, the eternal temples, the realized ideas of a new architecture, the groundwork of a new civilization. To the clergy the people cheerfully devoted tithes and a liberal share of the public property. As a branch of the learned body (*clerus*), physicians possessed church property : they were deans, prebendaries, abbots, bishops; in other words, they discharged the easy duties, and received the revenues of these lucrative offices."

Successive popes and councils, however, by decrees of growing stringency, had almost succeeded in separating the practice of medicine from the ecclesiastical function, when the Reformation, while breaking intellectual fetters, and clearing Christian worship of many superfluous ceremonies, at the same time afforded a tyrannical Monarch and his obsequious Parliament a plea for depriving the poorer classes of their rightful solace and help during sickness and infirmity, by confiscating for political objects the property by means of which these benefits had become their patrimony.

It is said that only two hospitals were spared for medical purposes in England—namely, the munificent foundations of St. Bartholomew on the north, and St. Thomas's on the south of the river in London; the first founded by Rahere, in the year 1102; the second by Richard, Prior of Bermondsey, and Peter de Rupibus, Bishop of Winchester, in the following century.*

§ 3. There was, however, a pretence for the care of the public health.

The earliest medical enactment in the reign of Henry VIII. premised " the grievous hurt, damage, and destruction of many

---

* At the dissolution of religious houses, St. Thomas's Hospital seems to have been purchased by the citizens of London, and re-opened by them for its present purposes.—Cunningham's *Hand-book of London*, p. 493.

of the King's liege people,"* resulting from the ignorance and incompetence of those who professed to cure disease. And, considering the rarity of materials then existing for the formation of a qualified body of practitioners, it would probably have been difficult to contrive a wiser measure than that which established in every diocese a Court of Examiners, presided over and nominated by the bishop (or his vicar-general out of the metropolis); and composed of "doctors of physike, and for surgery other expert persons in that faculty."†

No person could take upon him to practise as a physician or surgeon, unless he were first "examined, approved, and admitted" by this court; and a penalty of 5*l.* was imposed for every month's illegal practice, half to be paid to the King, half to the informer.

Whether such a system, under improvements which might have been gradually effected as science and civilization advanced, and with an efficient supervision of the diocesan courts, might not have been so worked as to supply the poorer classes adequately with medical care, can now only be a question for speculation.

It is certain, however, that the provincial bishops continued to grant licences for more than two centuries.‡

But the Act was soon virtually superseded, though not legally repealed, by the second great medical measure of that reign,—the establishment of the College of Physicians.

§ 4. In this matter, also, the influence of clerical physicians must still have been weighty; for Linacre and Chambre, both beneficed clergymen, and both court physicians, were the chief of the six to whom the King granted the College Charter.

* Act 3 Hen. VIII. c. 11.—Willcock's *Laws of Medical Profession*, 1830, "Records," p. vi.

† Ibid. p. vii.

‡ In 1687-8, a circular letter was sent from the College of Physicians to every bishop, to remind him that his power of *examining* candidates was transferred to the College by the act 14 & 15 Hen. VIII. c. v. The bishops were, however, still at liberty to *license.*—Ferris's *Estab. of Physic*, p. 24.

It is needless for my present purpose to show how greatly this learned corporation improved the position, raised the education, and promoted the dignity of English physicians.

Nor can one forget the invaluable additions to medical science made by many of its illustrious members.

The names of Harvey, Sydenham, Mead, Radcliffe, and Sloane, are imperishable.

But the College was founded in a reign during which patents of monopoly and exclusive privileges were daily granted; and more frequently for the purpose of replenishing the exchequer, and enriching individuals by the profits of the monopoly, than with a view to the public welfare.*

The political vice of the times infected the charter and constitution of the College, marred the noble design of its learned and generous founder, Linacre, and crippled its public usefulness.

Besides, in committing to a privileged corporation an irresponsible power of limiting the supply of practitioners for the medical necessities of the people, the Government forgot its responsibilities, and abandoned its rightful functions.

§ 5. The results, one would think, might have been foreseen. The standard of qualification for the fellowship, if not for the licence, was raised above the requirements of the public. The number of practising physicians was unjustifiably diminished. The cost of their services was unduly enhanced. If the College supplied the Court, the landed aristocracy, and the wealthy burghers of our principal cities, with a high order of medical attendants; the poor—the mass of the population—were left to their fate.

So strongly was the miserable condition of the poor, with respect to medical aid, felt, even before the termination of Henry's reign, that, when another Act had been passed, incorporating the surgeons with the barbers,† and conferring on that company like powers of limiting the supply of regular practi-

---

* Willcock, p. 36, Act 32 Hen. VIII. c. 42. Ibid. "Records," p. clxxi.
† Ibid. 32 Hen. VIII. c. 42.

tioners and punishing the irregular, three years did not elapse without an "Amendment Act,"* to exempt "divers honest persons as well men as women, whom God hath endued with the knowledge of the nature, kind, and operation of certain herbs, roots, and waters," from the penalties which the company of surgeons, "minding only their own lucre, and nothing the profit or ease of the patient," had sued for, under their charter.

The quaint preamble of this statute pleaded "for the ease, comfort, succour, help, relief, and health of the King's poor subjects, inhabitants of this realm, pained and diseased;" alleging that the prohibited practitioners "have not taken anything for their pains or cunning, but have ministered the same to poor people only for neighbourhood and God's sake, and of pity and charity."

Also, that it was "well known that the surgeons will do no cure, but . . . for a greater sum or reward than the cure extendeth unto, for in case they would minister their cunning unto sore people unrewarded, *there should not so many rot and perish to death for lack of help of surgery as daily do.*"

And again: "Altho' the most part of the persons of the said craft of surgeons have small cunning, yet they will take great sums of money, and do little therefor."

It was, of course, very easy for King, Lords, and Commons, after depriving the poor of their ancient sources of ease and succour, to turn round and abuse the surgeons for not relieving the sufferers gratuitously; quite natural for the appropriators, reeking with the spoils of abbeys and hospitals, to become acutely sympathetic with the miseries they had helped to create —at the expense of the doctors who would not, and of "divers honest persons" who would, work for nothing.

§ 6. When statutes had been passed and charters granted for the suppression of unqualified practitioners; when the charitable institutions from which the sick poor had derived more or less medical care, and at least a shelter, had been abolished,—what

* 34 & 35 Hen. VIII. c. 8. Ibid. p. clxxvii.

did the Crown and Parliament establish for their help? Nothing! No public grant was made, no stipendiary body of attendants appointed for the healing of their bodily ailments, or for their instruction in the laws of health.

"How much," says Dr. Farr, "is it to be regretted that the Government did not endeavour to suppress quacks by the *substitution* of educated physicians; that a part of the church property, formerly appertaining to physic, was not employed at the Reformation as a bounty upon medical education, in founding lectureships in London, ... ; that small salaries were not set apart from the monastic funds for the partial support of medical officers all over the country, upon the same principle as the Scotch system of schools ; . . . . and that the College of Physicians was not constructed upon liberal principles, including among its members all the medical practitioners in the kingdom !"*

But the opportunity was lost. We read of no public medical charity from the time of the Reformation until the early part of the 18th century, except the two old metropolitan hospitals.

Certain orders of Privy Council, and regulations of municipal corporations, during the prevalence of pestilential diseases—as plague or small pox—although admitted to be of legal force by subsequent Acts of Parliament,† can hardly be deemed a stated provision for the sick poor.

Nor did the incorporation of London Apothecaries by James I. supply the population at large with anything like a sufficiently numerous, still less with even a moderately-educated, class of medical practitioners. For the apothecary of those times knew less of the principles of his art than the ordinary druggist of our day. And many years passed before apothecaries were paid from the poor-rates to supply, on the barest scale, necessary remedies for the poor. The truth is, that the provision of medical attendance

---

* *Op. cit.* p. 176.
† For instance, by the Act 3 & 4 William & Mary, cap. ii. § 7. There was also an earlier "Act for charitable relief and ordering of persons infected with the plague." 1 James I. cap. 31.

for the mass of the people was then an impossibility. For not only had the State neglected the public duty of securing an adequate supply of instructed surgeons and physicians; but the examples of Italy and Germany, where public medical officers had been appointed, in towns at least for many years — the salaries in Germany being, at one period, charged upon the church revenues*—were lost upon this country. Yet the medical institutions of Italy were cited (whether appropriately may be questioned) in the charter of the College of Physicians as precedents for that incorporation.†

§ 7. It does not appear that the relief afforded to the destitute, under the famous statute of Elizabeth, included any sort of medical or sanitary care.

No one, indeed, can say how soon the overseers and churchwardens of parishes perceived that some kind of "healing"—some administration of remedies—was necessary in order to diminish the periods of illness, during which the sufferers had a legal claim upon the poor-rates for maintenance.

So obvious a discovery could not have been long delayed; but owing to the paucity of regular medical practitioners, it could have led to no practical results generally, for at least a century after the enactment of the Elizabethan poor-law.

Gale, a celebrated surgeon, who wrote during the reign of Elizabeth, says, that in the time of Henry VIII., he had helped to furnish out of London, in one year, seventy-two English surgeons, who served by sea and land, and were "good workmen." "At the present day" (1566), he adds, "there are not thirty-four of the whole company of Englishmen, and the greater part of them are in noblemen's service; so that, if we should have need, I do not know where to find twelve sufficient men."‡

After the great political changes of the seventeenth century,

---

* See a remarkable decree of the Emperor Sigismund. (Essay V.)

† "Itaque partim bene institutarum civitatum in Italiâ et multis aliis nationibus exemplum imitati."—*Vide* Charter, 10 Hen. VIII. in Willcock, "Records," p. viii.

‡ "The Office of a Chirurgeon," quoted by Dr. Farr, p. 141, *op. cit.*

physicians and surgeons of a more useful sort, and in greater numbers, settled in all large towns. And we may conclude, that, in addition to special arrangements during pestilence, a permanent medical provision, though of an inferior and partial kind, was here and there made for the sick poor; but we find no statute-law on the subject until the middle or latter part of the eighteenth century.*

§ 8. In the beginning of that century, however, an interesting and curious philanthropic project was put forth by one John Bellers.† From several passages in this tract, it may be inferred that the necessity for the public appointment of salaried medical advisers then began to be very distinctly felt.

After urging upon Parliament the establishment of hospitals, and *the registration of diseases*, &c., his seventh proposal ran thus :—" That in every hundred of a county and parish of a city, there be appointed one doctor or chirurgeon, or more if needful, to take care of the sick poor in them," and to " visit every parish once a week at least ;" " that they be paid by the overseers of the poor ; and that such whose illness may be chronical, especially if declared to be incurable, should be sent to the most suitable hospital."‡

He defended this suggestion by the consideration, that " it may be but little or no more charge to the parish than they are at now,‖ for the sooner the poor man is restored to his health, he will be the sooner able to provide for himself and his family, besides being a great advantage to the rest of the parish—the nobility and gentry—when they shall be sick."

As John Bellers seems not to have belonged to the medical

---

* In Sir G. Cornewall Lewis's evidence before the Medical Poor-Relief Committee, in 1844, he admitted that "one or two" enactments were made "in the early part of the reign of George III., which gave to justices some power of ordering medical relief to the inmates of workhouses." (Evid. 2.)

Probably, any enactment of the kind previous to 1790 was merely a *local* act.

† "An Essay towards the Improvement of Physic, in Twelve Proposals, by which the Lives of many Thousands of the Rich, as well as the Poor, may be saved Yearly. Humbly dedicated to the Parliament of Great Britain, by John Bellers. London : 1714."

‡ Page 7. ‖ Page 15.

profession, it is not unlikely that his "proposals" met with some favour; and we know that, within the next quarter of a century, several of our noblest hospitals were founded.

§ 9. In this great work, as in most others, personal and voluntary efforts took the lead.

The penurious, yet munificent bookseller of Lombard-street, Thomas Guy, was the first Englishman of modern times, to show by a grand example to owners of property and to Parliament itself, that the necessities of the sick poor were not to be subjected to the operation of peddling and parsimonious measures, nor to be met by imperfect attempts at succour in mean and inferior institutions.*

Whether or not the suggestions of John Bellers had anything to do with the event, ten years had scarcely passed before the most remarkable monument of individual beneficence since the Reformation—Guy's Hospital—stood side by side with its old monkish rival.

Many followed in the way which Guy had so nobly led. By spontaneous associations of the wealthy and charitable, other metropolitan hospitals were founded before the middle of the eighteenth century; and some of the larger county towns hastened to copy the example.

The cities of Winchester and Bristol were but little behind the metropolis, each contending for the honour of being the first in the provinces to establish a county hospital. This was in 1736.

Dispensaries were not instituted until the latter part of the same century. The Royal General Dispensary in Aldersgate-street, seems to have been the first of the kind in England. It was opened in 1770, and boasts of being "the parent and model from which all others have sprung."†

Thus, by the various methods of endowment, bequest, donation,

---

* The money with which he founded Guy's Hospital is said to have been realized in 1720 by the Great South Sea Scheme. He died in 1724, just after the hospital was finished.

† *Report of Royal General Dispensary, Aldersgate-street.* 1844.

and annual contribution, a steadily-increasing number of infirmaries and dispensaries have been established and maintained throughout England; so that, long ago, it was truly said by an aged philanthropist, that "there is scarcely a mode of inability, or a class of disorder or infirmity, that has not an appropriate charity, in some form, for its relief."*

And more than ten years have now passed since it was shown to a Parliamentary committee that the greater portion of the poor in the principal towns in England were supplied with the best medicines and superior medical aid, in charitable institutions, attended by honorary and unsalaried physicians and surgeons.

Whether such arrangements are in principle correct—whether much more good might not be effected, at the same cost, by more systematic arrangements—whether the resources of these charities are not in many instances worse than precarious—whether dispensaries, especially, may not be placed on a more generally useful foundation—are questions which must be considered by the nation at no distant period. But, in the meantime, their medical officers are entitled to ask, whether any class in society confer unpaid services upon the poor and helpless to an equal extent; and their honorary governors may reasonably doubt whether any paid official staff would direct the details of management with more zeal, kindness, and intelligence.

§ 10. With all these good works, the State had little or nothing to do.†

It seems that no general enactment, recognising the necessity of providing medical attendance even for the most destitute, was passed until 1790.

The very important Act of that year‡ set forth that the laws then in being for regulating parish workhouses, were "deficient and

---

* The late Dr. Storer, of Nottingham. See his *Hints on the Constitution of Dispensaries*. 1832. Page 4.

† Nevertheless, an Act of Parliament, in 1739, instituted the "Bath Hospital," for the reception of poor persons from all parts of the country, who might thus share with the affluent and luxurious the benefits of the ancient *Aquæ Solis*.

‡ 30 Geo. III. cap. 49.

ineffectual, especially when the poor in such houses are affected with contagious or infectious disease, in which case particular attention to their lodging, diet, clothing, bedding, and *medicines* is requisite." Accordingly, any of her Majesty's justices of the peace, or any physician, surgeon, or apothecary, or the officiating clergyman of the parish, authorized by a magistrate's warrant, were empowered to visit and examine into the condition of the poor in any workhouse, and to certify respecting it to the Quarter Sessions. That court was to make " orders and regulations for the removing of any cause of complaint," and to enforce the observance of the same by the parish officers.

Justices were also empowered to order "immediate medical or other assistance" for the inmates of workhouses, as well as their separation (as in contagious diseases) or removal, &c., when needed.

A great step was thus gained. Negligent or recusant parishes were now compelled to perform a duty, which must have been already fulfilled with manifest advantage in some better managed places; for, in England, compulsory legislation generally follows the performance of public duty.

In fact, it is the doing of the thing which suggests to the Legislature that it ought to be done. And it can hardly be denied that, in most parts of England, during the last hundred years, medical relief* has been practically looked on as a necessary item of parochial aid, which overseers were bound to provide.

§ 11. Miserably unsystematic, irregular, and without any foresight of consequences, were the methods by which a supply

---

* An error has prevailed, chiefly among official people, on this point. Because medical attendance on the *out-door* poor was not mentioned in any statute before 1834, they concluded that the law did not insist on its provision.

But for many years previous to the passing of the Poor-Law Amendment, the courts of law had interpreted the statute of Elizabeth as authorizing the provision of Medical relief, and had decided that, in default of such provision, the medical attendant of a pauper might recover reasonable charges for his spontaneous services in urgent cases.—*Admin. of Med. Relief*, London, 1842, p. 96.

of medical aid (frequently a mere empirical administration of drugs) was gradually extended among the poorer classes.

Sometimes churchwardens and overseers employed their favourite apothecary to "physic" the parish. Sometimes the vestry formally appointed the "doctor."

But, as general practitioners gradually superseded mere apothecaries throughout the country, the office became more definite in its nature, and more important in its relations to society.

The mode of payment was, at first, for each article of medicine supplied to the paupers, and for "journeys" in rural districts—by order of an overseer, churchwarden, or magistrate.

Annual contracts were, after a time, substituted in the larger parishes. It would be curious to ascertain when and where the nefarious custom originated of *contracting* for the cure of the suffering and destitute.

But the obvious saving of trouble and responsibility to all parties except the doctor, soon made it popular; and as no adequate protection existed against the grossest abuses, the sick poor were too often *farmed* to any apothecary who was ready to "undertake" them at the lowest sum.

These contracts applied only to such poor as, under the laws of settlement, belonged to the parish in which they resided.

A consentaneous arrangement among parishes for the care of their non-resident paupers was probably impracticable. At all events, if ever suggested, it was not carried into effect. So that the original mode of payment for items continued in force, with respect to this class of poor; and parochial authorities had no means of avoiding ordinary charges for attendance on their poor under suspended orders of removal in other parishes; although payment was very frequently refused where the surgeon, neglecting the formalities which would have legally entitled him to compensation, had acted promptly for the relief of the sufferer.

The liability, however, to these charges was made a common plea for a further reduction of the small annual sums paid by contract for the resident paupers; and no portion of the community more keenly felt or more strenuously opposed the abuses then prevalent, with regard to the care of the casual sick poor, than members of the medical profession.*

§ 12. Such were the methods of medical relief which had become general in the eastern, southern, western, and midland counties, by the early part of the present century.

The growth of pauperism at that time became alarming.

Not less than 13 per cent.† of the population, in 1815, relied for support on the poor-rates. And this condition of affairs, but slightly improved by 1834, formed an unanswerable plea for a Poor-Law reform of some sort.

But, while the number of persons depending on the public funds for maintenance had thus increased, the number attended in sickness by the parish doctors had augmented in a still more remarkable ratio; so that it is no exaggeration to say that, before the Act of 1834, throughout four-fifths of England, the majority of the inhabitants of those parishes which had not the advantage of charitable infirmaries or dispensaries, were attended under the parish medical contract.‡

Notwithstanding the mischievous tendencies of the old parochial arrangements, the better sort of medical practitioners had fairly obtained in their respective neighbourhoods an influence which led not unfrequently to their employment by parishes.

* "At a general meeting of the members of the Worcestershire Medical and Surgical Society, it was resolved:—

"That the present system of removing paupers, on account of application from the overseers of the parish in which they happen to reside, to that parish to which they belong, often deprives the poor family of the means of gaining a living, and frequently induces them not to apply for a suspended order; while if a medical man is called in, under such circumstances, to attend them, he has no legal means of obtaining any remuneration for his attendance."

Resolved,—"That petitions be presented to both Houses of Parliament, praying that some regulation may be introduced in the bill now pending, relative to the poor-laws, for medical attendance on the casual poor."—Dunn's *Suggestions*, 1817, p. 1.

† See *Companion to Brit. Almanac*, 1844, p. 183.

‡ The number of counties from which returns were received by the Warwickshire Committee in 1827, and by Dr. Kerrison in 1814, confirm this estimate.

So that, when annual contracts became the general rule,—and when consequently the doctor's services, time, and drugs were claimed by the public to the fullest possible extent,—the poor of most districts, and in unlimited numbers, were attended by those surgeons who enjoyed the highest local reputation, and who, in fact, could best afford to act generously, and without petty calculation, towards the suffering applicants.

§ 13. Soon after the commencement of the late forty years, when "the land had rest" from war, the abuses perpetrated under customary methods of medical poor-relief, attracted the notice of many benevolent and thoughtful men, chiefly belonging to the medical profession.

The author of an interesting *Essay on Medical Economy*, published in 1814, entered at some length into the necessity of a superior medical provision for rural districts.

His ideas were not unlike those of Mr. Bellers, in 1714; but his improved method of handling the subject shows how much a century had effected.

He seems to have contemplated anything but a "poor-law" provision. He saw no reason why an endowment, similar to that provided by the nation and by landed proprietors, for the moral and spiritual wants of the people, should not be extended to an organization for the care of their physical health.

It is said that the author of this pamphlet was the late Dr. Kerrison. At all events, that gentleman was soon afterwards engaged in an inquiry into the operation of the medical contract system,* under the presidency of Dr. (then Mr.) G. M. Burrows.

Some of the most striking facts elicited by that first investigation into the condition of the sick poor, were adduced, with considerable effect, by Sir G. Cornewall Lewis, in his evidence before the Medical Poor-Relief Committee, in 1844. His object was to place the former administration of medical aid in dis-

---

* Dr. Burrows's observations are also well worth perusal.
See his pamphlet *On Lunatic Asylums*, pp. 76, 77. 8vo. Lond. 1817.

advantageous comparison with that established under the Poor-Law Commissioners. On the other hand, Dr. Kerrison's forcible denunciation of the abuses was employed still more happily by Mr. Guthrie, in the same inquiry, to show how inexcusable those Commissioners had been in extending—" in making common through a great part of the country"—those flagrant though occasional evils which had thus been held up to public reprehension by an official report.

This, the earliest inquiry, was connected with that professional movement for the improved education of general practitioners, which ended in the passing of the " Apothecaries' Act," in 1815.

§ 14. The period between 1815 and 1827 was by no means wanting in valuable suggestions towards an organized system of medical attendance on the poor. Perhaps one of the most original pamphleteers was a Mr. John Dunn, a surgeon, of Pickering in Yorkshire.

He advocated a division of the kingdom into a suitable number of districts, the size of which he thought might be regulated by the number of " paupers" in each locality.*

He proposed the appointment of respectable and competent medical officers to these districts, and thought that their qualifications should be tested, and their appointments regulated, by County examining Boards. He urged the institution of proper authorities for superintending the performance of duty, and dismissing incompetent and negligent officers; and he suggested that these courts of inquiry should consist of twelve gentlemen, of whom three should be clergymen, and three magistrates.

Mr. Yeatman, of Frome, formerly an army surgeon, also made out a strong case for Parliamentary inquiry in 1818; offering many valuable suggestions towards a better system.

§ 15. But without attempting to enumerate all the writers on

* It may afford a hint to those who are now busy in such calculations, that for a population at that time not greatly exceeding half of the present population of England and Wales, Mr. Dunn estimated the total number of medical officers at 2000, and their salaries at 200,000*l*. (100*l*. for each), costing on the average not less than 6*d*. annually to each ratepayer.

RESULTS OF EARLY INQUIRIES.

the subject, at this period, I pass on to notice the second general inquiry into the state of the sick poor.

This took place in 1827, and was promoted by a mixed body of country gentlemen and clergy, aided by a few physicians and surgeons, residing in and near the county of Warwick.

The disclosures both of this and of former inquiries, may be thus summed up:—

i. In too many parishes the custom prevailed of contracting with medical men for the treatment of the sick, without reference to professional character or qualification; those who were ready to undertake the contract at the lowest sum were too sure of the offer; parochial jobbery was common; and continual inducements to mean and unworthy conduct were held out to the profession.

ii. Serious evils were thus inflicted on the sick poor; many were the instances of gross neglect—ignorant and mischievous practice—increased suffering and mortality—protracted sickness and permanent loss of usefulness—foundations laid for organic or hereditary disease—and fatal indifference to sanative care: all this winked at, if not promoted, by vestries and overseers, under the delusion that they were economizing parochial expenditure.

iii. There was no limit to the number of parishes or population, which might in this way be "farmed" by the medical contractor.

iv. There was no supervision, professional or other, with respect to the performance of medical duties among the poor, who were, without redress, under neglect and mismanagement, while the public were without security for the due fulfilment of the contracts.

v. Lastly—the objectionable corollary to parochial contracts already noticed—a portion of the doctor's inadequate pay depended on the great uncertainty of his recovering specific charges for attendance on the casual sick poor belonging to other parishes.

CHAPTER SECOND.

THE RISE AND PROGRESS OF SELF-SUPPORTING SCHEMES OF MEDICAL RELIEF.

§ 1. LEAVING, for a short time, the main current of this narrative, it may facilitate our subsequent course to show how the second of these general inquiries belonged to an effort to promote the extension of the Self-Supporting Dispensary project, devised a few years before by Mr. H. L. Smith, of Southam.

The Warwick Committee recommended the scheme as, in their view, the most hopeful way of escaping from the evils of an ill-managed parochial system. They also considered it, on general grounds, as a likely means of encouraging provident and self-reliant habits among the poor.

§ 2. Now, it should be remembered that something like an insurance for medical attendance had, for some years previously—probably from the commencement of this century—existed among societies of working people.* Benefit clubs, composed of labourers and artisans, had appointed, or rather contracted with, surgeons for attendance on their members when sick, at a small yearly and quarterly sum per head.

This practice led to most of the evils of parish medical contracts, and its main defects were exposed before the Parliamentary Medical Relief Committee, in 1844.†

They may be thus briefly stated.

The election of one surgeon to attend a large society of working people, in towns and places where several surgeons are in practice, limits, needlessly and vexatiously, the choice of the

---

* Societies among the poor for insuring a weekly allowance in sickness, a deferred weekly annuity, and a payment at death, were first proposed by Mr. Acland, in 1786. Baron Maseres had previously put forward a scheme for deferred annuities. The first Act of Parliament on the subject was, I believe, in 1793.

† Evid. 9089—9094.

members. The election, being scarcely ever unanimous, leaves a dissatisfied minority, which any accidental circumstance readily converts into a majority. Another surgeon is then named, and if the proposal is backed by the offer of lower pay—*e. g.*, if the candidate is willing to farm the club at 2*s.* per head, when the old surgeon required 2*s.* 6*d.*—the change is almost sure to be made! Complaints among the members of insufficient and careless attendance, under such wretched arrangements, are inevitable; and probably there is no physician or surgeon in full practice who does not continually hear them, and who is not frequently called upon for aid instead of the medical officer of the club.

The dissatisfaction of those members, who feel no confidence in a surgeon chosen during the Bacchanalian revels of a "club feast," may be often unfounded; but the consciousness that their medical contractor is underpaid, naturally renders them suspicious as to the proper fulfilment of the contract.

The exclusion of the families of the members of Friendly Societies from the assumed benefits of the medical contract, is another serious defect; which, in some cases, is imperfectly supplied by a private arrangement between the surgeon and the members of the club, securing his re-election at the annual meeting. Nor does any effective check exist upon this (almost gratuitous) supply of medical relief to persons, who may be fully able to provide for themselves in the ordinary way, but who, as members of the club, do not hesitate to avail themselves of their privileges.

The entire want of supervision, not merely by professional referees, but even by educated and philanthropic arbitrators, leaves the arrangements open to every kind of abuse and neglect.

Returns and reports of attendance, during sickness, and accident, form no part of the duties of the surgeon; and the results of the working of these arrangements are concealed.[*]

§ 3. Such was and is the system in lieu of which, as also of parochial contracts, Mr. H. L. Smith proposed to substitute self-

[*] See Evidence (1844), 9077.

supporting dispensaries; and it must be confessed that his original scheme was free from many of the abuses of benefit-club medical relief.

For instance, he proposed that all the surgeons in a district should join the institution; that the subscribers should have the right of choice, each surgeon receiving his share of the surplus fund, according to the number of cases attended; and that entire families and persons of both sexes and of all ages should be admitted.

He advised the separate provision of medicines in a dispensary, managed by a committee of honorary subscribers, who were to be empowered to receive complaints and rectify errors in management.

He proposed that the stability of the institution should be secured by a fixed annual sum to be paid out of the poor-rates, sufficient to meet all the medical expenses of the sick paupers in the district, who were to be attended from the same dispensary. And the plan further included a middle class of patients, neither parish paupers nor yet free subscribers, but "charity" patients recommended by the honorary governors.

§ 4. Nevertheless, the defects of this project, even in its most perfect form, were far from being few or immaterial. The rate of insurance premiums paid by the "free members," bore no relation to their respective liabilities. The aged, the sickly, and the infirm, paid no more than the young and healthy. Thus, as might have been expected, few of the latter entered, and the society consisted chiefly of the former class.* Thus, also, a rate of contribution, which afforded but a very scanty remuneration to the medical attendant, even when paid upon the average of a district, became absurdly inadequate when made, only or chiefly, for those who were always claiming his services and his drugs.

* The average *annual* number of cases of sickness in any body of persons, in an ordinary sanitary condition, should not exceed 50 or 60 per cent. Yet, in these societies, the ratio has been from 70 to 112 per cent., showing an enormous disproportion of sickly persons.—*Medical Relief on the Principle of Mutual Assurance*, p. 23. London. Parker. 1837.

Dr. Jenks, of Brighton, showed that out of 737 members, of whom 357 remained on the books, there had been 726 cases of sickness in a year!—*Sanitary Inquiry, Local Reports,*" 1842, p. 70. London. 8vo.

The want of an accumulating fund, such as exists in all other kinds of insurance, to meet the future liabilities and casualties of the younger members, was another discouragement to their entrance. The admission of children at a far lower rate than that paid by young and healthy adults, when their liabilities to sickness are known to be much greater, was an equally glaring blunder.

But when, in addition to those financial errors, inherent in and inseparable from Mr. Smith's project, other deviations from his original idea led to still more serious evils;—*when the fixed parochial stipends were withdrawn under the new Poor-Law;*—when the dispensaries were given up, the committees dissolved, and the members left to the uncontrolled management and care of the separate surgeons;—when the vast majority of respectable practitioners, observing the obvious fallacy of the arrangement, declined to co-operate, and left the appointments in the hands of a few, often needy men, seeking to obtain practice of a more remunerative kind by speculating in these clubs;—when the vile principle of pecuniary competition crept in, and several surgeons were to be seen in the same place, catering for poor patients, by various reductions upon the weekly penny and halfpenny;—this odious system began to stink in the nostrils of all sensitive and right-minded persons; the miserable societies were one after another broken up, and now exist in but very few towns and districts of England.

The Coventry and Derby Dispensaries, the Barham Downs Society, and probably a few more recent arrangements of the kind, may possibly have escaped the general deterioration, and may be still in operation; but, as shown by the inquiry of 1854, they are quite unlikely to lead to any extension of the system.

We shall soon see the use made of the "medical club" project, by the authorities constituted under the Poor-Law Amendment Act.

However applicable Mr. H. L. Smith's system might be to a mere supply of medicines and restoratives, under improved regulations, the result of a thirty years' unceasing effort to promote its extension has proved that it generally fails when applied to the remuneration of medical practitioners for the sanative care of the working-classes.*

While the self-reliant efforts of labourers and artisans, in matters within their reach, deserve every encouragement, it must be confessed that a mutual provision of *proper* medical care is beset with difficulties, and needs all the aid and guidance of an enlightened philanthropy.

* See Evidence upon Independent Medical Clubs, and upon the Provident Medical Institutions of Newmarket, Grantham, and Stratford-upon-Avon, pp. 107, 108, 109. Appendix to *Health and Sickness of Town Populations.*

CHAPTER THIRD.

From a.d. 1833 to 1843.

§ 1. Thus have I endeavoured to describe the preliminary stage—the original condition of this question, previous to those national and Parliamentary proceedings, which ended in the Poor-Law Amendment Act, and in a statutory connexion between the medical care of the poor and the administration of that Act.

Not merely Parliamentary committees, but also the Royal Commission, appointed to inquire into the working of the poor-laws—while adducing numerous reasons for the growing dependence of the labouring-classes upon the poor-rates—seem to have omitted altogether one of the most influential of these causes, namely, the grant of *medical* relief, as a branch of *poor-law* relief.

It was indeed perceived that a good poor-law ought to provide for the necessities of the destitute, in such a manner as to discourage mendicancy and pauperism; and that the welfare of society required judicious limitations upon the expenditure of the poor-rates, lest they should be applied in such a manner as to depress the wages of labour and to draw the poor into a condition of helpless reliance on the public funds.

But it was not seen that a law of this kind was wholly inapplicable to a national provision of medical care for those who were unable for various reasons—by no means merely on account of poverty—to provide it wisely for themselves.

Neither does it seem to have been fully perceived, that, beside the direct and obvious tendency of sickness and casualty to create destitution, by arresting man's capability for labour,—another more quiet, but scarcely less sure cause of pauperization was operating through the administration of an extensive system of medical aid, under contracts between parish vestries and parish doctors.

And certainly no official inquirers ever hinted at the possibility of so improving, extending, and confirming the provision made by hospitals and dispensaries, as to meet all the medical wants of the lower orders, and to relieve the poor-law of a most damaging and perplexing adjunct.

Still more Quixotic would it have been thought to bestow the slightest consideration upon historical and foreign precedents; whether those of antiquity, especially the complete medical organization for the benefit of the poor, under the Roman Empire—or those modern arrangements which provide so thoroughly for the population of most of the German and Italian States; all of which, be it remembered, were and are wholly distinct from any poor-law, in the English sense of that term.

Thus, while philanthropic societies and medical writers were exposing the "horrible evils of farming the sick poor to the lowest medical bidders," the political economists, with views still narrower, were only intent upon diminishing an item of public expenditure, most trifling when compared with the work actually performed, but one which never ought to have been charged upon the poor-law fund.

§ 2. It is worthy of notice, that, notwithstanding the magnitude and importance of this question, and its multifarious relations with other departments of civil administration, the Royal Commissioners of Inquiry, in 1833, despatched it in half a page of a Report containing 362 pages!! Notwithstanding repeated disclosures of mal-administration, numerous proofs of detriment to the public health, and many valuable suggestions towards the formation of a better system,*—the Poor-Law Commissioners—both those for inquiry, and those appointed under the Act of 1834—persisted in treating medical attendance merely as a department

---

* The Appendix to the *Report of the Commission of Inquiry* contains several interesting communications on these points.

of parochial relief, which it was their duty to reduce, with the rest, to the lowest possible cost.

Parliament interfered not either to correct the mistake, or to enlarge the view.

And thus, although the law itself made no distinct or methodical provision for medical relief,* the direction of the medical and sanitary care of the masses passed into the hands of those authorities, who, under that Act, succeeded to the administrative functions before exercised by magistrates, vestries, and overseers.

§ 3. It may be safely asserted, that a course more opposed to sound principles of public health and public economy,—to equity, reason, and humanity,—has been seldom pursued under official authority in this country, than that which was adopted with respect to the medical department by the Poor-Law Commissioners and their secretary, and by boards of guardians under their influence.

Large excuse and ample extenuation must, indeed, be allowed to those central and local boards, on the ground of the utter incompatibility of their main duties with the direction of a national provision for the health and sickness of the poorer classes; but no official mystification can get rid of the notorious fact—that most of the published and acknowledged evils of the former system, so far from being redressed or even mitigated, were for some time aggravated to a fearful degree.

i. More generally than before, medical officers were chosen without regard to past meritorious services, known competency, or full legal qualification.

Their appointment, in most cases, was determined by their readiness to accept the lowest amount of salary proposed for the district; and the former occasional practice of requiring " tenders" from medical candidates, became the common rule of

---

* The interpretation clause states that an "officer" may mean, among others, a "person duly qualified to practise as a medical man."

And by the 54th section, "any justice of the peace was empowered to give a similar order" (*i.e.*, for medical relief only) "to any parishioner or out-parishioner, when any case of sudden or dangerous illness might require it."

union administration,—hence facetiously called the "tender system."

An absurd plea for it, ignorantly or disingenuously set up* in the name of the Poor-Law Commissioners, was that they had no other means of ascertaining the proper rate of medical remuneration. But the fallacy of this pretext was soon obvious to the few who did not immediately see through the whole proceeding.

A common-sense view of the known objects of medical practitioners, whether in or out of employment in the locality for which "tenders" were required,† and some little experience of the results of this kind of competition under the old law, would have made it clear to any unprejudiced person, that these tenders could afford no guide whatever to a correct estimate.

Besides, it was known that the parochial authorities were in possession of full information respecting the previous amount of medical expenditure, which the Commissioners of Inquiry had pronounced to be economical.‡

If the total annual average of the former medical charges, in the several parishes of any English Union,‖ had been re-distributed according to the population, area, and distance from advice of each place or district,—low as that remuneration was,—it would have satisfied the profession, and provided for the needs of the poor, until opportunity for longer and wider experience had enabled the commissioners and guardians to rectify local anomalies.¶

---

* See *First and Second Annual Reports of the Poor-Law Commissioners*.

† S. G. O. asked, in the *Times*, "Why the Poor-Law Commissioners should so play off these contending parties (old practitioners and young competitors) against each other, that they may get out of the fears of the one or the hopes of the other, time, skill, and medicine, at a price *they know* to be virtually so unjust, that no upright man can claim them from the medical officer without blushing at the covenant on which he founds his claim?"

‡ "On the whole, however, medical attendance seems in general to be adequately supplied, and economically, if we consider only the price and amount of attendance."—*Report*, 1834. 8vo. p. 43.

‖ The northern parishes of England, and others in remote or peculiar districts, are exceptional cases, to which this process could not well have been applied without modification.

¶ The Provincial Medical Association, in 1837, petitioned Parliament for returns

ii. Numerous parishes were grouped in large and impracticable districts,* so as to tempt medical speculation, not only by a somewhat higher "figure," but by a smaller proportion of duty; it being obvious that the actual amount of service performed in any parish would, with few exceptions, vary inversely with the size of the district in which it was included.

In this respect, the former arrangements were greatly superior, as it was clearly the interest, personal and pecuniary, of the ratepayers of each parish to appoint the nearest or most conveniently located practitioner; the distance of the contracting parties increasing, generally, the cost of the supply,† and always the trouble of the poor parishioners.

iii. The number of medical attendants was reduced by the same process.

From facts on record in particular localities,‡ and from the extent of the professional movement at the time, it has been estimated that more than 2500 medical men were employed by parishes under the old system; each receiving on the average about 100*l.* a year, in salary and extra charges; or about 250,000*l. per annum* for the whole country.

Under the new arrangements, in 1836-7, the number employed had fallen to 1830;∥ and the total expenditure, in 1838, to 136,000*l.*

iv. Both of the last-mentioned changes must also have effected a considerable reduction in the numbers of sick poor attended.

---

of the average cost, and other particulars, of medical relief in each parish previous to the introduction of the new law; but the returns were vigorously opposed by official persons, and the demands of justice defeated.

* The immense extent and population of some of the new districts was proved before the Parliamentary Committee of 1838, (Evid. 14,763, *et seq.*; 15,703, *et seq.*); and more detailed information on this point will be found in the *Reports on Medical Relief of the Provincial Medical Association,* especially those of 1840 and 1841. (See note † p. 170.)

† Evid. 14,798. Parliamentary Committee. 1838.

‡ See Table, p. 49, *Administration of Medical Relief,* London, 8vo. 1842. In twenty-one Unions, the number of medical officers was reduced from 194 to 56.

∥ See *Third Annual Report of Poor-Law Commissioners.* (Appendix.)

There is abundance of unexceptionable testimony to establish this point.* But only two important witnesses need here be cited.

Mr. Gulston, the Poor-Law Inspector, said, in 1838, that in the more pauperized districts "not one half of the people were attended that used to be."†

Dr. Farr, of the General Register Office, referring with disapprobation to this withdrawal of medical aid, stated before the same Committee, that under the old system "*the great mass of the labouring population* have been led to expect a public provision of medical advice."‡

v. The process of diminution in the public supply of medical aid was, for a time, accelerated by the Commissioners' adoption of the "medical club" scheme, already noticed.

Neither the Warwick Committee of 1827, nor the originator of self-supporting dispensaries, while promoting a plan which they honestly believed would prove an important benefit to the labouring classes, could have guessed that it would be so perverted, both by those seeking employment, and by those in power, that the lineaments of the original project could scarcely be recognised.

* The fact of a diminution in the supply of medical relief, under the early operation of the Poor-Law Amendment Act, has been denied by parties interested in making the best of modern arrangements.

Thus, among other questionable statements attributed to Mr. Baines, during a debate, July 12, 1853, in the House of Commons, is the following:—

"Since that time (1834), the amount of medical relief given to the poor was, to use the words of an unexceptionable witness before the Committee of 1844, 'infinitely greater than before that time.'"

Now, it must be borne in mind that the distinguished metropolitan surgeon, who gave the evidence to which Mr. Baines refers, had no personal knowledge whatever of what was going on in this matter from 1834 to 1838; he depended on official statements; and I have the best possible authority—namely, his own—for saying that he then alluded to "medical relief being more general in *all* places, rather than in the same places where it had been given by the parish doctors." Now, it had been thus given in at least four out of five English parishes; and, as Mr. Gulston said, to double the number of people in most of those parishes.

See also Mr. Ceely's comparison between the supplies before and since the New Poor Law, in note ‡, p. 244.

† Evidence (1715) Parliamentary Committee.   ‡ Ibid. 15,787.

But the red-tape party had unfortunately adopted this dictum of a spurious political economy—that medical advice was a *commodity*, the price of which it was necessary to reduce in order to place it within the reach of the greatest possible number of the people. Accordingly, many local Boards acting on directions* from the Central Board proceeded to establish what they called—facetiously, it might be thought—" Independent Medical Clubs." The more thoughtful and far-sighted argued in vain against so preposterous an attempt.

Uninfluenced by protest or argument, the authorities required their medical contractors to form, and to attend upon, these clubs; the terms of contribution being fixed by the boards of guardians themselves, on the erroneous principles before mentioned;† with the threat of introducing by public advertisement, an unknown candidate for the private practice of the neighbourhood, under official patronage,‡ in the event of the medical officer declining to take part in his own further degradation.

Any correct notion of provident effort among the poor was of course hopelessly confused by what appeared to them only an arbitrary attempt to exact a sort of medical tax from their own small earnings, for the relief of the rate-payers.

The ill-contrived measure soon failed, especially where the establishment of the club was made a condition or part of the union contract; and the plan, if still lingering under a different

---

* See Circular from Somerset House, Feb. 1836.

† See pp. 160, 161. These ridiculous perversions of mutual insurance were carried to the extent of admitting all the children of large families *gratuitously!*

‡ The threat was carried into execution in several instances,—*e. g.*, in the Camberwell Union. (Report of Parliamentary Committee, 1838.) Dr. Kay—since Sir J. P. K. Shuttleworth—was the only Commissioner who seemed to understand the real drift of these clubs.

"I cannot deem it expedient," said he, " that by too low a rate of payment one form of assistance should be substituted for another, and that the dependence of the poor should be thus disguised."—(*Third Annual Report of Poor-Law Committee*, Appendix, p. 186.)

See also his forcible objections to the interference of the Commissioners and Guardians in such arrangements.—(Evidence 5,102—8, in 1838, quoted in *Administration of Medical Relief (Report Prov. Assoc.* 1842), pp. 57, 58.)

guise in a few districts, cannot now influence any conclusions of the statesman on the subject.

§ 4. The first two Annual Reports of the Poor-Law Commissioners contained remarks intended to justify their new medical arrangements. But the defence was singularly characterized by prejudice, inaccuracy, and sophistry, and did much more to damage themselves than to silence their accusers.

These attempts were conclusively answered by several professional bodies and individuals;* and at greater length in the Reports of the Poor-Law Committee of the Provincial Association.†

The discussion need not now be reviewed; yet before passing on, my readers should be reminded of a gross attack made by the Commissioners in their first Annual Report, upon the character of the former parochial surgeons as a body; accusing them "in the great majority of instances," of dishonourable collusion with the inferior parish officers, for the recovery of exorbitant charges for attendance on non-parishioners.

Whoever was the author of the slander, the object undoubtedly was to reconcile the Government, Parliament, and the public, to the unjustifiable proceedings of the newly-constituted Boards, by impugning the motives and injuring the good name of the whole professional body.

The libel was refuted, with very good effect, in the public documents just referred to.‡ The universal demand of the profession

* It would be impossible to give even the titles of the numerous pamphlets which appeared at this time on the subject. One, however, remains unrivalled: *A Letter addressed to Lord John Russell*, by the late amiable and accomplished Dr. Yelloly, in 1837. It contains a temperate yet conclusive defence of the parish doctors under the former system; an able exposition of medical duties and responsibilities; a calm and dignified appeal to Government for justice; and as the wise reforms which he proposed are still unaccomplished, it is, for the most part, applicable to present circumstances.

† The first Report—1836—was reprinted in a pamphlet, entitled *The Poor-Law and the Medical Profession*, London, 1837. The Reports for 1840 and 1841 were also reprinted in the pamphlet already referred to, *Administration of Medical Relief to the Poor*, London, 1842.

‡ The protests were printed in the Appendix—Part II. pp. xvii.-xxiv.—of the first edition of *The Report*, 1836, *of the Committee of the Provincial Association*.

See also *Poor-Law and Medical Profession, supra cit.* pp. 19, 20, 31.

to "name" the offenders was never complied with (though for the ends of justice they ought, if it were possible, to have been exposed); nor were the calumnious assertions again ventured upon.

§ 5. By their gradual abandonment of the most obnoxious and injurious of their medical arrangements, the Commissioners have virtually pronounced upon themselves or their predecessors a sufficiently strong condemnation.

Why then, it may be asked, stir up the embers of a waning controversy? Why denounce official mal-practices which no longer exist? For the following reasons:—

Public provisions for the medical relief of the poor, both before and after the enactment of the law of 1834, are of historical importance to those engaged in the sanitary movement.

They show the unsafe, one may almost say, the rotten, foundation upon which the administration of remedial and preventive duties among the poor still rests; and the radical evil of their connexion with the Poor-Law.

They show the injury deliberately inflicted on the cause of public health by late official authorities, acting under the influence of one, who has been held up by his partisans as the chief sanitary reformer of the age; and they serve to explain why, after his removal from the Poor-Law Board, the administration of medical relief so decidedly improved; and is now, perhaps, as free from gross abuses as is possible under any consistent poor-law management.

They explain the extraordinary difficulties which Boards of Health, central and local, have so often experienced, in endeavouring to obtain the efficient co-operation of the medical-aid department.

And they may serve to remove all doubts as to the real cause of the singular neglect and contempt with which the medical body has been treated in past sanitary legislation and administration.

§ 6. I now proceed to notice the principal investigations, which the medical department of the Poor-Law underwent from 1830 to

1844—before Parliamentary committees—by the Poor-Law authorities, and by philanthropic or professional advocates for reform; —as well as to mention the more important changes to which those inquiries led.

The vantage ground secured to the cause of science and humanity by the first Parliamentary investigation (1838), was mainly due to the courage and energy of Mr. Wakley, the sole medical member of that Select Committee.

To him, in no small degree, the profession and the poor owed that fairer recognition of their claims, and those reasonable admissions and recommendations,* which confirmed the truth of the chief complaints, and the justice of the principal demands, of the reformers.

The Select Committee, indeed, failed to show the "many respects" in which, they said—probably by way of courtesy to commissioners and guardians—the administration of medical relief

* " On reviewing the whole of the evidence connected with medical relief, your Committee are of opinion, that while most (?) of the witnesses called on this subject agree in representing many (?) of the evils of the old system to have been corrected, yet it does appear that the size of the medical districts is, in many instances, inconveniently large; and that in some cases the poor have been assigned to the care of too small a number of medical officers. They think, also, that it may be desirable to discontinue the practice of advertising for tenders from the medical men; this seems to have given offence to a profession whose feelings and wishes it is important to consult." . . . . (Here follow some suggestions as to remuneration.) . . . . .

" Your Committee, from a feeling of respect for the medical profession, and *believing that their attendance on the poor has been marked by great liberality and humanity*, are anxious that the suggestions which have been made by them should be favourably considered by those who are charged with the administration of the law. They recommend the evidence which they have received on this subject to the attention of the Poor-Law Commissioners; and they cannot but hope that arrangements may be made to remove some of the objections reasonably entertained to the present practice, and to put this branch of relief on a footing which shall be satisfactory to the medical men, and conducive to the comfort of the poor."

The resolution which the Committee came to is as follows :—

" That the administration of medical relief to the poor has been, in many respects, amended under the new law, but that there is still room for further improvement; that the medical districts, in some instances, seem to be inconveniently large; that they should be of such a size as to admit of an easy access of the medical man to his patients; and that the remuneration should be such as to insure proper attention and the best medicines."—*Report of the Select Committee on the Poor-Law Amendment Act.* Aug. 1838, p. 24.

had been "amended under the new law"; so that their report virtually amounted to a distinct repudiation of the miserable doings of the preceding four years.

§ 7. The necessity for great improvements became a question merely of time; yet, strangely enough, the very moderate changes indicated by the first Parliamentary committee, were entrusted to the same central and local Boards which had, (as I have shown,) aggravated original evils, and which soon manifested a disposition to delay, as long as possible, the required amendments in this department.

Instead of proceeding, however cautiously, to act upon Parliamentary instructions, they preferred, for obvious reasons, instituting an inquiry of their own, by means of their assistant commissioners, in the following year. Their Report, which appeared in 1840, *On the continuance of the Commission and some further amendments of the Poor-Laws,* contained the result of those partial investigations, together with the arguments and conclusions of the Central Board thereon.

Perhaps no clearer proof could be adduced of the inherent unfitness of such a Board to superintend a national provision of sanative care,—if not of their inability to form a correct theory on the subject,—than one of the introductory sentences in that report, headed in the margin—

" Objects of a System of Medical Relief."

" We must premise that the objects which we desire to attain are:— To provide medical aid for all persons who are really destitute, and to prevent medical relief from generating or encouraging pauperism; and with this view to withdraw from the labouring-classes, the administrators of relief, and the medical officers, all motives for applying for, or administering public relief, unless when circumstances render it absolutely necessary."

On this principle, medical advice is to be considered a sort of personal gratification, a luxury,* of doubtful if not of dangerous

---

* "If medical advice were a mere luxury, like fine clothes, delicate food, carriages, &c., the State might justly say—Let a man obtain it of the quality he can tendencies,—to be doled out sparingly, and to those alone who, in the opinion of *Bumbledom*, are "really destitute," and, to such, only when "circumstances render it absolutely necessary"!

Apply this meagre and limited idea of State Medicine to all the practical difficulties of public hygiéne, to precautionary measures against disease, to medical management during pestilences and epidemics,—and its mischievous inadequacy will be as immediately perceived as it has been lamentably felt throughout England since that report was made.

Holding, fundamentally, such opinions, how impossible was it for these commissioners to arrive at safe and correct conclusions respecting practical measures !

It is, however, but fair to observe, that they had, by this time, learnt one lesson. The manner and tone of their allusions to the medical profession were far more rational and conciliatory than those of their early annual reports.

But they abandoned their mistaken position slowly and reluctantly. They could not even decide on relinquishing their cherished "tender system," without producing "reasons" in its favour,*—mere reiterations, indeed, of inaccurate statements, and renewed attempts to justify the appropriation of the private means and resources of candidates for office,—all which had been repeatedly exposed and refuted.†

After the very general reprobation of their proceedings in this department, by humane and unbiassed observers, one might almost have suspected a joke in this their concluding remark:—" There is but little dissatisfaction‡ prevailing in reference to the existing

---

afford, or go without it; but it is assumed, as an axiom, that it is the *positive duty* of a state to take every necessary precaution to preserve the life and health of its subjects."—Sir J. Forbes, *Brit. and For. Medical Review*, No. XXXVII.

* See p. 46 of that Report.

† In their "Minute" of Oct. 31, 1840, they say that appointment by tender is less objectionable in the case of medical practitioners than in that of masters and matrons of workhouses, and of relieving-officers !—*Seventh Annual Report*, p. 126.

‡ The "little dissatisfaction" had, in the Commissioners' estimate, grown into "much dissatisfaction," by the time they had compiled their *General Order* of 1842. —See *Eighth Annual Report*, p. 139.

medical arrangements, and certainly none such as to call for any immediate general change."

The Reports, on the other hand, of the Provincial Medical Committee before referred to, may be fairly said to have finally disposed of the several erroneous statements and deductions contained both in the General Report of the Board, and in the district reports of the Assistant Commissioners.

§ 8. From 1839 to 1841, the name of a deceased ornament of the Bench and Bar appeared in the discussion.

Mr. Serjeant Talfourd's advocacy of the cause of humanity and civilization on this occasion did him the greater honour, inasmuch as a very considerable proportion of his learned brethren were at that time under Somerset House influence, and not a little disposed to look upon the medical faculty through Mr. Chadwick's glasses.

It has been supposed that warm-hearted alacrity in the defence of the oppressed, not less than devotion to elegant literature, is incompatible with the attainment of very high professional dignities and emoluments.

True or untrue as this notion may be,—good or bad as may be its effect, if any, upon society,—that lamented scholar, poet, and philanthropist, disregarded the conventionalism, and was deterred by no selfish considerations or professional prejudices from co-operating cordially with the medical associations in their efforts to secure a reasonable adjustment of this question by the legislature.

Nor did his exertions in this cause prevent his ultimately filling the exalted post of Judge of Common Pleas.*

§ 9. It would be useless to burden these pages with details, the interest of which has now passed away; but some of the proposals then made bear too closely upon the present state of the case to be passed over in utter silence.

* A portion of his correspondence is contained in the *Appendix to the Association Reports of* 1840 and 1841; it is well worth perusal. See *Administration of Medical Relief,* p. 124, *supra cit.*

The most prominent feature of the measure prepared by the learned Serjeant, was the appointment of a Medical Poor-Law Commissioner, who was to have equal power with the three other Commissioners in the supreme direction of the medical department, beside performing certain duties belonging specially to it.

Other objects to be obtained by the Bill were, limitation as to the extent and population of medical districts; the abolition of contracts and tenders, and the substitution of fixed salaries; an improved system of annual reports from the medical officers; greater permanence in their appointments; and as complete a legal qualification for future medical officers as the anomalous state of medical law in this country would permit.

The Medical Association had at first proposed to leave all details respecting the appointment, the duties, and the remuneration of medical officers, as well as the size of districts, to a sort of local arbitration; a medical assessor or referee to be elected by the physicians and surgeons of each locality, for the purpose of advising and aiding the Board of Guardians in their medical arrangements — any irreconcileable difference between him and the Board to be settled by the Medical and other Commissioners. But this simple suggestion having been set aside by Mr. Serjeant Talfourd's more complete project, the Association proceeded, in 1841, to recommend that the Legislature should define numerical limits within which the Guardians of every Union should be confined in their decisions upon all matters of detail.

That body also endeavoured, though with no better success than before, to obtain the insertion of a very carefully-prepared, yet by far too complex, series of clauses in the Bill then introduced by Government for the further Amendment of the Poor Laws.

These efforts, and especially Mr. Serjeant Talfourd's clauses, were effectual only to the extent of impressing upon Ministers and upon the authorities at Somerset House, a deeper sense of their responsibilities in this matter; and so far they probably contributed to the issue of the first " General Medical Order" of the Commissioners in the following year.

§ 10. It was not until March, 1842, nearly four years after the opinion of the Committee of the House of Commons had been distinctly pronounced in favour of a decisive change, that the Commissioners felt it necessary to enforce, even to some extent, and with several relaxations and exceptions, the recommendations of Parliament.

The General Medical Order of that date embodied provisions respecting most of the matters affected by Mr. Serjeant Talfourd's measure, with two or three additional regulations.

(i.) The invitation of tenders was prohibited, unless the remuneration were fixed and announced in the advertisement: but the Commissioners omitted any instructions for the calculation and determination of salaries; so that, as was shown by Mr. Guthrie, in 1844, the results of the "tender system" were left unremedied. Boards of Guardians might still beat down their medical officers by a species of pecuniary competition.*

(ii.) A qualification in both medicine and surgery was required of all future medical officers; but membership in a particular college of surgeons was to supersede the diplomas of all other colleges in the United Kingdom—a provision unsanctioned by precedent, since members of any "one of the Royal Colleges of Surgeons" were legally eligible to the appointment of surgeons to English prisons,† and to the army and navy.

This novel preference was the result of private conferences

---

* The Commissioners endeavoured to justify this omission, in their *Ninth Annual Report*, pp. 15, 17, by pleading (1) the wide diversities in the existing rates of payment to medical officers in different Unions, especially the very low remuneration in some northern counties; (2) the establishment in these counties of large dispensaries maintained by voluntary subscriptions; (3) the existence of numerous medical clubs in the mining districts. As there is apparent force in these pleas, it is hereafter shown how the difficulties might be met, without infringing upon the principle of a uniform standard of remuneration.

† Act 4, Geo. IV. c. 64, s. 33. The Commissioners omitted all reference to these precedents in their minute of May 12, 1842.

between the heads of the favoured college and the Commissioners.

It was, nevertheless, rescinded within two years; and members of the other colleges admitted on equal terms.

(iii.) A maximum area of 15,000 acres, and a maximum population of 15,000 persons, were required for medical districts in England; and thus a limit was very properly set to the extent of public duty which might be undertaken by any one officer. This clause was however soon confessed* to be inapplicable to many localities, and became almost a dead letter.† It was far inferior to Mr. Serjeant Talfourd's, which was based on a principle admitting of universal application—namely, that in proportion as the population of the locality was more scattered, so the number of persons included in a medical district should be fewer, —no extreme limit of area or distance being fixed.‡

(iv.) With regard to the specific payments directed in this General Order, to be made for certain severe surgical cases and operations, I have little to add to remarks made formerly on this point.‖ Its effects upon scientific surgical practice, if any, cannot be favourable. There should be no premium upon the operative method of treatment. Neither should the surgeon, who resists the double temptation of some personal *éclat*, and an addition to his scanty salary, and who cures the patient without an operation, nor he who sends the case to a hospital,—be in a comparatively worse position than their more adventurous and less scrupulous brother officers.

And with regard to the financial department, these payments,

---

* See *Ninth Annual Report*, p. 12.

† In Wales, the limit as to area was not applied; nor was it found practicable in the moors of Devonshire and the North;—the mountainous districts of the Lakes, &c.—*Report of Committee*, 1854, Cam. (48).

‡ Thus, where the area unavoidably exceeded 8000 acres, the population was not to exceed 4000; where the area exceeded 2000 acres, the population was not to exceed 6000;—and no district, however small in area, was to contain more than 10,000 persons. It is incredible that a population of 4000 should exist in any part of England and Wales, beyond the reach of a medical practitioner.

‖ See *Health and Sickness of Towns Population*, p. 59.

although generally acceptable to the medical officers, are almost universally disliked by the Guardians, and have proved a constant source of altercation and heartburning between the surgeons and the local and central Boards.*

(v.) Medical officers were required to name substitutes or deputies, to attend during their temporary hindrance or absence, " without cost to the Union."

The main defect of this regulation was, that the opinions and wishes of the inhabitants of the district were in no way consulted in the choice of a deputy.

This objection, be it observed, applies in a great degree to the election of medical officers by the Guardians.

(vi.) A mode of obtaining medical relief by the " permanent paupers," without the troublesome necessity of seeking an "order" in each case, was an improvement on the previous indefensible and dangerous practice; and had been, years before, urged by the medical body.

(vii.) Probably the most imperfect regulation of this order was the last, which professed to confer a sort of permanence upon the medical appointments—that is to say, the doctor might continue in office until his death, resignation, disqualification, or removal by the Commissioners; unless the period of his tenure of office were at first entered on the minutes of the Board of Guardians, or mentioned in a written contract.† Of course, Boards of Guar-

* The Commissioners very rightly insisted on separate payments for attendance in cases of midwifery,—curious as are some of their regulations on this point.

† The Provincial Association memorialized Government respecting the General Order of 1842, acknowledging the amendments which had been made, but soliciting attention to its manifest imperfections, and complaining especially of the continuance of *contracts*—"a mode of appointment (said they) which is unnecessary to secure the proper performance of duty, repulsive to the feelings of men of liberal education, and not imposed on members of the other learned professions, when appointed to any office in the Poor-Law Unions."—[*Documents relating to the Administration of Medical Relief in* 1842 *and* 1843, ordered to be printed by the Council of the Association, 1844.]

This appeal may have had a share in procuring the omission in the Order of 1847, of all reference to or recognition of "Contracts." In that Order, the medical appointments were placed, in this respect, on the same footing with those of the other superior officers of Unions.

dians, averse as they generally are to concede to their medical officers anything like independence, rarely omitted to enter or specify the period of service, and so the regulation for some time remained almost a nullity. But the number of permanent appointments slowly increased; until, by 1853, half the medical officers were so appointed, and the reform was enforced by the decisive and satisfactory order of 1855.

Thus may be said to have ended the first stage of a still pending controversy.

CHAPTER FOURTH.

PROSPECTS OF SANITARY LEGISLATION UNDER THE POOR-LAWS BEFORE 1844.

§ 1. BEFORE the second Parliamentary inquiry, in 1844, the administrative authorities, constituted under the Poor-Law Amendment Act, had acquired, under legislative sanction, a considerable accession of sanitary powers and duties.

We have seen how a public provision for curative medicine came to be directed by these authorities.

We may also safely assume that this was a ground (probably the main ground) for their being afterwards entrusted with the supervision and execution of certain matters belonging to preventive medicine.

There was, however, another reason. It needed not piles of "blue books," nor columns of questionable statistics, to prove to persons of common sense—that a considerable portion of the cost of pauperism arose from preventible disease,—that the charges of widowhood and orphanage upon the poor-rates were due, in no small degree, to premature deaths among adult labourers,—that the cost of sickness and mortality, of itself, was not trifling,—and that many "permanent" paupers, in and out of workhouses, had become maimed, or blind, or lame, from neglect of early symptoms, or from want of public precautions against disease and injury.

All this was notorious.

But since there were no sanitary courts of appeal in public emergencies—no organized medical police, and since the ratepayers were called upon to defray the expenses, direct or indirect, of whatever preventible sickness and infirmity, or excessive mortality, occurred in their respective parishes,—it is by no means remarkable that the Poor-Law Boards, central and local, were deemed responsible for carrying into effect measures, which—however foreign to their original sphere of action—were intended, nevertheless, to lower the rates and diminish the proportion of pauperism.

There might have been a third cause. Owing to a general misconception of the scope and objects of the healing and health-preserving art,—owing also to the singular prejudice against its professors, which appeared to actuate some of the leaders of poor-law reform,—the latter seemed to have concluded that the prevention of disease was a matter altogether extraneous to the province of medicine, and that among the many benefits which such prevention would confer on society, not the least would be a diminution in the number of doctors!

These various misconceptions and fallacies are now in process of correction,—slowly indeed, but surely,—and a future generation will marvel on looking back upon the blundering perversity of our recent sanitary legislation and administration.

Is it necessary to prove that such mistakes have been made?

§ 2. In the years 1840 and 1841, Parliament, moved by the warnings and entreaties of the very profession, which it so unwisely and ungenerously mistrusted, enacted a hygienic law, which speedily tested the correctness of the poor-law principle in medico-sanitary administration.

It matters not whether vaccination be termed a preventive or a palliative measure. Like all other public precautions against disease, it had been grievously neglected. Popular ignorance, prejudice and apathy, had rendered its application to the community very partial and irregular.

No adequate national provision, no organization, as in some continental states, existed for its diffusion.

The English Parliament, however, resolved that something should be done; and as the poor-law machinery was ready at hand and willing to be worked, our legislators deemed it quite needless to consider whether a more suitable machinery might not be devised, or whether so unheard-of a delegation of the sanitary

POLITICAL INCONSISTENCY.

functions of Government to a pauper-controlling department, was at all consistent with sound political philosophy.

In vain did physicians and surgeons throughout the land protest against the anomaly.* The medical colleges, true to their vocation, held their peace. Their sale of diplomas was not threatened. So the Poor-Law Boards were appointed, by a new law, to promote and direct (not the medical pauperization—be it observed—but) the vaccination of the whole working population.

The union contractor for vaccination was to operate upon every one who applied; the union contractor for medical aid was still to heal only the "really destitute"—and this only when the Guardians thought that "circumstances rendered it absolutely necessary."

Was it then a matter of less moment to the State to restore the health of the labouring population, in ALL diseases, by prompt and efficient medical care, and to maintain it by vigilant medical inspection,—than to protect that population against the ravages of only ONE disease?

Two opposite principles of civil administration in public medicine were simultaneously announced on State authority. Which was right?

The Vaccination Act of 1841 declared—

"That the vaccination, or surgical or medical assistance incident to the vaccination, of any person . . or of any of his family, under the said Act, shall NOT be considered to be parochial relief, alms, or charitable allowance to such person, and that no such person shall, by reason of such vaccination or assistance, be deprived of any right or privilege, or be subject to any disability or disqualification whatsoever."

On the other hand, the Poor-Law Commissioners, in the same year, after suggesting some judicious amendments in the medical-relief department, say :—

---

* "Vaccination is enforced and controlled in other countries by sanitary boards; but well-informed medical men are upon those boards. . . . The degradation of being subjected to a poor-law commission was reserved exclusively for the medical practitioners of England, *because*(?) they discovered and propagated the operation which other nations adopted."—*Lancet,* July, 1848.

"Before quitting this subject, we deem it right to remark, that although we entertain no doubt of our being able ultimately, and at no distant period, to establish a complete and effective system of medical relief for all *paupers*, yet its very completeness and effectiveness, however beneficial to those who are its objects, may have an influence, which ought not to be disregarded, on other classes of society. If the pauper is always promptly attended by a skilful and well qualified medical practitioner; if such practitioner is not only under the usual responsibilities of his profession, but is liable to reprimand or dismissal from office in case of neglect or error; if the patient be furnished with all the cordials and stimulants which may promote his recovery; it cannot be denied that his condition, in these respects, is better than that of the needy but industrious ratepayer, who has neither money nor influence to secure equally prompt and careful attendance, nor any means to provide himself or his family with the more expensive kinds of nutriment which his medical attendant may recommend.

"This superiority of the condition of the pauper over that of the independent labourer, as regards medical aid, will, on the one hand, encourage a resort to the poor-rates for medical relief, so far as it is given out of the Workhouse, and will thus tempt the industrious labourer into pauperism: and on the other hand, it will discourage sick clubs and friendly societies, and other similar institutions, which are not only valuable in reference to the contingencies against which they provide, but as creating and fostering a spirit of frugality and forethought amongst the labouring classes."*

Now, for the present, passing over the last question mooted in this paragraph,—it may be fairly asked how, on their avowed principles, the Commissioners could carry the Vaccination Act into execution? Why "tempt the industrious labourer—the needy ratepayer—into pauperism," by encouraging him to get his children vaccinated gratuitously by the Union contractor?

Perhaps it might be replied that one of the conditions of a perfect system of medical relief, assumed by the Commissioners —namely, " IF the patient be furnished with all the cordials and stimulants which may promote his recovery,"—does not apply to cases of *variolæ vaccinæ*, constituting an important difference in the two public provisions. But such a distinction would involve

---

* *Annual Report*, p. 16.

a professional discussion, in which the economist would probably be defeated, but into which I am not now to be drawn.

That particular condition has, indeed, a very important economical bearing upon the whole question of *poor-law* medical aid, and will be of use in future deductions.

In another Essay, I notice the practical consequences of committing public vaccination to the poor-law authorities, as regards the prevention of small-pox. It is enough here to have shown the bearing of this enactment on the medical-relief question.

§ 3. The first of that series of sanitary inquiries, which led to the Public Health Act, was committed by direction of the Secretary of State to Mr. Chadwick, when Secretary to the Poor-Law Commissioners.

Had he retained that office, there is reason to conclude that the Poor-Law Board of London would have been selected by Parliament, as that of Dublin has been since, for the central direction of sanitary administration.

It is far from certain that the able compiler of the "General Sanitary Report" intended that Boards of Guardians should be the local executive authorities, in the management of the public health : yet this may be inferred from the general tenour of his very valuable suggestions towards an amended organization of the *corps* of Union medical officers, under medical inspection, for sanitary purposes. For instance ; while noticing the advantages which the Central Board had derived from the occasional employment of physicians and surgeons of repute in local inquiries as to the health of particular establishments or epidemic outbreaks, he says :*—

"The results of such occasional visits appear to prove the necessity and economy of an increase of the permanent local medical service, and to establish a case for the appointment of a superior medical man for a wider district than an ordinary medical officer, for the special aid and supervision of the established medical relief."

* *General Sanitary Report,* p. 350.

And after describing many important duties which might be performed by his proposed " district physician or [inspecting] officer of public health," he remarks, in a concluding paragraph :*—

" The business of a district physician *connects him more immediately with the Boards of Guardians*, which, as having the distribution of medical relief, and the services of medical officers, I would submit, may be made, with additional aid, to do more than can be done by any local boards of health, of the description given, separated from any executive authority or self-acting means of bringing information before them."

That an extension of functions in the direction of State medicine had long been a cherished design of the Poor-Law Commissioners, may be gathered from the following evidence given by Sir J. P. Kay Shuttleworth, in 1838 :—

" As respects the services of a medical assessor, in relation to the physical condition of the poorer classes, and the sanitary state of the neighbourhood, I am aware that the Poor-Law Commissioners entertain the strongest opinion that the medical officers of unions will become most important agents and functionaries for the attainment of the objects which have been proposed to the committee,—and that application has been made to the Secretary of State, who is supposed not to be averse to the proposition, *to confer additional powers on the Boards of Guardians and medical officers*, for the purpose of improving, especially, the condition of some of the town districts which are inhabited by the pauper population."†

And my inference on this point seems to be confirmed by Dr. Southwood Smith's culminating evidence before the Health of Towns Committee, in 1843—more than a year after Mr. Chadwick's propositions :—

" A suggestion to this effect, which appears to me to be deserving of notice, has been made in the Report on the Sanitary Condition of the Labouring Population,—namely, that an increase should be made to the permanent local medical service *under the Poor-Law Commissioners*, by the appointment of a superior medical officer, for the aid and supervision of the medical relief at present afforded to the poor."‡

* *General Sanitary Report*, p. 356.   † Evidence, 16,074.
‡ *Health of Towns Commission First Report*, folio, p. 85.

§ 4. Such, then, were the strong probabilities that the sanitary management of the people would become an integral part of poor-law administration.

The prospect was now viewed with no little alarm by the few, who, knowing what *State medicine* means, were at the same time free from the trammels and bias of office.

That prospect, however, was not fully realized in England, owing, as has been supposed, to the removal of Mr. Chadwick from the Poor-Law Commission, and his appointment as virtual chief of a distinct Government department, modelled, if not on his own plan, yet for the realization of his sanitary projects.

On the advantages or disadvantages of the course adopted by the Legislature in 1848, I have nothing to say at present.

For the sake of those who may still be in doubt, I shall, both in a future section of this Essay and in remarks upon Boards of Health in the Fifth Essay, adduce some indisputable evidence of the evils resulting from the committal of sanitary powers to Boards of Guardians, under the " Nuisances-Removal and Diseases-Prevention Acts."

The efforts of the Poor-Law department, previous to 1844, to obtain from the Legislature the power of administering the projected code of sanitary laws, have appeared to me to deserve particular notice, because they exerted an important influence upon the next stage of the medical-relief discussion.

CHAPTER FIFTH.

From a.d. 1842, until after the Second Invasion of Cholera in 1849.

§ 1. Those who had fancied that Boards of Guardians were generally ready to carry into full effect the few improvements made by the General Medical Order of 1842, were speedily undeceived. Little as that Order was calculated to accomplish, still less was practically secured by it.

Hence the radical defects of the system,—those which no orders from a Poor-Law Board could touch,—led to a revival of agitation on the subject.

On this occasion the movement began in a high professional quarter. Mr. Guthrie, then President of the College of Surgeons, put forth, in 1843, a stirring appeal to Members of Parliament, characterized by his usual warmth of expression and earnestness of purpose.* His vivid and faithful description of existing abuses showed how completely the central and local Boards had failed to put in force the recommendations of the Select Committee of 1838.

And he steadily pursued his object until he had induced the then Lord Ashley to propose another Parliamentary inquiry. This was granted; and a Committee of the House of Commons on "Medical Poor-Relief" sat for some months in 1844. The noble chairman's patience, diligence, and urbanity in the conduct

---

* *Facts and Observations relating to the Administration of Medical Relief to the Sick Poor in England and Wales.*—London: printed by Manning and Mason, 1843.

This pamphlet affords some information respecting conferences between the Council of the College of Surgeons and the Secretary of State, in the earlier of which, it is well known that the late Sir Astley Cooper took an active part. Those proceedings led to no successful result, except, perhaps, as regards the surgical qualification of Union medical officers.

of this investigation, fully sustained his well-earned reputation for zealous interest in the moral and physical welfare of the poorer classes.

§ 2. Few would have leisure, and still fewer courage and endurance to wade through the mass of evidence taken before that Committee; nor is a fresh analysis* of it required; but time will not be lost in a brief notice of one or two groups of facts.

The intervention of relieving officers in the grant of "orders" for attendance, was shown, by an immense amount of incontrovertible evidence, to be the cause of serious evils in a professional point of view; and of disastrous consequences to the unfortunate sufferers from delay in the administration of aid.†

When the case of sickness or accident came (as the majority of such cases did) under the provisions of a contract for attendance at a fixed annual sum, the relieving officer was seldom applied to; his intervention might be dispensed with by the Guardians; but then it was no less needed as a protection to the medical officer against improper demands upon his time and remedies by persons not entitled, as paupers, to his services.

In one way or another, then, the system was shown to hold out a direct inducement to defer prompt relief.

It was admitted that commonly-received maxims of medical ethics would lead the doctor to disregard official routine, and to do his duty to the sufferer; but, on the other hand, it was pleaded that the authorities had no right to shelter themselves behind esoteric principles of action, especially when the claims of the faculty to consideration and confidence on that account were ignored and repudiated.

---

* The evidence has been reviewed twice already. The *Times*, of Dec. 26, 1844, devoted four columns to an abstract—of course, incomplete—of verbal and documentary matter occupying nearly 1000 pages, and containing nearly 10,000 questions and answers. And an examination, more at length, of this evidence, forms the second part of the author's pamphlet, entitled *Health and Sickness of Town Populations*. In this may be found the principal points mooted, the facts elicited, and the views of the leading parties called before the committee.

† The Rev. S. Clissold instanced some lamentable effects of this method of limiting relief in cases of injury to the joints and eyes.—(9202.)

But as to the relieving officer, he was shown to be a local impersonation of the anti-pauperism principle; and in that capacity the main question with himself, on being applied to for an "order," would probably be, and perhaps ought to be—

"Shall I make this man a pauper? Shall I inflict upon him civil disabilities, and deprive him of his social independence, because he seems to have a bad cold, or because his child complains of a stomach-ache?"

It was, therefore, urged that, to combat effectively insidious attacks of sickness, under such regulations, was impossible.

The sanitary principle of anticipating the development of disease—of preventing those permanent lesions which result from neglected casualty, and of quickly restoring the sufferer to his previous condition of capability for work—was proved to be wholly irreconcileable with the Poor-Law principle of withholding relief, except in cases of destitution, lest the "industrious labourer or needy rate-payer be tempted into pauperism."

As to midwifery, Mr. Guthrie marshalled an alarming array of evidence to prove the distress and mischief,—in some cases even mutilation,—suffered by poor women, from the necessity of an "order" from a reluctant relieving officer, before they could obtain professional aid.

Yet, on the other hand, it was urged that, of all kinds of medical relief, that afforded in ordinary cases of parturition is one which the mass of the population ought to be chiefly encouraged and enabled to provide for themselves.

Again, the continued enormous extent of medical districts,—and this even in localities where there was ample opportunity of providing medical aid in small and manageable districts,—was established by unimpeachable testimony; and the evils resulting from the intervention of the relieving officer were proved to be fearfully aggravated by the circumstance of his residence being, in many cases, at a considerable distance from that of the medical officer; so that the sick and hurt poor, for whom no messengers or porters are provided by the public, were often unable to procure aid until it could be of no avail.

In defence of the relieving officer's functions, the Commissioners could only reply, that, if these were abrogated, the law must be altered, and *another system of medical aid substituted by the State,*—the very conclusion at which the advocates for a comprehensive reform had already arrived.

§ 3. It is a disagreeable duty to notice the weak points of a good cause, especially when one honours the advocates. But the object, and I hope the character, of this narrative, forbid anything like concealment of the narrator's opinions with regard to the course pursued by either of the parties in this controversy.

Thus, as it appears to me, the main, perhaps the only, mistake in Lord Shaftesbury's and Mr. Guthrie's conduct of their case, was their undue reliance upon the Poor-Law Board, and their belief that the Commissioners, if backed by the Government and Parliament, were both willing and able to correct evils the existence of which were so clearly proved.

Influenced, not unreasonably, by the desire expressed, and doubtless really felt, by Mr. Cornewall Lewis (now the Right Honourable Sir G. C. Lewis), to provide, if possible, some better securities for a just and humane administration of the medical department, the movers for this inquiry neither advocated an entire change in the central and local direction, nor acknowledged even if they perceived the fundamental incompatibility of a comprehensive provision of medical and sanitary care, with the precise and limited objects of a system of Poor-Law relief.

Hence Mr. Guthrie's grand remedy was the appointment of a Medical Commissioner and Medical Inspectors under the Poor-Law Board; very disinterestedly offering to fill the former office without salary.*

§ 4. It will be recollected that a medical commissioner was originally proposed by Mr. Serjeant Talfourd and the Provincial

* Evidence, 3773.

Association; but those who had been chiefly concerned in conducting the several investigations, and in framing the reports of that Society, had gradually come to a very different conclusion, which they, in their turn, laid before the Parliamentary Committee.

Certain suggestions contained in the *General Sanitary Report* of 1842, to which reference has been already made, the recent Vaccination Enactment, and the current which the Public Health movement appeared to be taking,—had thrown new light upon the whole question, and had led the last-mentioned witnesses to conclude that no benefit was likely to arise from the appointment of any medical authorities by and under the Poor-Law Commissioners.

Beside pointing out to the Committee the connexion, then developing, between medical relief and preventive measures,—they urged that sanative duties among the poor, considered separately, were only in part a poor-law affair; by far the greater portion* of such relief in towns being supplied by medical charities, and other voluntary associations; and that for all these reasons public medical attendance required to be dealt with either as an independent department of the State, or as a branch of the public health administration. They were also the first to call attention to the wide difference, in principle, between medical relief afforded to the inmates of workhouses (of which they admitted that the Poor-Law authorities, with the aid of medical inspectors, were obviously the natural directors), and the care bestowed by sanitary advisers upon the poorer classes in their own dwellings; a difference analogous to that between the duties of a workhouse chaplain and those of a parochial clergyman,†—a difference also exemplified by the separate offices of workhouse teacher and national schoolmaster.

§ 5. When these views,‡ so opposite to those of Mr. Guthrie

---

* See Tables, App. to *Health and Sickness of Town Pop.*, pp. 78-89.   † Evid. 9371.

‡ HEADS OF THE PLAN submitted to the Select Committee of the House of Commons on Medical Poor Relief, in 1844, by the Representatives of the Provincial Medical and Surgical Association.

That the provision of medical aid for the *out-door* poor be separated from the and his numerous medical witnesses, were laid before the Select Committee, and when Sir G. C. Lewis was again called upon for his reply, the Committee must have felt something like perplexity; for, while the Commissioner admitted that great and beneficial improvements in the local medical arrangements might be effected under an entirely new system, distinct from the Poor-Law, he proved by a simple and clear illustration that the appointment of a medical commissioner, acting with and controlled by the other Commissioners, was altogether unlikely to secure such an amendment as the philanthropists desired.

He thought therefore that, so long as the Legislature was satisfied with a Poor-Law system of out-door relief, it had better be left to the existing lay authorities to amend in their own way, gradually, and as they were able.*

After this, who can wonder that a committee, consisting partly of a minority disposed to support the views of the noble Chairman and the President of the College of Surgeons, with a majority clinging to Somerset House traditions, should have declined to report in favour of any of the proposed reforms? After so full a substantiation of many crying abuses and flagrant errors in the working of the established system, it is scarcely credible that the Committee expressed no opinion, because† "there was no special

---

administration of the Poor-Laws; with the reservation of certain powers to the Poor-Law Commissioners and the Boards of Guardians.

That the administration of medical aid be combined with the regulation of the sanitary condition of the labouring population, and be committed to authorities, central and local, to be constituted expressly for the management of this department.

That an adequate remuneration, equitably adjusted, be paid to a sufficient number of medical officers, appointed to take care of the poor, in conveniently-arranged districts.

That medicines be supplied to the sick poor by the proposed authorities, at the public expense; and that in places where the separate provision of medicine may be impracticable, the medical officers be paid, at a fixed rate, for the supply of the same.

That the poor, when sick or hurt, be provided freely and promptly with medical aid, no official check being interposed between them and the relief they need; and that the receipt of medical relief shall not constitute them paupers.

* See Supplementary Note B.
† See *Speech* by Mr. Baines, July 12, 1853, in the House of Commons.

grievance on which they could make a recommendation." It may therefore, be safely concluded that the diversity of the two leading plans before the committee, and the quasi-conservative opposition prevailing against that more novel and startling change, which alone was justified by Sir G. C. Lewis—were the main causes of the evidence being reported without comment to the House.

§ 6. Little as seemed to have been gained by this laborious investigation at the time, it is probable that some subsequent changes of greater moment resulted from it.

For example, the measure of national finance, brought forward by the late Sir R. Peel in the beginning of the Session for 1846, included a provision, which, if viewed as a precedent for future legislation in the same direction, may be considered the most important of all amendments hitherto made in the administration of this department.

In charging half the cost of medical relief throughout England and Wales upon the Treasury, that far-sighted statesman recognised the responsibility of the State in a matter which had been heretofore held to be of merely parochial concern.

The greatest defect of his measure was that, while he left only a moiety of the cost to be defrayed out of the poor-rates, he permitted the whole of the management to remain in the hands of the Poor Law authorities, and thus lost the opportunity of securing to the Government a share in the control of State Medicine, proportioned to the share of the cost for which it became liable.

Another scarcely less obvious defect was, that he roughly halved the expense of medical relief, without reference to the different nature of the matters included in the total estimate; and thus he also lost the opportunity of separating the pay of the Medical Staff from the cost of the materials required for the treatment of the sick. For, as the charge was to be partly local and partly national, the expense of medicines, appliances, and dispensing should have been left, as in continental States, to be defrayed by the inhabitants of the district in which they were consumed, while the salaries of the medical officers, as servants of the State, would in like manner have fallen upon national funds.

It is the more singular that this course was not adopted, as the *whole* of the salaries of the workhouse schoolmasters was, by the same measure, charged upon the Treasury.

§ 7. In 1847, the Poor-Law Commissioners revised the Medical Order of 1842, and embodied it in their "Consolidated General Order"—the code by which the medical arrangements of Boards of Guardians are at present regulated.

The several clauses of the order of 1842, were re-distributed under various heads, which included a vast amount of other matter relating to the general management of parochial Unions; so it is now more difficult than before to determine the precise nature and extent of the medical regulations. But, on making a careful comparison of the two orders, it will be found that the amendments in the more recent one are mostly verbal. Many useless legal phrases were judiciously struck out in 1847. A few important practical details were also simplified. The "qualification" clause stood as corrected in 1844. Boards of Guardians were permitted (but not compelled) to make "gratuities" to medical officers for extra services,* not contemplated under their original appointment,—*e. g.* for arduous duties during epidemics, or under sanitary enactments.

But, viewed as a whole, the medical regulations of 1847 are open to the general strictures already made on the order of 1842. Virtually, the system continued the same.

The authorities looked upon this consolidated order as an act of finality with regard to medical relief, and thus displayed their intention to maintain as far as possible, the integrity of the principle of "medical relief for paupers only," at the expense of the principle, that "the safety of the people is the supreme law."

But this, indeed, was beyond their province.

---

* See Evidence, 1854, Mr. Cane, 183.

§ 8. The philanthropists and doctors were, therefore, soon again in the field.

Lord Shaftesbury, after his two years' absence from the House of Commons, seized an early opportunity in the session of 1848, to propose a series of resolutions embodying the principal reforms before recommended by Mr. Guthrie.

As the issue of the tedious inquiry in 1844 could have given that benevolent nobleman but little encouragement to proceed with the matter, the steady earnestness with which he again brought it under consideration of the legislature did him very great credit.

It might, indeed, have been regretted that higher and broader ground was not taken on this occasion.

If Lord Shaftesbury hoped, by diluting the strength of his remedy, to mitigate parliamentary resistance and to soften official obduracy; if he expected, by a moving appeal, to effect a sudden conversion of the majority of an assembly like the House of Commons; he was deservedly disappointed.

Had he on the contrary asserted those clearer and more comprehensive principles, which he might have supported by Sir G. C. Lewis's admissions, he would have arrested and riveted the attention of an unprejudiced and reasoning minority, and thus have contributed to the future settlement of the question on a firm and defensible basis.

Lord Shaftesbury's propositions need not here be given *in extenso.** Four of the seven related to the mode in which medical assistance might be claimed and granted in certain urgent cases.

The first related to attendance in midwifery, under peculiar circumstances; and, though the discussion would have more befitted a jury of matrons than a body composed of lawyers, merchants, country gentlemen, army and navy officers, and youthful scions of nobility,—the motion somehow or other, obtained the support of a large minority.

---

* They were given at length in the *Lancet* of Feb. 12, 1848; and reviewed in the *Medical Gazette*, N. S. vol. vi. p. 507. 1848.

§ 9. The two propositions, which alone touched the general control and administration of this department, were far less successful. That relating to the appointment of *medical* inspectors—one to each Poor-Law Inspector's circuit—for the superintendence of public medical relief, was the most important. The wide extent of the functions* suggested for those inspectors, and especially the "other sanitary duties of every kind," which were to be committed to them, involved the whole question of a permanent medical organization for the protection of the public health.

But was it reasonable to propose the subjection of such superintendents of State hygiéne to a Poor-Law Board?

Whether such a doubt occurred to any member of the House, we are not informed. It was doubtless the *argumentum ad crumenam* which ensured the rejection of the motion.

The chief (then recently appointed) of the re-constructed Poor-Law Board, in exerting himself to defeat these imperfect but well meant resolutions, is reported to have taken very much the same ground as his predecessor Sir G. C. Lewis. He acknowledged that "he had felt the want of medical aid as soon as ever he got into office;" but it was "his deliberate opinion, that if the House wished to have a larger and more complete system of medical aid for the poor, *it must not be administered through the Poor-Law,* nor by a charge upon local funds, but through some system of central administration for providing medical attendance from the general funds of the country."

After this bold (and it may be prophetic) declaration—originating in a plan which, as we have seen, was laid before the Parliamentary Committee in 1844†—who would have supposed, that the very assembly, which apparently assented to Mr. C. Buller's view of the case, would have created, in the third fol-

---

* Some were not very judiciously expressed, *e. g.*—"to report on the *fitness* of the medical men appointed to the Unions;"—"to *regulate the treatment* of the sick in the Union Workhouses."

† See note p. 192, "Heads of Plan, &c."

lowing session, *five* such medical inspectorships, *under the Poor-Law Commissioners,* for Ireland?

It is also worth notice that, in opposing another of Lord Shaftesbury's propositions—for the greater permanence of medical appointments—Mr. C. Buller merely postponed an improvement, distinct from any theory or system, which was afterwards recommended by a parliamentary committee, and is now in full operation. So imperfectly do the wisest see what is before them!

The remaining resolutions were withdrawn by the disheartened mover; and nothing further occurred in Parliament with reference to medical relief in England and Wales, until 1853.

§ 10. The interval was not passed without renewed agitation.

Where the question was left by the Provincial Association, it was taken up by a "Convention of Poor-Law Medical Officers" formed in 1847. Much was done by the latter society in the way of correspondence and consultation. The zeal and energy with which their able secretary* conducted the proceedings deserve special notice. The committee collected not only statistical returns of medical duties and remuneration, with other useful information, from the medical officers of more than a fourth of the districts in England and Wales, but also proofs of the miserable evasions by which too many Boards of Guardians escaped full compliance with even that stinted measure of justice contained in the general orders of 1842 and 1847.

Among their printed proceedings may also be seen reports of important conferences with successive heads of the Poor-Law Board; and a clear statement of the objects sought for by the Convention.

These efforts, nevertheless, failed to enlist the same amount of sympathy among disinterested persons, which some previous professional movements had obtained. The "convention" consisted almost exclusively of those whose pecuniary interests were concerned in a more equitable adjustment.

It was not a scientific association taking up the matter inci-

* Mr. Lord, of Hampstead.

dentally; nor was it a philanthropic body occupied in promoting the advance of civilization and humanity in any direction; nor was it an ancient corporation exerting conventional influence upon the profession and the public.

Then, again, with regard to the objects of this new society; its main demand, as might have been expected, was a fair and uniform scale of remuneration for the several services required of the Union medical officers, on the ground that the poor could never be properly attended until their attendants were properly paid.

The repetition of this truism, in various forms and with various illustrations, lost much of its moral force when urged by parties who were to profit by the proposed amendment.

It was, nevertheless, always courteously admitted by the official respondents, none of whom probably (excepting Mr. C. Buller) ever intended to bestir themselves for its practical adoption.

Those great principles, on which mere administrative reforms in this department should be based, and which, if adopted, would lead to a proper consideration of the claims of the medical *employés* of the State, were omitted in the scheme of the convention; while the hackneyed proposition—*a Medical Director-General and Inspectors under the Poor-Law*—was revived.

It must, however, have gratified the leaders of this movement to perceive that some tried friends of their cause, having no personal interest in its success, rallied to their support.

Such was the learned and philanthropic Dr. Hodgkin, who accepted the office of their President. Lord Shaftesbury also took the chair at one at least of their meetings. The chief officers of the College of Surgeons accompanied a deputation of the convention to Sir George Grey, and "warmly pleaded its cause";* while among the Committee were found the names of more than one distinguished for large and liberal views on the subject.†

---

* See *First Report of the Convention*, p. 19.

† For instance; Mr. Liddle, of Whitechapel, well known for his efforts in the

§ 11. About this time, new and powerful supporters of right principles appeared in the field.

A pungent yet fair critique of existing arrangements, by the Hon. and Rev. S. G. Osborne, appeared very opportunely in the *Times*. None but a master-hand could have so vividly described the predicament of the Union doctors, or so clearly indicated the practical reforms which the system then needed, and which are yet unaccomplished.*

Mr. Disraeli also announced his intention of endeavouring to remove the remaining moiety of the cost of medical relief from local taxation and to include the whole in a charge upon national funds, and thus of completing the judicious change which a greater Statesman had commenced.

Whilst the then Lord Morpeth's Bill of 1848 was under discussion, not a few were cherishing the hope that a comprehensive view of public medical aid would be adopted by the Legislature, and that this department would be included, with all other provisions for the public health, and placed under the proposed General Board of Health. It was thought that this council might be so judiciously constituted and so ably assisted by a permanent organization of circuit medical inspectors, as to qualify it thoroughly for directing the medical provision for the poor out of workhouses; and that, by this means, the pauperizing tendency of such medical relief might be abolished, and the Poor-Law

---

sanitary cause, who also contributed some very excellent papers on medical poor-relief, to the *Journal of Public Health* and the *Health of Towns Magazine*, in 1848. His objections to a *poor-law* provision may have again to be noticed.

* "The Report of the Committee that sat upon the subject of medical relief ought to have led to some improvement; but the mere setting forth of a list of fees for extra services—the cumbering the medical officers with new forms of returns—is but poor fruit of such labour. The whole system of 'orders' needs revision—the medical officer ought to be paid the real value of his services ;—*he should be made subordinate, in the first instance, to a board of medical inspection; he should be paid for attendance and prescribing, not for drugs and appliances ;* he should have *these* liberally supplied him from sources which would secure their being the best of their sort, or at least as good as his purposes required. The present system gives us no security, either for proper attendance, or the administration of proper remedies. *It makes boards of guardians authorities in matters they do not understand.*"

Boards relieved of a troublesome and unsatisfactory portion of their duties.

Such were the views not of mere theorists. Some of the most practical writers of the day took the same ground.*

The defeat of Lord Shaftesbury's merely palliative propositions, and Mr. C. Buller's indication of a larger and better scheme, fostered these hopes; but they were soon crushed by the Public Health enactment—a measure originally limited in scope and design, and further maimed in its passage through Parliament.

The year 1848, so eventful in sanitary legislation, had not closed, before Mr. C. Buller's hopeful official career was cut short by his premature death. With him sank all immediate prospect of a wise and liberal reform of the medical relief department.

The succeeding chiefs of the Poor-Law Board have rested as quietly as they were permitted to do on the fundamental errors of their system—" letting evil principles work themselves out at the expense of the public, and applying the rule—*Never to act until you are obliged, and then do as little as you can.*"†

§ 12. The medical staff, under the Poor-Law, had now to experience additional perplexities and responsibilities.

On the approach of pestilential cholera, the General Board of Health was empowered to require very important duties of Union Boards and officers; but it had no power to secure the full and efficient performance of such duties, either by adequate means of contest and inspection, or by awarding proper remuneration to the district officers.

The evils of divided authority were soon severely felt.

What the General Board of Health ordered by way of medical *prophylaxis*, Boards of Guardians were generally loth to carry into effect, and still more unwilling to pay for; while the central

---

* In particular, there appeared an admirable article among the "Topics of the Day,"—in the *Spectator* of Oct. 23, 1847,—in support of this view.

† Mr. Chadwick. *Papers on the Re-organization of the Civil Service*, p. 190. 1855.

Poor-Law Board on the one hand, and the district medical officers on the other, were too desirous to propitiate both the other official parties to make their course of action very smooth or clear to themselves. The Poor-Law Board and the Board of Health were alternately and fruitlessly appealed to for redress, and for direction in these local dilemmas. The doctors of course had the worst of it. And the public derived all the benefit which such imperfect organization could afford, from the zealous though unsystematic and unrequited exertions of the medical staff.

The first General Board of Health bore honourable testimony to those acts of courage and devotion, and candidly confessed the incurable faultiness of the very machinery which the acting members of that Board, when connected with the Poor-Law Commission, had so strongly recommended for purposes of sanitary administration.

I shall have again to notice more particularly the utter incompetence of Boards of Guardians to direct the execution of comprehensive measures of palliation and prevention, during times of unusual sickness, and such times are the only safe test of their competency in ordinary circumstances. But here it seems necessary only to cite a passage from the Report of the General Board of Health on the cholera of 1849—including statements from their two chief inspectors—which may give some idea of the sacrifices made by the medical officers in that epidemic, and the manner of their reward:—

" In conclusion, we would call attention to the unanimous testimony borne by all classes, to the exemplary manner in which the medical officers of the parishes and unions, and the medical visitors specially appointed for this service, have performed their difficult and dangerous duties. Our own Superintending Medical Inspectors have had the best opportunities of forming a judgment on this subject.

"With reference to the medical service of the metropolis, Mr. Grainger says:—'At a time when all who were able, quitted even the healthiest parts of London; the medical officers, often debilitated by their incessant labours, and even suffering under unmistakeable symptoms of the disease, never quitted their post, though that was of necessity in the very focus of the pestilence. Many among their number were, after the exhausting fatigue of the day, disturbed in their rest at night for weeks and weeks together. One surgeon did not change his clothes for eight or nine days, sleeping at intervals on a sofa: another for eighteen days had not two hours' consecutive sleep. And all these great services, it should be recollected, were, for the most part, performed amidst the obscurity of dark alleys and pestilential dwellings, unseen by the public eye, frequently undervalued, even where known, and always miserably underpaid. Examples are not wanting of surgeons who, after a year of such labours and such services, have received for their recompence actually less than would defray the additional outlay caused by the enormous amount of expensive medicines, and by the provision of an extra assistant. In other instances, no extra remuneration whatever was granted.'

" Dr. Sutherland reports :—' I would bear the strongest testimony to the self-denying zeal and ability with which the medical officers so nobly discharged the highly responsible duties confided to them during a great public emergency.

" 'The question of remuneration for services rendered by medical officers, though not coming under the regulations of the Board, nevertheless arises out of the recommendation that they should be liberally dealt with, on account of the heavy additional duties thrown on them. I know a number of instances in which a suitable payment has certainly been made; but the complaints of the miserable remuneration afforded have been so numerous, that I question very much whether it would be wise to encounter another epidemic such as the last, without other arrangements. I feel satisfied that in the majority of instances which have come under my own observation, nothing but the dictates of humanity would induce the medical officers to undertake the work anew, with the chances of being similarly paid for it.' "*

* *Report of General Board of Health on Cholera,* p. 142.

CHAPTER SIXTH.

Rise, Revolution, and Present Position of the Medical Charities in Ireland.

§ 1. It would be almost impossible to form a correct notion of the third and last Parliamentary movement for a reform of medical relief in England, without a previous survey of the very striking changes which had been then recently effected in the administration of the corresponding department in Ireland.

For many years preceding these changes, the sick poor, in most parts of the Sister Island, had been treated in county infirmaries, fever hospitals, and dispensaries, instituted and maintained under a series of Acts of Parliament.

The infirmaries of Ireland were the older institutions; but as the present sketch refers primarily to the *extern* class of poor patients, we must first notice the dispensaries,*—those institutions to which, in fact, the important enactment of 1851 was finally limited.

If we except the inmates of the new workhouse infirmaries (parts of Union Workhouses set apart for the sick and infirm), and those of the still newer Union Fever Hospitals, established under recent Acts for the relief of the poor in Ireland,—the destitute, and indeed the labouring classes generally, were aided by a State provision of medical care wholly unconnected with a Poor Law.

---

* Dispensaries in Ireland were established by Acts of Parliament, in 1805 and 1818, which empowered Grand Juries to originate "Dispensaries in parts of counties too distant from the infirmaries to allow the poor of those districts the advantages of immediate aid and advice . . and to supply medicines and medical and surgical aid and advice to the poor *of the place and its neighbourhood* wherein they were established."

For this and other information I am indebted to an able pamphlet by "Medicus," Dublin, 1851.

But beside the precedents for a change in the superintendence of medical relief, which were established by the last-mentioned institutions, the thin end of the wedge which was to shiver in pieces the old system of medical charities, was inserted by the first Irish poor-relief enactment (1838). By this, the Poor-Law Commissioners were empowered to "inspect and examine into the administration of" the Irish medical charities.

The Poor Inquiry Commission in 1835 had already made out a very strong case for Parliamentary intervention; and the Poor-Law Commissioners, in their elaborate Medical Charities Report of 1841, while confirming previous exposures of inefficiency and mismanagement, recommended, as they were probably expected to do, that the principal share in the management of these charities should be vested in themselves.

Nevertheless, two Parliamentary Committees* thoroughly re-investigated the subject; and their reports will be found to contain many materials of great value towards a settlement of this difficult question, without handing over the management of sanative institutions to central and local Poor-Law Boards.

Indeed, the Medical Charities Bill of 1850,—a measure which disappeared among the usual "droppings" at the close of the session,—would have vested the government of infirmaries, fever wards, and dispensaries, in a separate Board, to be styled "Commissioners of Health."

Had a judicious constitution been devised for the Central Board (although in that case it would probably have become too good a measure to pass into law†), we might possibly now have been able to refer to medico-sanitary legislation for Ireland, as a plea for "Justice to England."

But official influence, professional misconceptions, and government prejudices, combined to deteriorate the character of the

---

* One of the House of Commons in 1843 and one of the House of Lords in 1846.
† "The late Sir Robert Peel, speaking of the Encumbered Estates Act, said it was 'so very good a measure that he really wondered how it had ever passed.' "— Chadwick *On the Civil Service*, 1855, p. 221. *Papers*, &c. *Supra cit.*

Bill; and the Act of the following session (1851) brought all the dispensaries of Ireland under Poor-Law direction.

§ 2. Let it not be forgotten that the medical charities of Ireland constituted a national provision for the public safety, which by no means involved the reliance of the recipients and administrators of medical aid upon poor-rates, parish-officers, or Boards of Guardians; nor had it the slightest tendency to *pauperize* those whom it benefited.

Whatever defects there might have been in the old system, and they were many and serious, experience leaves no doubt of the superiority of that one great principle,—a principle which was unfortunately sacrificed in order to solve temporary difficulties, and to cure some acknowledged abuses in practice.

It was quite true, that the localization of those institutions was capricious and irregular; that the boundaries of their respective districts were either imperfectly or not at all defined; that their benefits were very unequally supplied to the island at large; and that the poor in many places were entirely beyond the reach of aid.

It was also proved—that the funds of the dispensaries were uncertain, and failing year by year; that the "county cess," on which the main burden lay, was raised solely from occupiers, and left wealthy absentee proprietors free from liability; that medical officers were frequently reduced to the degrading, if not demoralizing, position of being compelled to solicit from the gentry of their districts, a sufficient amount of annual subscriptions to secure a corresponding grant from the county grand jury; that a more safe, honest, and uniform method of maintaining these charities was essential to their efficiency; and that a compulsory tax, fairly levied upon the whole community, without absolutely excluding voluntary contributions, ought to form the financial basis of their support.

It was further shown, that they were lamentably in need of control and inspection by specially qualified medical authorities, men of "character and standing," unfettered by private or professional bias, and rendered as independent as possible of corrupting influences.

Such were the premises, generally admitted; but these by no means justified the conclusion at which the Legislature arrived —namely, that the whole medical and sanitary care of the poorer classes, not merely of workhouse paupers, should be controlled by Boards of Guardians, or committees of such Boards, under the Poor-Law Commissioners; that the entire cost of this provision, including the salaries of the medical officers in each district, should be defrayed exclusively by poor-rates raised in that district; and that all voluntary aid, hitherto afforded by the independent and educated classes of society in the support and management of these institutions, should be rejected.

On this last point, indeed, a stand was made in the House of Commons. A proposition was made by Mr. Vesey, that an annual subscription of 1*l.*, or a donation of 10*l.*, should entitle the donor or subscriber to serve on the committee of management.

The objection urged by the Government was, that the amendment, if adopted, would limit the power of the Board of Guardians over the Dispensary Committees; the very reason why it should have been passed.

Mr. Sidney Herbert, with his usual comprehensiveness of view and nobleness of purpose, supported the amendment. But the pauperizing party were too strong, and the amendment was defeated by a small government majority.

§ 3. The question naturally occurs—Why were the dispensary surgeons so clamorous for the Bill of 1851.

Drowning men, we are told, catch at straws. But probably no class had suffered more than the dispensary surgeons from that aggravation of national distress which was caused by the great famine, and two successive pestilences, devastating the island, from 1846 to 1850. They also apprehended, and not without reason, a total failure of resources for the maintenance of their dispensaries.

They had, moreover, endured with vexation and disappointment, the peddling and oppressive operation of the three temporary Fever Acts, by which, in succession, the Legislature had endeavoured to mitigate the horrors of those calamitous years.

A stranger medley of incongruous administrative machinery was perhaps never before created by sanitary legislation, than that which struggled, miserably and ineffectually, in 1847 and 1848, to do something by way of relief and prevention, at the expense chiefly of the doctors; for they suffered personal risk and loss in addition to their share of the public burthen : while the last of those temporary measures, by concentrating certain powers in the Poor-Law Commission, served, at least, to check abuses, and to favour an approach to order and efficiency.*

These circumstances may partly account for the almost unanimous support which the Irish doctors† gave to a measure for converting the national dispensary system into a branch of poor-law relief.

Like the frogs in the fable, not being content with the *log* of a grand jury system, they were, in reply to their complaints, handed over to the *stork* of a poor-law government.

The bait of a *medical* commissioner and five *medical* inspectors, was too enticing to be withstood; and the unsatis-

---

* "The two first *temporary Acts* proved inadequate, as was apparent in Dublin and in other cities and large towns; but in rural and remote districts, where means were crippled and resources were unavailing, disease pursued its course—the people perished through want of proper relief, and their medical attendants fell from the effects of contagion. Adverting to the incongruous materials for working the second of these Acts, it is not difficult to account for such results ; that machinery comprised Relief Commissioners, Relief Committees, Finance Committees, Boards of Guardians, and the Board of Health. Every proceeding under the Act, to be complete, required the united action of these distinct bodies, whose co-operation was demonstrated by endeavours to shift and shake off responsibility; ' while the Board of Health, although complaints were constantly pouring in, had no power to prevent the greatest extravagance on the one hand, or the greatest cruelty to the poor on the other.' They had no legal power to enforce or even to superintend the carrying out of their own recommendations."—Observations by "Medicus," Dublin, p. 34. 1851.

† " With a shortsightedness for which," said an eminent Irish surgeon, "I could never account."

factory experience of Union medical relief in England made little, if any, impression.

> *Segnius irritant animos demissa per aurem*
> *Quam quæ sunt oculis subjecta fidelibus* . . . .

§ 4. Many decided improvements, nevertheless, resulted from the operation of the new law.

The "General Rules and Regulations" of the Poor-Law Board, and the personal superintendence of the Medical Inspectors, introduced order, method, and attention. Responsibilities and duties were defined and enforced. The cost of each dispensary was explicitly stated, under separate heads. The medical officers were relieved from the discreditable necessity of advancing or procuring the requisite funds.

"The benefit of medical relief was extended to the sick poor in many districts of Ireland, where the absence of resident gentry formerly occasioned a total destitution of such aid, otherwise than by resort to the workhouse."*

Domiciliary visitation, which under the old system was casual and defective, was strictly required, and in general well performed, under the new.

Reports of cases, and returns of attendance and relief afforded, though grievously complained of by the surgeons, were doubtless of use to themselves in inducing systematic habits of record, while they promoted punctual attention to the sick, and enabled the Commissioners to compile periodically a mass of information respecting the statistics of sickness, the sanitary state of the population, the administration of medical relief, and the operation of palliative and preventive measures, such as probably no country, however civilized, had before witnessed; and which contrasts singularly with the meagre and unsatisfactory information afforded by the English Poor-Law Board.†

---

* *First Annual Report on Medical Charities*, 1853, p. 15.

† The third of these *Annual Reports* (1855) ought to be read by every one concerned in preventive medicine.

The country is much indebted to the Medical Commissioner and Inspectors for

§ 5. If such were the advantages of the change,—what were its evils? Such, I reply, as are inseparable from any *Poor-Law* provision.

In carrying into effect any new system of administration throughout a country, it is inconceivable that some cases of hardship to individuals, and of inconvenience to communities— some anomalies and inconsistencies,—should not occur.

But the operation of the Irish Dispensary Act seems to have created an extraordinary amount of needless annoyance and just dissatisfaction.

Nor were the doctors by any means the sole murmurers. The invariable and inevitable result of planning districts for the medical care and sanitary management of the poorer classes, upon the basis of parochial Unions or districts already formed for pauper relief, is to disturb the natural tendencies and to cross the inclinations of the people in their demand for medical advice; while it subverts arrangements which have been tested by time and corrected by experience.

This was the case, as we have seen, in England. Parochial districts were formed for other objects than those of the public health; and parishes which had previously grouped themselves into what were virtually, though not nominally, "medical districts," according to popular preference and convenience, were arbitrarily re-arranged by Commissioners and Guardians, in order apparently to accommodate the boundaries of such districts to their territorial divisions for general purposes, and without respect to the habits and wants of the people in sickness.

The same arbitrary interference with long-established arrangements took place in Ireland. The change was doubtless sometimes for the better: often for the worse.

For example. Towns, as every one knows, are the centres and sources of medical aid to the surrounding rural population, and

their arrangements respecting the last cholera epidemic, and for the really philosophical method in which they treat disputed questions as to the origin and propagation of that pestilence.

ought to be regarded as such in any new sanative arrangements. But the following case was as common as in England:—

The boundary of the new Union B approached very near to the town A in Union C, and all the poor inhabitants of that part of Union B, which heretofore depended on A for medical advice, were driven in sickness and accidents to a distant centre devised for them in district D of Union B.

It also often happened that some old dispensary had supplied the medical wants of the poor in portions of two or three unions in its immediate vicinity.* But, as the Guardians of each Union planned their own dispensary districts irrespectively of their neighbours' arrangements, the former dispensary was too often abandoned, and its dependent poor unmercifully dispersed to seek aid in different directions from more remote sources.

Again, Boards of Guardians are notoriously prone to diminish the number, and thus increase the size, of medical districts.

But the enormous extent of some dispensary districts in Ireland would astonish even those who complained of the size of medical districts in the Northern counties of England. The Commissioners' tabular view of the population and area of the Irish districts† contains at least seventeen with a population exceeding 20,000; and no fewer than ninety-seven, the area of which exceeded 40,000 acres!

Yet, the influence of the Commissioners seems to have been generally exerted in the right direction.‡

---

* *E. g.*—Annadown.   Killaloe. Ibid. Oct. 15.
Medical Press, Sept. 15, 1851.   See remarks by Rev. W. Edwards,
Killane, Ibid. Oct. 22.   Portarlington, Ibid. Jan. 21, 1852.

† The average population in each district is 9060
 ,,   ,,   ,,   to each medical officer 8440
The average number of acres in each district 28,000
 ,,   ,,   ,,   ,,   to each medical officer 26,180
—*Second Annual Report*, p. 209.

‡ "In a small number of Unions (ten), we found ourselves under the necessity of overruling the propositions of the Guardians, and taking into our own hands the division of the Unions into dispensary districts.—§ 8.

"In a much larger number of cases, we objected on account of the *number* of districts proposed being too small."—§ 9, *First Annual Report*.

If the total number of dispensaries in Ireland was somewhat augmented under the new system,* (beside a further increase in the number of medical officers, and the addition of several drug-stations or depôts); this increased supply of medical attendance was by no means commensurate with the increased extent of country provided with dispensary relief; and in districts previously so provided, the number of dispensaries was, on the whole, reduced.

These features of Poor-Law medical relief in Ireland, if not loudly complained of by the doctors,—for, as has been observed in England, large medical districts are not always professionally disadvantageous,—were grievously felt by the sick poor, and not unregretted by the gentry and clergy.

§ 6. The surgeons, however, had further and valid grounds of complaint.

If the actual amount of salary was not, on the average, much reduced,† its general ratio to the duties performed was very greatly diminished.

The additional labour imposed on the medical officers,—especially the case-books and the statistical returns,—would have justified, on an economical estimate, the addition of one-third to their salaries, raising them to an average of 100*l*. a year.

The change, even as to remuneration, was therefore felt severely by the great majority; while the change of masters, from their

---

* In 1849 there were 668. (In 1850 some of these were dropped in expectation of the new system.) Under the Poor-Law Board there are 720.

† It appears from returns of County Cess that 76,000*l*. was spent on the maintenance of 668 dispensaries in 1849.—*First Annual Report on Medical Charities*, 1853, § 38. Each dispensary thus cost, on the average, nearly 114*l*. per annum; though the proportions expended on the medical officers, drugs, and other matters, are not specified.

In 1853-4, there were 722 dispensary districts (968 drug stations) and 777 medical officers; and the total cost 88,439*l*.,—which, calculated in the districts, gives 121*l*. to each, and, on the medical officers, nearly 114*l*., as before; but of this only 73*l*. on the average came to them as salary, the remainder being spent in drugs, appliances, and official experiments.—*Second Annual Report*, p. 206.

The last (third) Report shows a reduction of districts to 720—the number of medical officers remaining the same—and the total cost is slightly increased, so as to give 75*l*., on the average, to each medical officer.

educated and philanthropic neighbours to persons (however respectable) elected by the rate-payers for merely fiscal purposes, proved in many instances most galling to men of liberal views and cultivated minds.

This deterioration in the managing body was but partially compensated by the controlling influence of the Medical Commissioner and Inspectors, themselves hopelessly fettered by connexion with a Poor-Law Board.

Any one might have foretold the result of the plan devised in 1851, for the constitution of dispensary committees. Composed of sections of the Boards of Guardians, with the addition in some cases of a few local rate-payers nominated by the same Guardians, —they evinced, in too many instances, an absence of those higher motives which generally actuated the governors and voluntary supporters of the former institutions.

Hence, it proved very difficult to ensure a sufficient attendance at the meetings of the new committees,* for the transaction even of ordinary business, and for the proper revision of the grants of medical relief.

Nevertheless, however defective the composition of these committees, and however imperfect their working in some districts,— it is asserted that their efforts to provide adequately for the wants of the sick poor, and to act fairly by their medical officers, were commonly thwarted and crushed by the Boards of Guardians under whom they acted. The doctors evidently preferred the district committees to the Union Boards, and not unreasonably urged that larger powers in the administration of sanitary matters

---

* The Commissioners, in their *Second Annual Report* (§ 5), confess the difficulty, and hint, as plainly as they can, that the Guardians do not select proper persons for the committees. Mr. Power, also, the Chief Commissioner, in his evidence (603) on Medical Relief in 1854, confessed that the Dispensary Committees did not meet as often as they ought; yet that the General Order for them to meet "once a fortnight," had been relaxed to "once a month," in cases where the assent of the Commissioners might be obtained.

"It is a well-known fact that months have elapsed in some dispensary districts without a single meeting of the Committee having taken place."—Mr. Ellis's *Lecture on the Working of the Medical Charities Act*, p. 3.

should be conferred on these committees, to be checked only by the Central Board and its inspectors.

§ 7. This seems to be the proper place to notice one very important particular, in which the administration of external medical relief in Ireland differs from that in England.

It does not involve dependence on the rates for the supply of nourishment and cordials in sickness.

It is reported,* that Boards of Guardians had been asked for "wine, brandy, and other stimulants; beef-tea, arrow-root, and other articles of nourishment, and even groceries, for the use of dispensary patients."

The Commissioners, however, "after a careful consideration of the Medical Charities Act, arrived at the conclusion that it was not the intention of the Legislature that articles of this description should be provided at the expense of the ratepayers for dispensary use."

They said further—

"We have uniformly opposed ourselves to the establishment of this new form of out-door relief, and refused our sanction to the supply of these articles under colour of their being to be regarded as medicines or medical appliances."

If owing to absolute destitution, the patients were unable to procure or provide such articles for themselves, the workhouses and fever hospitals were open to them, "where stimulants, nourishment, and all other requisites can be legally supplied."

There was also, as the Commissioners explained, a provisional power vested in the relieving officer, "to relieve, out of the workhouse, destitute persons in cases of sudden and urgent necessity."†

These regulations, as we shall see, contrasted singularly enough with the English custom of medical "orders" for mutton and porter, &c.

Whatever opinion may be entertained as to the completeness and efficiency of any system of sanative care, which does not provide suitable diet, as well as drugs, for the sick,—it must be obvious that, with reference to the repression of pauperism, the Irish arrangements in this particular are far superior to the English.

* *First Annual Report on Medical Charities*, 1853, § 10.

† In Ireland there is a distinction between "destitute poor" and "poor persons." The former are entitled to receive *general* "in-door" relief; the latter receive only medical relief at the dispensaries, and are not considered paupers as in England.

But, although based on more correct principles of political economy, the Irish method is far less satisfactory to the medical officers, not only because it deprives them of important remedial aids in the treatment of disease, but for the following reason.

In England, the liability to supply "medical comforts," as they are called, has acted in some measure as a check upon the indiscriminate grant of medical relief. In Ireland, where no such check exists, a very extensive and occasionally a profuse distribution of "tickets" for dispensary aid is customary.*

§ 8. It appears that some of the dispensary committees endeavoured to define the circumstances or condition of the class, just above the "poor," which should not be entitled to gratuitous public aid.†

But these attempts, sometimes whimsical enough, seem to have been unsuccessful; and the Commissioners, perhaps wisely, declined "to give any more precise definition of the persons who would be fit objects for receiving medical aid, than that afforded by the Act itself," namely, "any poor person resident in the district."

"The Legislature," said they, "appears to have relied on the exercise of a proper discrimination on the part of those individuals who are authorized to afford medical relief by the issue of tickets, and subject only to *the power of the Dispensary Committee to cancel orders or tickets* given to persons who may be improper objects for such relief." ‡

How unfortunate, then, was it that the Legislature had not fixed upon a superior and better qualified class of "individuals" to exercise such "discrimination."

* See Mr. Power's Evidence (572, 573) before the Select Committee on Medical Relief in 1854.
† One committee wished to limit tickets to those whose ground was not worth more than 5*l.* a year, or who had not more than three cows!
Another fixed the standard at a 12*l.* rental, for relief at the dispensary; and a 6*l.* rental for relief at home.
A third decided that no persons (nor the families of such) valued at above 2*l.* per annum should receive medical relief!
The Commissioners judiciously advised these committees to reconsider their resolutions.—*Medical Press,* Oct. 6, 1852.
‡ See an important letter from the Central Board to the Kiltoom Dispensary.—*Medical Press,* Dec. 8, 1852.

The doctors complained, and with fairness, that, while their remuneration was strictly limited to an amount barely sufficient to meet the claims made upon them by the very poorest class of the community, there was no sort of limitation or restriction of their official services to that class. And they ultimately requested, though without effect, that they might be empowered to recover by legal process the cost of medical relief bestowed on improper objects.*

The Commissioners, on the other hand, reminded them of "an abuse most fatal to their interests, which prevailed extensively under the former system, whereby many contributors to the funds were permitted to look upon themselves, their families and dependents, as peculiarly the objects of the charity; and which led them to expect attendance and advice in return for their subscriptions."†

It was, however, fairly rejoined, that the members of dispensary-committees and others, to whom the Legislature had granted the power of issuing " tickets," made quite as unscrupulous a use of their privilege, at the expense of the medical officers, as any of the former subscribers or cess-payers; and that such acts, on the part of official authorities, were far more morally and socially injurious than demands made, even unreasonably, upon medical benevolence, by influential neighbours or patients.

§ 9. Within less than two years from the passing of the new law, the medical profession in Ireland had discovered painfully the extent of their blunder in promoting its enactment.

The late President of the Irish College of Surgeons, Mr. Ellis, in a published lecture‡ on the subject, forcibly denounced both the measure and its administration.

* See *Report of the Council of the Irish Medical Association*,—and the resolutions of that body,—at its anniversary, June 6, 1854.—*Medical Press,* June 14.

† The Commissioners added (§ 40, *First Report*):—"We trust that all tendency to abuse of this nature may, under the present law, be effectually suppressed by a judicious and firm exercise of the power possessed by Dispensary Committees, to cancel tickets for medical relief given by the individuals authorized to issue them to persons not entitled by their position to receive it, and by the publicity which may be expected to arise from discussions in the Committee on such occasions."

‡ *Lecture on the Working of the Medical Charities Act,* by Andrew Ellis. Dublin, 1853.

CONCLUSIONS FROM THE DISCUSSION.

Following the example of Mr. Guthrie in England, he had procured information from a large number of dispensary surgeons; and his description of their wrongs and grievances deserves to be read by all who wish to know what the medical attendants of the poor had to say on the subject. It was "unusual," as Mr. Ellis observed, for one in his position to commence a collegiate session with a "stormy narrative" of injuries inflicted on the profession by the State; and nothing short of a very serious accumulation of grievances could have led to such a course.

However partial might seem his view of the case, he was doubtless correct in the following inferences:—

"It is my firm conviction that so long as the medical officers be paid *out of the poor-rate*, through the different *Boards of Guardians*, —neither contentment nor good feeling are likely to be reciprocated between these parties" (p. 25).

"The medical officers of dispensaries, *being employed in the service of the public*, should, through the public bodies to which they respectively belong, assert their claim to be paid out of the Consolidated Fund, as in the case of the Officers of the Army and Navy" (p. 27).

§ 10. Granting, fully, the advantages obtained by the more systematic management of the district dispensaries (advantages which have been already distinctly enumerated) —it is impossible to escape the following main conclusions from the published accounts of the working of this Act:—

First, that the dispensary arrangements, as to their number, and localization, and as to the size of districts, were characterized by singular instances of irregularity* and of inconsideration for the wants of the poor;

Secondly, that the local administrative authorities, being originally appointed for a specific object—viz., the control of pauperism,—and having thus to do only with the poorest class of the people, were very improperly selected by the Legislature

---

* Mr. Power, the Chief Commissioner, is reported to have acknowledged to a professional deputation, in June 1853, that "there certainly appeared to be very great discrepancies, and that they should be attended to."—*Medical Press.*

for the direction of medical aid, which necessarily applied to a much larger proportion of the community. For the same reason, they were still less fit to execute measures for the prevention of disease and the mitigation of pestilence, which apply more or less to the whole population, and which ought to be administered by persons of cultivated minds and special qualifications;

Thirdly, that the new arrangements have borne oppressively upon a majority of the medical officers; and that the mere addition of a medical commissioner and medical inspectors, acting in subordination to a Poor-Law Board, affords little real security, either for a correct medico-sanitary management of the lower orders, or for just treatment of the district medical officers; and

Fourthly, that, as regards the mass of the people, the tendency of the present system is to familiarize them with pauperism,—though to a less degree in Ireland than in England, owing to medical aid there not necessarily leading to the receipt of relief in money or in kind.

§ 11. Here we might have left the consideration of State Medicine in Ireland, had not the Parliamentary Session of 1854 afforded more than one remarkable illustration of the aggressive character of a Poor-Law provision,—of its tendency to spread among other classes of society, and to invade other institutions than those to which it ought to be strictly confined.

County Infirmaries were founded in Ireland not many years after their rise in England. They were established by an Act of the Irish Parliament, in 1765, and were confirmed and regulated by several succeeding enactments. They were maintained by voluntary contributions, Grand Jury presentments, and grants from the Consolidated Fund.

They were officered by a very superior body of surgeons, necessarily members of the Dublin College, and often University Graduates, men of considerable influence among all classes of society, and able to make themselves heard in the Legislature.

Now, it had been for many years, a design cherished by many in and out of the profession, to bring all the institutions for supplying public medical aid in Ireland under ONE system of administration, central and local.

The task of proving that many and great national advantages were likely to result from consolidating this department of State medicine, under highly qualified and scientific direction, was an easy one.

But it was unhappily undertaken by certain official persons, whose object, as we have seen, was to connect all medical institutions with the Poor-Law administration.

The reforming party, although tolerably united so long as Boards of Health and medical authorities were talked of, split as soon as Government selected the Poor-Law machinery.

§ 12. Whilst Dispensary managers and surgeons, anxious for any change, eagerly accepted the Act of 1851, the Infirmary doctors, supported by the Grand Juries and by their Parliamentary representatives, rejected it. They perceived that the benefits provided for the working classes by means of hospitals and infirmaries, differed wholly in principle from Poor-Law relief; they urged the policy of discouraging "a familiarity with pauperism"; they saw no reason for delivering over these institutions to the management of parties, who certainly had not proved successful in conducting establishments for medical relief elsewhere; they protested against rejecting or discouraging voluntary contributions, which secured for these hospitals and infirmaries, the superintending care and patronage of many of the most respected and trustworthy members of the community.[*]

These reasons were deemed satisfactory: the opposition succeeded; and the Legislature struck out from the Bill all but the Dispensary clauses.

Thus the advantages which might have been secured by a

---

[*] See Report of Meeting of County Infirmary Surgeons, at the Dublin College, in November, 1850.—*Medical Press.*

good medico-sanitary administration were indefinitely postponed; the blame fairly resting upon those who proposed a machinery wholly inapplicable to a national object of so great importance.

§ 13. Though the attempt failed, it was not abandoned. The second Report of the "Dispensary" Commissioners, put forth in 1854, while acknowledging in terms of high commendation the utility of the infirmaries, and the benefits which they conferred on all classes of the community, recapitulated the objections already made to their management and organization.

These objections were answered with great spirit and ability by Dr. Little, Surgeon to the Sligo Infirmary; and, although the Commissioners were a second time defeated, there are reasons for calling attention to the several allegations, with their respective replies.

It was said of the infirmaries:—

1stly. "They are inadequate to the wants of the entire country."

An argument, it was replied, for their extension and increase, but not for the entire subversion of an approved and popular system, and the substitution of a doubtful Poor-Law experiment.

2ndly. "They are badly distributed:"—

"An overstatement," was the rejoinder; since the principal county towns, being the centres not of "imaginary circles," but of the most populous districts, were the natural localities for these establishments, and had been selected, as such, on valid grounds, by the legislature.*

3rdly. A large proportion of the country "derives little or no practical benefit from them."

This was shown to be only another form of the first objection; the right remedy for the admitted deficiency, being to establish a second or even a third infirmary, in the larger counties, on the principle of

* "The bulk of their populations constantly employed in occupations—in breweries, distilleries, mills, and factories of different descriptions—where accidents are frequent, and the elements of a sanitary condition wanting, the mode of life and the habits of the lower order of tradesmen and artisans in such towns much less favourable to health than those of the rural population, and the natural disinclination of medical men of high standing to settle elsewhere—all point out such towns as the fitting sites for such institutions, and on such very sufficient, and one would suppose such unimpeachable grounds, they were, no doubt, so selected by the legislature of the day; the specific reason assigned for such choice being, in the words of the Act, because it had placed them 'convenient to the best inhabited parts of the country.'" (See 7th and 8th Geo. III. chap. 8.)—*Dr. Little*, p. 7.

the original enactment, and in the midst of thickly inhabited districts.

4thly. "The mode of supporting them by taxation, which bears as heavily on the large portions of the counties which derive no benefit from them, as on those limited portions that enjoy the whole of it, is inequitable."

It was replied that the so-called "limited portions" of population surrounding the infirmaries by no means engrossed the whole benefits, twenty per cent. of those relieved, coming from beyond a ten-mile radius; that the parties taxed made no complaint, but, on the contrary, continued spontaneously to vote an increased amount* of county cess for their support; and that the small farmers of Ireland who pay this assessment, not amounting to a halfpenny per acre were the very persons most benefited by the system.

5thly. "A complete want of uniformity in every important particular relating to their general management."

This merely showed the necessity for a well-devised system of medico-sanitary inspection and reports, with moderate powers of control,—and by no means indicated the propriety of incorporation with the poor law arrangements. Absolute "uniformity" was truly said to be as undesirable, as it is visionary and impracticable, if an attempt were made to enforce it in different localities, varying as to character, habits of population, climate, and produce.

To the last objection, Dr. Little retorted by a curious picture of the "want of uniformity" which characterized the "reformed" dispensary system, already under poor-law management.

Those who wish to refer to particulars, will not regret devoting an hour to Dr. Little's amusing pamphlet.† If there appears to be a little exaggeration on some points, (arising out of the circumstances—that the arrangements were barely completed when he wrote, and that the expenditure of the first year was not a criterion for the regular annual cost of any dispensary,) there can be no doubt of the fidelity of his statements and the general correctness of his deductions.

§ 14. But if the Commissioners were worsted in the discussion about County Infirmaries, they made out a better case for proposing to take charge of all *Fever Hospitals*.

* Progressive amounts of County Cess granted to the infirmaries, at septennial intervals:—
    1838......... £17,480   1845......... £20,649   1852......... £23,547

† *The County Infirmaries of Ireland;* a Letter, addressed to the Editor of the *Dublin Medical Press,* by W. S. Little, A.B., M.D. (T.C.D.) &c. &c. Reprinted, Sligo. 1854.

This description of medical charities was instituted by Parliament, in 1807; in the first place, as *County* Fever Hospitals, supported wholly by Grand Jury presentments.

Afterwards, *District* Fever Hospitals were established by the same authority, and maintained partly by subscriptions and donations, and partly by contingent grants from the county. But the uncertainty of their income, the precarious nature and decline of subscriptions, and certain defects in distribution and arrangement, which they shared with the dispensaries, had contributed to their gradual absorption into a new class of Fever Hospitals, established under the Poor-Law.

For, in 1843, Boards of Guardians had been legally empowered to provide hospital accommodation for "poor persons" affected by "dangerous contagious disease."

At or soon after the period of that enactment, the Grand Jury Fever Hospitals are said to have exceeded 100.* Within ten years they had sunk to 37.

On the other hand, no fewer than 146 "Union" Fever Hospitals had been established within the same period. A remarkable change had thus been quietly going on. And it was obvious that these hospitals throve better under Poor-Law than under County support.

When the "Union" establishments had attained the proportion of four to one of the former class, there was a show of reason in suggesting that all had better be placed under one system, and that those districts which contributed both by county cess to the old hospitals, and by poor-rate to the new, should in future be spared a double taxation.

§ 15. We are now led to a closer view of the more serious and objectionable features of the Commissioners' project.

They confessed that "persons above destitution" (called in official phraseology "poor persons") whose relief from the poor-rates was "not contemplated by the present Poor-Law,"

---

* 110 in 1816.—See *Second Annual Report on Medical Charities*, p. 12.

were sometimes admitted into workhouse infirmaries and fever wards; and that this practice was on the increase, especially in districts most remote from any county infirmary.* They deemed it "most difficult, if desirable, to control" such admissions.

Such being the case (ran their argument) why not also place under their care, the County Infirmaries and the other Fever Hospitals, which profess to be reserved for the same class—that above "paupers?"

Thus, they first broke down the barrier between pauperism and comparative independence, and then made their own act a pretext for including *all* public medical aid in one department, under their own direction.

In offering to cater for a respectable class of society, industrious and generally self-supporting, but with incomes insufficient to purchase medical attendance, the Irish Commissioners ignored principles which had always been asserted by the wisest economists in England—namely, that this portion of the population ought never, if possible, to be brought into contact with the Board of Guardians, or with the officers and regulations of such Boards; and that it is a class for which hospitals—not being workhouses—are specially adapted, as having no tendency to weaken habits of frugality and self-reliance.†

Yet it was a favourite notion of the Commissioners to admit artisans, domestic servants, small farmers, shopkeepers, the constabulary, &c., into these Union hospitals, under a separate registration, and on the condition of their contributing "the whole or some part (according to the judgment of the managing committee in each individual case) of the average personal cost of maintenance in the institution."‡

---

* See their *Second Annual Report*, § 31, p. 13.

† It was well said by the opponents of the Poor-Law plan, that "the Irish infirmaries have their analogies, in similar institutions, in every civilized country in the world, quite irrespective of pauperism" (London Correspondent of *Medical Press*, May 31, 1854); and that "institutions, which now, as county infirmaries, are active and successful agents in keeping down pauperism, would, as Union hospitals, become *negative causes or incapable spectators of its extension.*"—Dr. Little, *sup. cit.* p. 21.

‡ *Second Annual Report*, § 35.

Surely, the authors of this project were not oblivious of the vitiating influences of workhouse association, nor unconscious of the danger of accommodating in the same wards, and subject to the same official management, a class of persons who can afford to pay the cost of their own maintenance, with those whose utter destitution too often arises from idleness, waste, intemperance, and vice!

What was this scheme in principle but another phase of the attempt made by the English authorities, in 1836—8, to interfere in the organization and management of "independent" medical clubs?

There was this difference, however, between the English and Irish manœuvres, that the first applied only to *out-door* medical attendance, while the second comprehended *in-door* maintenance, —a more important and dangerous experiment.

§ 16. One more feature of the Commissioners' plan for converting the old county infirmaries into "Union" hospitals, deserves notice.

Small committees of management were to be appointed by the several Boards of Guardians.

But—as a compliment, perhaps, to those whose munificence had endowed or helped to maintain the former institutions—in case any seats in the proposed Hospital Committee were left unoccupied by the Guardians themselves, or by resident rate-payers, the ancient governors (the aristocracy of Ireland, be it remembered) might, by conciliating the favour of the Guardians, be honoured with leave to occupy the possibly vacant places!

A free and easy method, doubtless, of dealing with the rights of founders!

Subscribers of twenty guineas to the new institutions might be favoured in like manner; and thus the privilege of talking and voting on these "Union" committees, might be purchased of the Guardians on moderate terms.

Now, without further animadversions on the patent absurdity of *such* an offer to voluntary benefactors, of representation in the governing body of their own institution, it may be fairly asked—If the principle of combining voluntary support with taxation were utterly wrong, as the Government contended when the Dispensary Act was under discussion,—why was it thus admitted into the Infirmary Bill?

§ 17. Notwithstanding the vigorous defence made by the Infirmary surgeons and governors, and their unanswerable objections to the poor-law scheme, a measure* founded on the Commissioners' recommendations, was brought into Parliament for the second time during the session of 1854, but only to be again speedily abandoned, though perhaps not finally shelved.

Intimations of official designs often creep out when and where they are least expected. In a nice little "explanatory analysis" of the Nuisances Removal Bill of last session (1855), the ingenious and anonymous author, referring to the modifications necessary to accommodate this measure to Ireland, says:—

"The administration of dispensary relief in Ireland is already under the same authorities [the Poor-Law Boards], *and it is likely that* HOSPITAL *relief throughout the country unions will soon be entirely charged, as it is now in great measure, on the poor-rates, and made subject to the Union Boards and Poor-Law Commission.*"† —p. 9.

To be forewarned is to be forearmed. I do not hesitate to predict that, if the Irish Hospitals, at any future period, should be handed over to the management of Poor-Law Boards, it will be time for the governors of the Provincial Infirmaries of

---

* In its chief provisions, this Bill corresponded with the Dispensary Act.

Support from County Cess to cease. Expenses of each hospital to be defrayed by poor-rates raised in its own Union. Unions to be hospital districts. Board of Guardians to appoint a Hospital Committee, of not less than nine, nor more than twenty-one members—either themselves, or ratepayers of 50*l*., or Life Governors of the *old* infirmary, or donors of 21 *l*. to the *new.*

Old infirmary building might be appropriated for new hospital, or the Commissioners might sell or exchange it. Committee to appoint the medical officers at salaries approved by the Commissioners.

† In the last Session, 1855, an attempt was made, by a clause in an Irish Poor-Law Amendment Bill, to legalize the admission into workhouse infirmaries of "poor persons"—that is, *not* paupers.

England, and the managers of our County Lunatic Asylums, to look to their own unsafe position, and to set their houses in order.

§ 18. The just fate of the Irish Infirmary Bill was probably hastened by a most complete and interesting inquiry, made by a Committee of the House of Commons, in the same session, respecting the hospitals of Dublin; and this is the last movement, bearing on State Medicine in that part of the kingdom, which need be noticed in this historical sketch.

Anything like a narrative of the origin of the noble metropolitan institutions of Ireland would be irrelevant here.

It is enough to say, that all of them seem to have been founded in the course of the last century.* Although three or four owe their establishment to private beneficence, and several have been from time to time aided by voluntary gifts, they have always depended, more or less, on grants voted by Parliament.

Three great hospitals attached to the House of Industry (now one of the Dublin workhouses) fell under the control of the Poor-Law Commissioners a few years ago; and it had been actually proposed by some meddlers in office, to bring the other metropolitan hospitals under the same baneful influence, and to maintain them by poor-rates! This was, indeed, the climax of bureaucratic presumption. But the idea was too monstrous for production on this side of the channel.

However, it was thought that something might be effected by a starving process; and a Parliamentary Committee, in 1848, having recommended, without sufficient investigation and under the influence of false notions of public economy, that the national grants should be gradually diminished and ultimately extin-

---

* "From the year 1188 till the Reformation, a large amount of medical relief was afforded to the poor of Dublin, through the medium of monastic institutions, particularly that of the Priory of St. John's, in Thames-street. When religious houses were generally suppressed, the property belonging to the Dublin monasteries was sold, while that of St. Bartholomew's and St. Thomas's, in London, was re-granted by the Crown."—*Report Dublin Hospital Committee*, p. viii. referring to Mr. Wilde's very valuable evidence.

guished,—this ridiculous experiment was actually tried. The Whitworth Hospital was, in consequence, closed in 1849; until the Lord Lieutenant, struck with the inexpediency of shutting up such an establishment, ordered it to be re-opened in three weeks, on his own responsibility.

§ 19. The Committee of 1854, after a most searching and carefully conducted inquiry, recommended an entire reversal of the previous miserable policy.

Entering fully into the circumstances and condition of every hospital in Dublin,—its foundation, means of support, particular objects, and amount of utility,—the Committee furnished ample proofs of the necessity of maintaining those institutions in full efficiency, as indispensable sources not only of admirable relief to the poorer classes, but of the very best medical instruction.

Seldom, indeed, among the dreary pages of a "blue-book" does one come upon so refreshing—so fair and hearty an acknowledgment of the claims of scholarship, science, and humanity, as in the concluding paragraph of this Committee's report.

Practically, they recommended an increase of the Parliamentary grant from less than 13,000*l.* to 16,000*l.* annually.

They were of opinion "that it is not desirable that these hospitals should be placed under the control of the Poor-Law authorities."* They even recommended that the Hardwicke, Whitworth, and Richmond Hospitals should be "entirely separated" from the Workhouse establishment, and that the Poor-Law Commissioners should thus "be relieved of a charge which in the opinion of the Committee, does not fairly come within their department."†

This bold recognition of public medicine, as a matter totally distinct from the legal provision for paupers, was in no small degree due to the evidence of two chiefs of English surgery.

Mr. Guthrie, in 1844, had proposed to place his Medical Commissioner and Medical Inspectors under the Poor-Law Board; but, in 1854, when consulted about metropolitan institu-

* *Report*, p. viii. † Ibid. page vi.

tions, he appears to have advised, " not to leave them, as they are, *half supported, and most certainly not to put them under the Poor-Laws.*"

It is reported, also, that Mr. Guthrie judiciously suggested that the grant should be conditional on the maintenance of the Medical School and clinical instruction,—and that Sir B. Brodie, whose clear-headed practical judgment makes his opinion invaluable on any subject, after liberally acknowledging that " the Dublin School produces as eminent men as there are in the profession in Europe," recommended the Government to take "this view of the question, and *not a Poor-Law view.*"*

It is almost impossible to over-estimate the importance of such principles in the administration of public medical aid, as were laid down in the Report of the Dublin Hospital Committee. This† and the rejection of the Irish Infirmary Bill were omens of a brighter æra in the relations of the profession with the State.

* See "London Correspondent" of *Dublin Medical Press,* May 1854.

† The Irish Executive Government has since issued a commission "for further inquiry;" as a preliminary measure to the permanent endowment of the Dublin Hospitals, and the correct distribution of the Parliamentary grant.—*Medical Times and Gazette,* March 1855.

The allocation of the sums to these hospitals was said to be completed in September last.—*Medical Press,* Sept. 1855.

CHAPTER SEVENTH.

FROM A.D. 1853 TO 1855.

§ 1. RETURNING to medical attendance on the poor in England, we may now complete this historical review.

The third and last Parliamentary inquiry arose, apparently, out of a movement in Bristol. It will, therefore, be as well to preface an account of that inquiry with a brief notice of the Bristol provision of parochial medical aid.

The management of the poor of that ancient city was under a local Act, and thus exempt from the operation of the New Poor-Law.

A population of 64,000, out of workhouses, was entrusted to the care of only one medical officer, residing at one of the workhouses (St. Peter's Hospital) and receiving 150*l*. per annum, with his "board." Such an extent of duty necessarily occupied his entire time. Although many thousands of the Bristol sick poor were attended at the Dispensary, at the General Hospital, and chiefly at the Infirmary;*—and although the workhouse duties of the resident medical officer were lightened by the Honorary Physicians and Surgeons of St. Peter's Hospital,—

"he complained of enduring great bodily fatigue in attempting to discharge his duties; as well as of the large number of sick poor, who were very inefficiently attended, owing to the difficulty of his reaching them.†

The drugs and a dispenser were provided by the Board of Guardians.

* Evidence Medical Relief Committee, (1854.)—844.
† Evidence, ibid. 690. "Frequently, after he has considered his day's duty done, there are numerous sudden calls, perhaps from the extreme end of the city, to which either he is obliged to go, or the next day we have found that the parties have sunk under the disease before they could be seen."—692.

Every poor person applying to the relieving officer for an order for medical aid, became a pauper, and thus lost many privileges to which the industrious classes of Bristol are entitled.

§ 2. As far as a separate supply of medicines and a comparatively accurate registration* of cases went, the system was superior to that in force under the Poor-Law Amendment Act; but the invasion of cholera, in 1849, severely tested the inadequacy of the public provision; and it was then found necessary to form five medical districts, identical with the registration districts, a dispensary station and a medical officer being attached to each.

The medicines were freely supplied to all poor applicants, without depriving them of their civic privileges, or herding them with paupers at the Relief Office. The results of these extended arrangements were highly satisfactory and encouraging; and Dr. Wallis, who had watched them closely, put forth a pamphlet at the close of 1850, in which he advocated the establishment of National Free Dispensaries throughout England. This plan, taken principally from the Irish system, was also warranted by Mr. Miles, the member for Bristol.

Dr. Wallis, having zealously entered into the question, pursued his useful inquiries, and collected many facts and opinions, bearing chiefly on the pauperizing tendency of the present system of Poor-Law medical relief.

§ 3. Mr. Miles afterwards† brought the subject before Parliament. He complained of the large number of persons who became annually chargeable on the poor-rates, from the circumstance of their being unable to obtain medical relief at the public cost unless they became paupers.

He showed that there was no competent supervision of such medical relief; and he recommended a separate provision of

* The returns of cases from Bristol in 1843, at the request of the Provincial Association, were singularly explicit.—Appendix A, *Health and Sickness of Town Populations.*

† July 12, 1853.

drugs, to be freely and promptly administered to the sick poor, without involving the further grant of nutriment and general relief, and without any communication with the relieving officer. His proposals were, in short, identical, on many points, with the dispensary organization of Ireland.

Mr. Baines and Sir John Trollope, on that occasion, undertook the defence of the arrangements over which they had, in turn, presided. They ingeniously avoided a direct reply to Mr. Miles's principal statements and suggestions, as involving " certain new principles hitherto unknown to the law of this country."

They dwelt, with great complacency, on the improvements which had been of late years effected in their medical department; the increased number of medical officers; the higher nominal qualification required of them; the increased cost of medical relief; and the remarkably few official complaints of neglect or malpractice, against their medical staff. They also urged the non-necessity, and the expense, of a corps of medical inspectors. Indeed, their statements on this point were so specious and so positive, that one could only wonder how the Irish doctors succeeded in obtaining their *medical* commissioner and inspectors two years before.

§ 4. Mr. Miles must have perceived that nothing would be gained by then pressing the matter. But, in the next Session (1854), he co-operated with Mr. Pigott, the Member for Reading, in procuring the appointment* of another Committee of the House of Commons, " to inquire into the mode in which medical relief is now administered in the different Unions in England and Wales, and to ascertain whether any additional facilities might be afforded the poor in obtaining medical aid."

The nomination of the Committee, and the choice of Sir John Trollope as Chairman, at once showed the course which the inquiry was likely to take; but there seemed no other way by which Parliament could escape from the troublesome con-

* May 9, 1854.

clusions to which a full and impartial sifting of the question would have led.

The Select Committee sat for about six weeks, and examined twenty-four persons; four of whom were connected with the Poor-Law Board (two of these being Inspectors, and one the Chief Commissioner for Ireland); five were members of Boards of Guardians (one of these a chairman, another a vice-chairman, and a third an active clerical magistrate); two were parochial clergymen unconnected with Boards of Guardians (the observations and opinions of such distinguished men as the Rectors of Barham and Eversley could not fail to command attention); three other witnesses were overseers or relieving officers, affording much practical information from Bristol, Clifton, and Liverpool; one more was governor of a County Infirmary, testifying to the undue pressure of the present system upon the medical charities of the country;—and lastly, nine were members of the medical profession,—three of these being district medical officers, two others having lately held that post, and four (including Dr. Wallis) being unconnected with Union arrangements, and having no personal interest in them.

§ 5. The Report,* it is needless to say, represented the opinons

---

* Resolutions of the Select Committee, 5th July, 1854 :—

1. That no sufficient evidence has been adduced before your Committee to justify their recommendation of an entire change in the present system of medical relief as administered under the General Consolidated Order of 1847, by means of which the poor have derived greater facilities in obtaining medical aid than they were enabled to do previous to its promulgation.

2. Your Committee, however, recommend that the Poor-Law Board should continue to direct their attention to the extent of the medical districts, to the reduction of their area where they are found to be inconveniently large, and to the appointment of additional medical officers in such cases.

3. Your Committee also recommend that every medical officer to be appointed after the 25th of March, 1855, should continue in office until he may die, resign, or become legally disqualified to hold such office, or be removed therefrom by the Poor-Law Board.

4. They also recommend that the Poor-Law Board should direct their attention to the salaries of the medical officers, which, in some cases, appear to be inadequate to the duties they are required to perform.

5. Your Committee further desire to call the attention of Parliament to the facts given in evidence, that a considerable number of poor persons have been placed on

of the majority of the Committee, rather than legitimate conclusions from the evidence taken.

With reference to their first resolution, it was hardly to be expected that a conclave so pledged, would recommend " an entire change in the present system." It should, however, be observed, that no evidence had been adduced to prove that the consolidated order of 1847 afforded any greater facilities to the poor in obtaining medical aid than had been granted by the previous medical order of 1842. The gradual increase in the number of medical officers mainly effected by the limitation to the size of districts contained in the order of 1842,—and the formation by the same order, of lists of "permanent" paupers who might obtain relief at all times, without the formality of an application to the relieving officer,—were the only assigned or assignable causes of the alleged " greater facilities."

The second resolution recommending a reduction in the area of some of the medical districts, shows, as indeed the rest do, a sincere desire on the part of the Committee, to make the " present system " as efficacious as possible.

The third resolution has led to the recent promulgation of an order * from the Poor-Law Board, which seems to have been

the pauper list through the receipt of medical relief in cases of sickness or accident, and from that cause alone; they therefore recommend, that persons so circumstanced should be enabled to receive such medical assistance as their cases may require, without being placed on the list of paupers, but that it should be left to the Boards of Guardians to decide in what cases medical relief shall be so given to persons who are not otherwise in want of, or in the receipt of, parochial relief.

6. That evidence has been given before your Committee respecting purely medical clubs, the contributors to which are entitled to attendance and medicine alone, with the option of selecting their medical attendant; that in some districts, where provident habits are encouraged among the industrious classes, the existence of such clubs, mainly maintained by their contributions, evinces at once the value they attach to prompt medical attendance, and an honest desire on their part to maintain their independence.

* Order, Feb. 15, 1855 :—Art. 1.—" Every medical officer of a workhouse duly qualified according to the regulations of the Poor-Law Board in force at the time of such appointment, and every district medical officer duly qualified as aforesaid, and residing within the district in which he is appointed to act, shall hold his office until he shall die, or resign, or be proved to be insane by evidence which the Poor-Law Board shall deem sufficient, or become legally disqualified to hold such office, or be removed by the Poor Law Board."—*Medical Times and Gazette*, March 10, 1855.

hailed with almost universal satisfaction by the medical profession; for, although permanent appointments had been already adopted voluntarily by more than half the local Boards, there were good reasons for the change being made imperative on all.* This is probably held by the Union Surgeons to be the greatest improvement in the medical department of the Poor laws, since the general order of 1842. But some persons still doubt, and with reason, whether a septennial tenure of office, as proposed by Dr. Wallis, under medical inspection, would not have conduced more to the public interests.

From the fourth resolution may result a further augmentation of the medical salaries. This may foster the *vis inertiæ* of the medical staff, and perhaps tend to prolong, for a time, the existence of political and social evils, inseparable from a public provision of medical aid, under Poor-Law management.

The fifth resolution is most questionable. The Committee recommend that poor persons, not being "paupers," should be enabled to receive—of course, through Relieving Officers and Boards of Guardians—medical assistance without being placed on the list of paupers.

Although this has doubtless been the practice already, in a large proportion of Unions, a general licence to that effect, by authority, could hardly fail to impair the fundamental principle of the English Poor-Law, while it will extend the most objectionable feature of the vaccination laws, and include a still greater amount of medico-sanitary duties, under a department which ought wholly to be relieved of them, except as regards workhouses.

The sixth resolution, containing a complimentary notice of the better sort of Medical Clubs, the contributors to which have "the option of selecting their medical attendant," may be left to its probable fate.

* "I cannot help having a great distrust of the motives of *Local Boards* in making any man a permanent officer."—Rev. C. Kingsley, Evid. 1593.

POSTSCRIPT.

Sir G. Nicholls's *History of the Poor-Law*, has come under my notice since the completion of this Essay.

In that large and no doubt useful work, the subject of medical relief occupies nearly three pages.* And in these passages, I believe it may be truly said that there are not ten consecutive lines which do not contain some often refuted statement or some manifestly incorrect assumption.

It would have been better had he altogether omitted his meagre allusion to this controverted question; for, as it stands, it displays something very like the *suppressio veri*, if not the *suggestio falsi*. But I think the error is not wilful; for it really seems as if the author were helplessly fettered by the effete notions and hackneyed phraseology, which characterize the earlier ventures of the Poor-Law Commissioners on this subject.

Concerning the efforts and opinions of such distinguished men as the late Dr. Yelloly and Sir T. N. Talfourd, and of many living writers from whom it would be invidious to select a name or two,—concerning also three successive Parliamentary inquiries of no trifling importance,—and concerning the several very decided changes which the Commissioners have already been compelled to make in their mistaken arrangements,—this " History" saith nothing!

The idea of medical aid for the poor, as a distinct national provision, and not necessarily or even generally connected with any poor-law system, seems never to have crossed Sir G. Nicholls's mind.

So contracted a view of the case probably arises from his official confinement *inter mænia*,† where he could scarcely be

---

* See vol. ii. pp. 338—391.

† See passage from Taylor's *Statesman*, selected as a motto for this Essay.

cognizant of the progress of opinion and the social movements around him.

The health and sickness of the poorer classes, constituting the bulk of the population, is treated by him as a mere matter of quarrel between parochial surgeons and Boards of Guardians, upon which the Commissioners' duty was simply to arbitrate by conceding something to both parties.

In order to examine and answer his remarks in detail, it would be as well to compare each with one or more of the previous sections of this Essay, and with the works to which they refer; perhaps also, with the conclusions to which they lead in the following pages.

But this may be done as fairly by any considerate reader of both historical statements as by myself.

ESSAY IV.

THE MEDICAL CARE OF THE POOR IN ENGLAND, WITH NOTICES RELATING TO IRELAND.

PART II.

ITS PRESENT CONDITION AND REQUIREMENTS; ITS RELATIONS TO POLITICAL ECONOMY AND SANITARY MANAGEMENT.

" QUOT regiones urbis sunt, totidem constituantur Archiatri. Qui scientes annonaria sibi commoda a populi commodis, honestè obsequi TENUIORIBUS malint, quàm turpiter servire DIVITIBUS.

. . . .

" Quòd si huic Archiatrorum numero aliquem aut conditio fatalis aut aliqua fortuna decerpserit, in ejus locum, non patrocinio Præponentium, non gratiâ Judicantis, alius subrogetur, sed horum omnium fideli circumspectoque dilectû, qui et ipsorum consortio, et ARCHIATRIÆ IPSIUS DIGNITATE, et Nostro Judicio, dignus habeatur.

" De cujus nomine referri ad Nos protinus oportebit.

" Dat. III. Kalend. Feb. Triu. VALENTINIANO ET VALENTE III. AA. Coss."

[*Cod. Theod.* lib. xiii. tit. iii. lex 8.]

ESSAY IV.
PART II.

§ 1. Upon the rit ordering of a State Provision for the medical care of the poorer classes in their own dwellings, depends the stability and efficiency of the whole superstructure of Medical Police.

And I say CARE of the poor, because it is now pretty generally acknowledged that any such provision, to be permanently useful, must not be limited to mere routine attendance on cases of actual illness and accident, to a perfunctory supply of pills and potions, with a bald return of names, diseases, visits, &c., from uneasy officers to incompetent Boards.

A far higher order of duties and responsibilities appertains to the true *status* of this intrinsically noble office. And if it can be shown that under practicable reforms, and without an unjustifiable increase of public expenditure, the anomalous conditions and relations of the corps of union medical officers can be reduced to order, and reconciled with reason and precedent, one of the greatest difficulties of the sanitary question in the United Kingdom will be solved.

In offering suggestions towards the formation of a comprehensive scheme for future legislation, it seems desirable to look a little more closely into the present condition of the Medical Relief Department; and, with this object, to examine not merely some of the evidence taken in 1854, but other documents containing information on the subject.

I.—*As to Statistics of Medical Relief.*

§ 2. The number of Medical Officers in England and Wales increased from 2530 in 1842,* to 3151 in 1853; an addition considerably beyond the increase of population, and therefore accompanied by a diminution in the size and population of districts.

Of these 3151, however, not less than 110 were either officers of workhouses, infirmaries, and schools, or mere dispensers, so that the districts amounted to 3040.†

This, according to a "Return of the Area and Population of Medical Districts," made to Parliament in 1853, allows an average population of 5700, and an acreage of 11,250, to each district.

§ 3. The salaries and other remuneration, not including vaccination fees, had increased during the same period from 154,054*l.* to 215,054*l.* a-year.

But these sums include payments for workhouses and other parochial institutions. Now the salaries of 108 (of the above-mentioned 110) medical officers of workhouses and schools, amounted in 1853, to 7260*l.*‡ There were also more than 586‖ workhouses and union establishments *included in district appointments.* Estimating these at the average country salary¶ of 49*l.* 7*s.* for each establishment, and adding the above 7260*l.*, we have to deduct a trifle more than 36,000*l.* for workhouses, &c., from the 215,000*l.*, leaving 179,000*l.* to be divided among the 3040 districts—*i. e., nearly fifty-nine pounds for each.*** For

---

* Mr. Cane, Parliamentary Evidence, (1854.) 40.

† Several medical officers hold a second district in the same, or in an adjacent Union, so that the number of *district* surgeons probably does not exceed 3000.

‡ See Parliamentary Return, 1853.

‖ 594; but seven or eight of these held not more than thirty inmates, and are therefore not reckoned.

¶ This is the average of the salaries for those sixty Workhouses with separate appointments, which remain when the vast establishments of the metropolis, Liverpool, Manchester, Birmingham, and Portsmouth, are struck out.

** Nearly 2¼d. per head on the population.

IN-DOOR AND OUT-DOOR CASES. 241

this sum, medicines and all appliances are to be furnished by the medical officer.

§ 4. With regard to the number of cases of sickness and accident attended; as there is no available registration of such casualties in England and Wales, we can only approximate to the fact.

The official party, at the last inquiry, wished it to be inferred, that the total number of cases among the poor attended by the Union Medical Officers, during the year, did not exceed the number of actual paupers returned on a certain day of the year, to the Poor-Law Board as in the receipt of general relief.*

The several fallacies in this assumption would be obvious to any statist; yet the estimate of the "Convention" in memorializing Sir G. Grey was probably an error equally wide of the mark in the other direction.†

There are fair grounds for concluding that the *in-door* cases, occurring in the course of a year, amount to more than twice the number of paupers resident on a given day.‡ This would allow more than 200,000 cases annually in workhouses and other Union establishments.

The *out-door* cases coming annually under the care of the district officers cannot be fewer than 1,400,000.‖ Thus, the

---

* Sir John Trollope, Q. 3315.—Evidence (1854,) and Appendix No. 6, p. 246.

It was asserted by persons practically acquainted with the working of the Poor-Law, that many sick poor are attended by the medical officer who are not returned by the relieving officer as paupers;—such, for instance, as were not ordered "medical comforts," or other kinds of relief.

See Mr. Lord, Ibid. 3303. Mr. Gray, 1135. Mr. Wooldridge, 1800.
See also Return from Tewkesbury—Appendix, p. 244.

† "They would remind you that 3,000,000 of her Majesty's subjects are entrusted, in the hour of sickness and suffering, to their professional care and skill."— Memorial, 26th March, 1848. *Appendix to Report of Committee*, p. 245.

‡ See *Returns from Metrop. Workhouses*, 6 July, 1855. See also column A, Table 30, p. 121, *Appendix to Seventh Annual Report of Poor-Law Board*, 1855.

‖ It was ascertained by returns from 805 medical officers to the Convention, that the average rate of payment for each case attended, in country districts, is 2s. 7d. Applying this rate to all the districts of the kingdom, the salaries for which, as has total number of cases of sickness and injury attended by the present Union Medical Officers, is at least 1,600,000 annually.

The *out-door* cases only, divided among the 3040 districts, give an average of 460 cases to each district.

§ 5. All the preceding facts, relating to *extern* patients in Ireland, are precisely and accurately stated by the Commissioners in their Annual Reports. The comparative position of the district doctors in England and in Ireland would, according to the previous estimate, stand as follows,—

Average.	Medical Salary and Cost of Medicines.	Annual number of Cases.	Population.	Area in Acres.
England... ...	59*l*.	460	5700	11,350
Ireland	105*l*.*	890	8443	26,178

The charge on the rates is greater in Ireland. Mr. Power showed that the total *medical* expenditure in Ireland, including workhouses, &c., is about half that of England, the population being only one-third.† The working classes are thus more liberally supplied with medical relief from the poor-law in Ireland. But the Commissioner omitted, in this comparison, any notice of the large and costly provision made in England, by charitable dispensaries.

§ 6. When the "Convention" obtained their returns from 805 districts, the remuneration of medical officers exhibited great want of uniformity. The rate per case varied from 3*d.* in some, to 14*s.* 4*d.* in others.‡

The size of districts also varies extremely. In Wales, the irregularity is necessarily great; but, in England alone, there were, in 1853, no less than 560 districts, the area of which

---

been shown, are 179,000*l.*, we arrive at 1,367,900 cases—a result below the mark, because the metropolis and other large towns pay a lower rate per case.

* Namely, 75*l.* for medical salary, and 30*l.* for drugs and dispensing.

† Evidence (1854), 585.   ‡ Ibid. 3269.

exceeded the acreage sanctioned by the general order of the Poor-Law Board; and in more than 180* the population exceeded 15,000.

The extent of many of these districts was extravagant and unjustifiable.

II.—*The Social Economy of a Provision of Medical Relief in connexion with the Poor-Law.*

§ 7. It has been shown† that on the introduction of the new Poor-Law, a very great diminution in the number of poor receiving parish medical aid, took place throughout the southern three-fourths of England; and by referring to the Reports of the Commissioners, we find that *pari passu* with that reduction, the poor-rates diminished for three or four years. A "heavy blow and great discouragement" was then given to pauperism.

In 1838, however, simultaneously with the first Parliamentary inquiry, the supply of medical relief began again to be somewhat extended. At the same time, as shown by published official tables,‡ the total expenditure on the poor again mounted upwards. The cost of both medical and general relief continued gradually to increase for ten years, but since 1848, the extension of medical relief has been unaccompanied by a general rise of pauper expenditure; and this may be due partly to the greater demand for labour, caused by enlarged commerce and emigration, and partly to successive epidemic visitations, which have increased the demand for medical services.

The cotemporaneous fall and rise in pauperism and in medical relief, before 1848, are probably more than simple coincidences; and from such general facts alone, it might be inferred that a widely extended grant of medical relief from Boards of Guardians and parish officers, tends to pauperize the working classes, and to check that desire for independence which many thought would

---

* Parliamentary Return, 1853. † See p. 168.
‡ See Table No. 20, p. 101, *Appendix to Seventh Annual Report of Poor-Law Board*, 1855.

have been restored by the operation of the Poor-Law Amendment Act.

§ 8. Local and personal observation serve to establish this inference. Mr. Inspector Weale said, that a willingness to apply for parochial relief of all kinds prevailed as much as ever in the agricultural districts.* He also thought that medical relief in particular was often given too freely;† and that quite as many persons were benefited by the Poor-Law supply of medical relief, " as ever received it under the old system."‡

In Bristol and Manchester, the wish to retain the elective franchise was said to operate against the parochial grant of medical relief, which, as involving the necessity of an order from the relieving officer, deprived the recipients of their political rights.‖ Thus, the effort to preserve social independence and civil privileges was believed to be the cause of much personal suffering and peril, aggravation of disease, and even increase of mortality.¶

This may also be the case in other Parliamentary boroughs; but it may reasonably be doubted whether the elective franchise, *per se,* had much to do with the matter,—whether the loss of certain material and tangible advantages, which not unfrequently accompany that privilege, even in the most virtuous constituencies, had not a more direct effect.

At all events, it was shown that in Bristol and Clifton, the recipients of parochial medical aid were deprived of a share in some comfortable endowments and local charities.**

---

* Evidence (1854), 465, 466. See also Oxenden, 1562. Ellison, 2568.
† Ibid. 342.
‡ Ibid. 454. This admission tells against Mr. Baines's inference that a *larger* grant of medical relief was made under the new than under the old system. (See note, p. 168.) "I am quite sure," said Mr. Ceely, in 1854, "that *more* medical relief was given under the old parochial contract system *than is now*. I am not less sure, however, that the more limited supply given now, is far more regular and efficient, and more costly of time and means, than when a greater number were attended."

‖ Evidence (1854), 709. ¶ Ibid. 676—8, 712, 2201.
** Ibid. 699, 1061, 2468.

But there was almost unanimous testimony to the fact, that, after passing the threshold of the Relief Office, the spell was broken, and any previous repugnance to dependence on the poor-rates rapidly vanished.*

Mr. Weale informed the Select Committee that " medical relief was generally only the forerunner of other kinds of relief." † " Parochial relief always follows upon an application for medical relief."‡ And it was the opinion of the Guardian from Bristol and others, that two-thirds of those who apply in the first place for medical relief become habitual paupers.||

§ 9. That medical aid, granted by the local administrators of Poor-Law relief, leads the working classes to depend on the same source for other necessaries of life, was indeed too clearly shown before Lord Ashley's committee ¶ to need further confirmation. Dr. Wallis, however, explained to the last Select Committee how this tendency operated far more strongly in the rural districts than in cities and towns.**

The artisan in populous places can often obtain the aid he needs at some infirmary or dispensary; and this, he feels will not degrade him.†† The agricultural poor have no such alternative. The noble " subscription " dispensaries of Liverpool, in which upwards of forty thousand poor‡‡ are yearly relieved, are thus the means of preventing a vast extension of the pauper roll.|||| The *quasi* public character of the hospitals and other

---

* Evidence, 624, 702.   † Ibid. 350.   ‡ Ibid. 383. || Ibid. 701, 3020.

Dr. Wallis had endeavoured to found on these and similar statements a numerical average of "paupers," made so by coming first upon the rates on account of sickness. But the calculation was open to criticism, and probably involved fallacies, some of which were indicated by the chairman (2750). The reality of Dr. Wallis's ground, however, would be admitted by any candid observer, without his statistics; while the attacks of uncandid objectors would be merely strengthened by the obvious uncertainty of the numerical method in such a case.—See Austin, 296.

¶ See Evidence (1844), 9702, 9281, *Pauperizing tendency of Medical Relief.*
** Evidence (1854), 2790—2792.   †† Ibid. 2238.
‡‡ Beside patients relieved at the hospitals and other medical charities. The total number of cases relieved in all the medical charities of Liverpool in 1843 was 64,112.—See Appendix A, *Health and Sickness of Town Populations*, p. 85.
|||| Ibid. 1164.

medical charities of our large towns, removes from the benefit which they confer, any sense of depression or shame on the part of the recipient,—any stigma of pauperism. And it was rightly judged by an impartial witness in 1854, that the same kind of medical aid provided

"by public taxation, would work exceedingly well; it would not at all lower the recipient in his own opinion or in that of others; it would enable him to be much more independent of other circumstances." *

But then, the Poor-Law authorities must have nothing to do with it; for there was a firm substratum of good sense in opinions, which some would call harsh, expressed by two other gentlemen,† who protested against the removal of the pauperizing condition of medical relief, *so long as it was bestowed by the Boards of Guardians* with which they were connected.

§ 10. When the abolition of that pauperizing condition was recommended by Mr. Ceely and myself, in 1844, it was in strict conformity with our general scheme of separating the public sanative provision from the Poor-Law administration.

But the proposal of Dr. Wallis and Mr. Miles to effect the same object, at the same time leaving the grant and control of the provision in the hands of pauper-managing authorities, was inconsistent with itself, and opposed to every sound principle of policy.

The social danger of such a system of relief, during epidemic visitations, was well stated by Dr. Sutherland, who, as chief Inspector of the Board of Health, had received complaints "of the pauperizing tendency of the relief measures in the hands of parochial authorities." He had also been informed

"that it was found to be very difficult to make persons return to their usual independent habits who had received parish medical relief for the first time perhaps in their lives."‡

* Evidence, 1460.   † Ibid. 1957, 2613.
‡ Appendix A, p. 139, *Report on Epidemic Cholera*, 1850.

In the epidemic of 1854, the objections to Poor-Law measures of relief were equally strong. The fatal neglect of the premonitory diarrhœa was ascribed, by

He then strongly and sensibly expressed his own opinion on the subject:—

"It must be confessed that the very placing of any portion of our population, except actual paupers, under a system of pauper medical relief, appears to be a proceeding of so entirely an objectionable character, that nothing but the most pressing necessity could have justified its adoption. No conveniences of existing machinery could make up for the mischiefs likely to accrue from it, or from the hardships to which it was likely to have exposed the applicants for relief. Whatever provision was contemplated for the protection of the lives of the working classes, during a period of pestilence, *ought certainly not to have been a pauper one.*"*

This statesmanlike and correct view of the subject was wholly ignored by the fifth resolution of the Select Committee in 1854.

§ 11. It is not public medical aid, in the abstract, any more than public vaccination, which tends to pauperize the recipients. It is the administration of any such benefit by pauper-controlling authorities.

And on this sound distinction, the Legislature (perhaps unconsciously) acted, when, in the Municipal Corporations Act, it decreed that gratuitous supplies of medical assistance and of education, out of Borough Charities, should not disqualify those who received these advantages from the exercise of municipal privileges.†

Here then we have public healing and public teaching placed in the same just relation to political freedom.

The analogy is too important to be neglected. It was pointed out by Dr. Yelloly, nearly twenty years ago.‡

the late Mr. Walsh, partly to the medical relief of cholera having been made a parish matter, for, said he, the numerous respectable working population of Bermondsey, who were the chief sufferers, naturally held anything connected with the parish "in the greatest abhorrence."

* Ibid. p. 137.

† Municipal Corporations Act, § 10 :—"That no medical or surgical assistance given by the Charitable Trustees of any borough shall be taken to be such charitable allowance as shall disqualify any person from being enrolled as a burgess aforesaid ; nor shall any person be so disqualified by reason that any child of such person shall have been admitted and taught within any public or endowed school."

‡ "I am very averse to consider as paupers persons who merely receive medicines

Sanative care, as well as instruction, are beyond the means of half the population. Both are imperatively necessary for the safety of the Commonwealth—for the health and happiness of the people. Both may be bestowed gratuitously, from a right source, without causing pauperism. Nay, they are the best means of preventing it, by promoting health and longevity, and by enabling the sick and the ignorant to work usefully and profitably. Both therefore should be brought home to every working man's family;* and both need to be directed and administered by specially qualified authorities.

III.—*As to the Persons, or Official Authorities, from whom the Poor obtain the right of demanding Medical assistance.*

§ 12. The ordinary practice under the English Poor-Law, as every one knows, is still—that all, not on the "permanent pauper" list, should apply for "orders" to the relieving officer, or some other parochial functionary. In the vast majority of English hospitals and dispensaries, "recommendations" from subscribers or medical officers are required. In the public provision of medical aid in Ireland, "tickets," as we have seen, are granted.†

The evidence taken by the three successive Parliamentary Committees, on this subject, has been remarkably accordant.

No room now is left for doubt, that the interposition of *any* economical check between the sick man and his medical adviser,—creating obstacles, delay, and uncertainty in the administration of aid,—must, and does in many cases, produce increased suffering, prolong disease, and not seldom lead to fatal results. It matters not whether that check consists in

---

or instruction from the public," said Dr. Yelloly to Lord John Russell.—" *Letter,*" *supra cit.* p. 36.

* See Sir G. C. Lewis's remarks on my suggestion of an aggressive policy—a medical house-to-house visitation. Note, p. 53, *Health and Sickness of Town Populations.*

† Dr. Wallis asserts—and not without reason—that the "tickets" will cause the failure of the present Irish system.—Evid. 2655.

"orders" from Poor-Law officials,* or in "tickets" from governors and guardians of medical charities.†

Stronger and more trustworthy testimony on this point has never been given than by the Rev. Mr. Oxenden;‡ nor is there any apparent escape from his conclusion that the first application should invariably be to some person conversant with disease; for it may be that the applicant is a malingerer and in no need of medical advice, and he will then be sent about his business with a salutary warning; but if it be a real case of illness, as it generally is, the sooner the patient is relieved, the better for all parties.|| Hence the advantage of a primary application to the medical officer.

§ 13. Some witnesses went so far as to attribute the frightful mortality among children in large towns, mainly to the want of a system of "free" medical aid.

Those, however, who know anything of the condition and localization of the dwellings of the poor—of their habits and temptations,—who have traced out the many social causes for the prevailing neglect and mismanagement of the young, in crowded communities,—will assign but a small share of this excessive mortality to the mere want of prompt medical attendance.

But there are sad facts, which cannot be lost sight of, in such an inquiry. For example:—half the children born in large towns die before they reach five years of age;—in Manchester, out of 2179 deaths (including children) 726 had no medical attendance;¶—in Bristol, one-tenth died without it; and these cases would have been more numerous, were not medical men

---

* Evidence, 2652, 3023. † Ibid. 2192, 2245.
‡ Ibid. 1381—1387.
|| The late Mr. C. Buller is reported to have said in Parliament, that he, for one, thought that very little ought to be left to the discretion of the relieving officer, who ought not to be allowed to be a judge as to whether a poor man was sick or not. That was a matter in which he was wholly incompetent to give an opinion.—Dr. Wallis's evidence, 2729.
¶ Ibid. 2198.

continually asked to see dying patients, just in time to secure a certificate of the supposed cause of death.*

The lamentable extent to which the working classes, to their great injury, resort to unqualified practitioners, is often owing to their praiseworthy desire to maintain their independence.† This seems to be especially the case in the north.

That these circumstances—beside their manifest influence on the average health, effective force, and longevity of the population—also produce pauperism, has been asserted by every intelligent observer.

§ 14. The defence made for the *order and ticket* system is twofold; first, that it acts as a check upon the too great extension of gratuitous medical relief; and, secondly, that it fixes the responsibility of the medical attendant.‡

The first of these objects can, however, be attained far more simply and easily; as has been repeatedly urged. The investigation into the condition and circumstances of the applicant should be a subsequent act. Any medical man engaged in visiting the poor must be competent, generally, to judge, not only of the medical requirements of the case, but also (especially if engaged in private practice), of the ability of the patient to procure medical aid for himself;—and a protest from him or others against a gratuitous supply, in any case, should always be followed up by special inquiry:|| and if this should terminate in proof that the recipient is able to make a self-provision, the local authorities should be empowered to recover the cost and all expenses, by a summary legal process.¶

Dr. Wallis considered that the public and the profession might

* Evidence, 713. † Ibid. 2467.
‡ Sir G. C. Lewis, in 1844, 9820—1.
 Sir John Walsham ,, 9718.
|| Mr. Power showed how this inquiry worked in Ireland.
Out of 690,411 tickets granted in the year ending September 29, 1853, the Dispensary Committees, irregularly as they met, cancelled no fewer than 5256, on objections being raised to the grant by medical officers or others.—Evidence, 520—2, 603.
¶ Evidence, 2063, 2137.

be sufficiently protected against fraudulent demands, by authorizing each Board of Guardians to define the circumstances and income of the class to whom they are willing to supply attendance and medicines.* He advised that these conditions should be publicly announced at each dispensary; so that every one might know whether or not he were entitled to the benefit of the State provision. Then, he also recommended that the cases should be liable to the same subsequent investigation, as has been just suggested. And he thought that persons obtaining medical aid under false representations of their circumstances or wages, should be fined, as well as made to pay for the benefit they had received.†

This proposal is somewhat similar to one which has been made for the prevention of indiscriminate bounty in Ireland.‡

But in a free and industrious population, persons will be so constantly rising above the line drawn,—while, from misfortune, often unavoidable, others in comfortable circumstances, will be as constantly falling below it,—that a revision of the list, however frequent, would scarcely keep pace with the vicissitudes of life, while it would become almost as troublesome an affair, and lead to as many disputes and attempts at imposition, as special inquiry into each case.

Besides, the nominal amount of wages, and the apparent condition of working people, *primâ facie*, are but very imperfect tests of the real extent of their necessities. Very useful as a general published statement of conditions might be found in each locality, a register appears to me to be undesirable; and the right of recovering the assumed value of the aid granted,

---

* Evidence, 2653. † Ibid. 2654.

‡ The *Medical Times* for Jan. 1854, contains the following plan:—A register of persons entitled to medical relief to be made by Dispensary Committees,—persons to prove their claim to be entered on register, some reasonable standard of house valuation or rateage being assumed, as a limit above which no one should be entitled to registration. Medical officers or any one else to have a right of appeal against the continuance of any name on the register, which should be subject to a weekly revision. Medical officers to be furnished with a copy, in form of a pocket-register, to be also corrected weekly.

would constitute the real solution of the difficulty. No injury to persons or to the community will be inflicted, if the power of decision could be vested in local authorities unconnected with the Poor-Laws.

For the second object intended to be secured by "orders," we require a system which defines the responsibility of medical men on surer grounds, and holds out higher and better inducements for the performance of duty, than the uninformed eye of a relieving officer, or the ineffective supervision of a Board of Guardians.

IV.—*As to the class or proportion of the Community for which the public may be expected to provide Medical aid.*

§ 15. So far as that is a Poor-Law provision, in any sense of the word, it should be confined to paupers;—on correct principles, to those only who are maintained in workhouses and pauper schools.

But when separated from Poor-Law relief, and given on grounds of public policy, not less than *half* the population should be thus aided gratuitously;* those, in short, who constitute what are called the "working classes."†

The safety and expediency of a more extensive grant of curative aid, under a different system, was thus pointed out by Mr. Power, the Chief Commissioner in Dublin:

"In Ireland, it is purely *medical* relief, ... in no way connected with the *general* relief of the poor;"—while in England [as he put the case], claimants for medical assistance are, in the first instance, entered on the books of the relieving officer, who, in his turn, becomes

* Evidence, 2070.

† Dr. Wallis relied on Mayhew's estimate of four millions. But by referring to the "Occupations" of the people in the last census, it will be found not less than that number are actually employed in productive labour. Accordingly we must add the family dependents, the infants and the superannuated, those also who may assist in domestic labour, but "do not work at money-getting employments." This class, as shown by an able writer in the *Companion to the British Almanac* of this year (see pp. 64, 65), numbers about half of the population.

We have still to add paupers and others maintained by the rest of the community. We may therefore safely say nine millions.

responsible for administering the "comforts" ordered by the medical officer. "We can afford," said he, "more liberality about our medical relief, because we are guarded from the general relief."

And so, if the curative provision could be separated from the "general" system of relief in England, he saw not why a dispensary organization, analogous to that of Ireland, might not be applied with equal advantage to this or to any other country.*

§ 16. The number of those entitled to receive medical aid under a sanitary organization, has been estimated, I repeat, at a moiety of the entire population; and this estimate is borne out by local observations.

In large manufacturing towns, the number of the working classes has been calculated, by accurate and independent inquirers, at *seven-tenths* of the entire population.† But, probably, two of the seven-tenths might be enabled to procure medicines, sick diet, and restoratives, for themselves; leaving five-tenths of the population incapable of providing safely for all the wants of sickness.

In some rural districts, where wages are lower and facilities fewer for procuring medical assistance, it is probable that more than half of the community ought to be thus provided for.‡

Dr. Sutherland must again be pressed into the service. His opinion as to the danger of relying on a pauper-controlling machinery for the direction of sanative and sanitary measures during pestilence, has been already cited. In the following quo-

* Evidence, 572—4.
† See Dr. Duncan's estimate for Liverpool; and Mr. Baker's for Leeds,—with comments thereon,—in the *Minutes of Evidence* (1844), 9120.
‡ Mr. Oxenden recommended that the members of any family, whose united earnings amounted to 25s. a week,—or single persons earning more than 10s. a week,—or persons occupying houses rated at 10l. and upwards, or having an income from property of 20l. a year—should be excluded from the public provision. All below should be attended gratuitously, although not all of them need be supplied with "sick comforts."—1390.

Dr. Wallis's proposed limit of income or wages—for individuals—was also 10s. or thereabouts, leaving the precise line to be drawn by each Board of Guardians.—2653.

tations, his experience of the necessity of a wide extension of such aid among the working classes, is shown with equal force:

"It was apparently the intention of the Contagious Diseases Prevention Act, that the medical relief to be afforded during the continuance of the epidemic cholera, should be considered as an extension of the ordinary parochial medical relief; whereas, the real necessities of the case required that the Boards of Guardians should, as far as possible, divest themselves of their parochial character and assume the office and responsibilities of *Local Boards of Health*, to exercise all those important functions which were required not only for the protection of the parish poor, but the lives of the entire community. Had the great majority of cases of cholera occurred among paupers, there would have been some show of reason for the parochial arrangement of relief being adopted; but it was very soon discovered that the force of the epidemic fell not on the paupers, but on the working classes and small tradesmen. It was no uncommon thing for the Registrar's Report to exhibit a mortality *twice as great* as the Surgeon's Return; and in the City of Bristol, where an account was kept of the classes who suffered from the disease, it was found that out of 15,529 epidemic cases in all stages, not above one-fourth occurred among the paupers, *the remaining three-fourths taking place among the independent working classes*, who were thus thrown upon the parochial medical relief, with no other alternative than to take it as the law had provided, or run the risk of death."*

Again:—

"The deaths from cholera in the metropolis, during the epidemic of 1849, were 14,590. Of this, 329, or little more than 2·2 per cent., were gentry; 1989, or 13·6 per cent., were tradesmen; and 10,332, or 60·8 per cent. of the total mortality, fell to the lot of mechanics and their families; and 1940, or about 13·2 per cent., were undescribed."†

It would be worse than folly to shut one's eyes to the social peril of trusting longer to so inadequate, so fallacious, a public provision of medical care, and especially at such a time.

§ 17. Let us, then, look carefully for a clue to guide us out of the difficulty.

If half the population is to be supplied with medical aid—it

* Appendix A, p. 136, *Report*, 1850. † *Report*, p. 63, 1855.

has been asked—will not the whole of the working classes be led, step by step, to depend for the ordinary necessaries of life on the other moiety of the community? This question, as I have endeavoured to prove, would never have arisen but for the *poor-law* connexions of the existing provisions. But, admitting that the poor are easily induced or tempted to abate their efforts at self-reliance,—the simple refusal of medical relief will neither cure their destitution, nor prevent their improvidence.

Is it not safer to grant freely and promptly, from an unexceptionable source, that protection which the working classes cannot be trusted to procure for themselves? And can we not, at the same time, place before them judicious plans, which may enable them to meet those other demands, arising out of casualty, which are not utterly beyond their means and capabilities?

It is, I think, obvious that a larger proportion of the population may be reasonably required and encouraged to provide restorative diet, clothing, fuel, and other such "comforts" in sickness, than that which is expected to provide drugs and other medical appliances; and that the latter class, again, is greater than that which can be safely left to a self-provision as regards medical advice.

To reverse the statement. The State may prudently provide medical skill and superintendence to an extent which might be politically unwise as regards the supply of drugs,—the *materia medica* being more easily procured than the services of the professors and practitioners of the art. On this principle, the public regulations of Berlin, and other German towns, entitle a class above the very poor to medical aid, who are nevertheless obliged to make some arrangement for the purchase of their medicines.*

Still more obviously, the *materia medica* may be supplied,

* The opposite practice has prevailed in England. Thus a sagacious Guardian, examined before the Committee in 1854, thought it best to encourage "independent" medical clubs by a *gratuitous* provision of medicines at a public dispensary (Evid. 1843); that is to say, he was ready to "find the physic," and to let the poor man settle with the doctor as best he might!

without impairing social independence, to a more numerous portion of the community than it would be wise to supply publicly with the ordinary necessaries and comforts of life, even those of special use in sickness.

Here, then, we are led on to the next question.

V.—*As to a self-provision of Medical Attendance and Medicines by "Clubs."*

§ 18. If the preceding remarks are based on correct principles of public economy, Clubs and Provident Societies among the working classes ought, in the first place, to raise funds (or to supply weekly allowances) for the purchase of "sick diet," cordials, and other articles of domestic and personal use in sickness.

Where and when working people are able to contribute insurance premiums larger than are necessary for the above purposes, a supply of medicines, &c. might be provided by arrangements between the managers of their common fund and a public dispensary or proper pharmacists.*

Supposing, then, that any considerable portion of the working classes should succeed in making judicious arrangements, not only for what ought to be their first concern—the weekly allowance in sickness, the deferred annuity, and the reversionary payment at death, secured by good Friendly Societies—but also for a supply of sick diet and nutriment, restoratives, and medicines, when needed; we may be quite sure that no further insurance-premiums (as for medical advice) will be in the power of any but skilled artisans and other persons, who, though operatives, are rather in the circumstances of employers.

§ 19. Very little remains to be said on the subject of "Clubs." In the first part of this Essay, I mentioned their entire failure to provide reliable medical aid. The balance of evidence in 1854 was also decidedly against them.

---

* Before arrangements with pharmaceutical chemists would be generally advantageous in England, they ought to be placed under scientific inspection, as on the Continent.

The two Poor-Law Inspectors spoke of them in very disparaging terms.* Even the ordinary "benefit clubs" were not considered by them as really advantageous to the community.

"I do not think pauperism is much affected by these things"—said Mr. Austin.†

Persons "are not made independent by joining benefit clubs"—said Mr. Weale.‡

Their mysterious connexion with great brewers was shrewdly pointed out by the author of *Yeast*, who also referred to the atrocious frauds so commonly practised upon the older and more infirm members of these societies by rampant junior majorities.‖ The same popular writer affirmed, with truth, that by means of these clubs, the poor generally "pay out of their own pocket for disease brought upon them by the neglect of others"¶—disease which might have been prevented by those capitalists, owners, and public bodies, who are morally responsible for the site and structure of the dwellings of the poor.

§ 20. By far the most important evidence relative to *purely medical* clubs, was that given by Mr. Oxenden, the founder of perhaps the only reasonable and successful society of this kind which has been formed in the rural districts.

The Barham Downs' Society had existed for twenty years, and was still in favour and in active operation, providing a fund for medical relief half as large again as the total union salaries in the same district,** the members numbering one-sixth of the whole population, and having the privilege of freely choosing their own medical advisers, who were said to be "perfectly satisfied."††

---

* Evidence, 363, 365, 366.   † Ibid. 316.   ‡ Ibid. 422.
‖ Ibid. 1605. No one has more powerfully exposed these abominations than the Rev. J. B. Owen, of Bilston, in his paper entitled *Popular Investments*, contributed to Lord Ingestre's first series of *Meliora*.
¶ Ibid. 1606.   ** Ibid. 1414.
†† Ibid. 1416. The medical attendants receive scarcely 4s. per head per annum on the total number of members, yet the contributions from single persons are far higher than any society of the kind that I have heard of.—1413, 1405.

Yet with this exceptional specimen under Mr. Oxenden's own paternal care and protection, he had the candour and moral courage to acknowledge its inferiority to a good public provision. He deemed it less advisable to maintain this "self-supporting institution,"—to which by the bye there were large honorary contributions,—than to allow the working classes to depend on a gratuitous supply, by means of national dispensaries.*

By confessing that "many members were hurting themselves very much, *in other respects*, by continuing their contributions," he indirectly supported the doctrine laid down in these pages,— that medical aid ought to be the last thing left to the poor to provide for themselves.

The Barham Downs' Society is the only club in which the medical attendance is well spoken of. "Club patients do not get anything approaching the attendance which the paupers get from the medical officers of the Unions,"—said Mr. Inspector Weale.†

Even the sturdy Yorkshire Guardian who thought it as well to "punish" paupers,‡ and recommended giving the poor patient a shilling or two to find a doctor to his own taste,|| nevertheless honestly avowed that the benefit clubs, containing, on his estimate, two-thirds of the working classes,¶ did not obtain as satisfactory and efficient attendance as the paupers; and he confessed that he had heard many complaints of medical neglect from the members of those clubs.**

§ 21. The only justification for encouraging or even permitting arrangements of this kind is that offered by the proviso contained in the last resolution of the Parliamentary Committee, —*i. e.*, "with the option of selecting their medical attendants." Yet greatly as this privilege may be prized, it is far too dearly purchased, if made a plea for withholding a comprehensive public provision for medical care and sanitary advice in every parish and district of the land.

* Evidence, 1448, 1454.   † Ibid. 369. See also Dr. Wallis 2843.
‡ 2570. || 2516.   ¶ 2594.   ** 2606.

When that national benefit shall have been fully and fairly established, it may be advisable for the State to promote well-considered arrangements for mutual insurance,—in which, after adequate funds for the supply of all other necessaries in sickness are secured, some facilities may be offered to larger contributors for the free selection of their medical advisers.*

VI.—*As to the power, exercised by the Medical Officers of Districts, to direct the supply of Necessaries (not being Medicines) in sickness, at the cost of the Rate-payers.*

§ 22. The promoters of the late inquiry assented fully to that feature of the Irish system, which in a social point of view, constitutes its main difference with the English law.

The almost unlimited power possessed by the medical officers here, of recommending—or as some call it, ordering—articles of diet, vinous and alcoholic stimulants, even fuel, flannel, and other personal comforts, for the sick, was stated not only to be a source of constant altercation between these officers and Boards of Guardians, but to offer direct temptation to the poor to make use of the doctor as the key to the parochial relief-chest.

The notions of some medical officers, as to their duty in this matter, were rather extravagant. One gentleman thought that the relieving officer ought to obey the directions of any and every medical practitioner who might be willing to give them.†

Another admitted that, when he had an average of forty poor persons at his surgery in a morning, he usually wrote twenty or twenty-five orders for "medical comforts."‡

He avowed that he took upon himself to judge of the destitution of applicants,|| and that he considered it his duty to attend to their wants.¶ So that on hearing the common complaint—" I have no means of support—I must have some relief

---

* Certain conditions or regulations considered essential to a sound system of mutual assurance for medical relief, are stated in Supplementary Note C.
† Evidence, 2381. ‡ Ibid. 1285—1297. || Ibid. 1299—1301. ¶ Ibid. 1344.

—some bread and meat," he, not doubting the truth of the statement, and without the right or possibility of making proper inquiry, at once gave them " orders" for food !*

No wonder that so complete an usurpation of the functions of the relieving officer kept the two officials in a constant state of antagonism. Whether the doctor might not have performed this duty better than the officer legally appointed for the purpose, is quite another question.

§ 23. The Boards of Guardians, however, are, and must continue to be the ultimate courts of appeal in the matter;† and after such unsatisfactory discussions with their officers, these Boards must be fully excused for their general impression, that the doctors order " dietetic tonics to save their own drugs."‡

When the cost of these " extras" nearly amounted to the sum of the medical salaries,||—when the supply had " doubled within the last two or three years"¶—the local authorities cannot be justly blamed for their suspicions.

Mr. Kingsley might have been justified in saying that, " the notion with rural Guardians is, too often, that medicine is to cure everything, when, in fact, food is what is required;"** but he also testified to the " continual jealousy and irritation" prevailing in most districts " about medical officers ordering too many necessaries;" " substituting them for medicines."††

Mr. Oxenden, whose disinterested position and knowledge of medicine entitle his opinion to much weight, stated that these recommendations are given " a great deal too often;" that a free provision of medical aid‡‡ ought to be wholly unconnected with power to interfere in the grant of other relief.

---

* Evidence, 1306—7. See also Rev. E. J. Howman's evidence :—" They (the medical officers) constitute themselves into irresponsible deputy relieving-officers.—1875.

† Mr. Inspector Weale's evidence, 419.   ‡ Ibid. 352.
|| Ibid. 1783.   ¶ Ibid. 2875.   ** Ibid. 1560.

†† Ibid. 1555. See also his story of a medical officer who was turned out for ordering too many of these good things, but being re-elected in three years, the Guardians found that they had not taught him the lesson they intended, for "he is as liberal as ever."—1558.

‡‡ Ibid. 1472.

§ 24. The present practice is doubtless* one of the main causes of the pauperizing effect of English medical relief.

It would, in itself, almost justify an entire change of system. And as has been shown, it might be superseded, to a great extent, and with great benefit to society, by a well-regulated mutual provision of those "comforts" by means of provident associations.

If drugs were supplied by local Boards, even though a reduction in the cost of dietetic adjuvants did not follow,—the district surgeons would no longer be liable to such diagreeable imputations. And this leads us to the next point.

VII.—*As to the parties by whom the Medicines for the Poor are, or ought to be, provided.*

§ 25. Every one knows that, with few exceptions, drugs and other appliances are at present furnished by, and at the cost of, medical officers, under the Union contract. The reform proposed long ago, and still urged with increasing force, is, that articles of the *materia medica*, like nutriment and cordials, should, in general, be provided by local Boards.

If medical officers are subjected to accusations, by interested parties, on the last head—*i. e.*, sick diet,—their contracts (to furnish medicines) lead no less to unwelcome calculations, by other parties totally disinterested, as to the possibility of their fulfilling such engagements, without loss to themselves, yet with full justice to their patients.†

For instance, Mr. Kingsley, after an extensive inquiry, came to the conclusion that costly medicines, such as cod-liver oil,

---

* Evidence, 1378—9, 1445.

† One of the medical officers examined in 1844 was too communicative on this point. He acknowledged that instead of supplying leeches and expensive drugs, which he could not afford, he got rid of the cases as soon as possible, by sending them to hospitals and dispensaries. (Ans. 2317.) Or if he had a doubt whether to order medicine or food, he should prefer ordering food to ordering medicine which he could not afford to provide.—2348.

quinine, and sarsaparilla, "cannot be given except in charity," at the average salary of the medical officers.* One surgeon, it was reported, feeling his inability to incur the expense, applied to the Board of Guardians for a grant of cod-liver oil, in a case where it was much needed.

The Guardians referred the application to the Poor-Law Commissioners, who replied—that, if the oil were given *as a medicine*, the medical officer was bound to pay for it; if *as food*, it would be a different case. They might as well have asked the patient, after swallowing it, which he considered it. Of course, the Guardians gave themselves the benefit of the doubt, and at once refused to grant the request.†

It appears however that the Poor-Law Board has decided that cod-liver oil *is a drug*. A medical commissioner was not needed to enable them to arrive at this remarkable verdict. They, however, left the special supply of this remedy to the discretion of the local Boards. The liberal Guardians of Kingston (and they alone) actually agreed to include it among medical "comforts," at their own cost! *O si sic omnes!*

§ 26. It was the opinion of Mr. Cane, of the Central Office, that a supply of drugs from dispensaries, to be established by the local authorities, would be advantageous in places where the population is not widely scattered, and where economical arrangements could be made for dispensing.‡

The Inspectors however differed with their official colleague. They advised leaving the matter as it is, in the hands of the medical officer, on the ground that he has a pecuniary interest in supplying good drugs, since by so doing he economizes time; ‖ a view of the case in which the medical staff generally concur.¶

On this subject Mr. Cane was at issue, also, with a former Commissioner, who assured Lord Ashley's Committee** that they had never been able to find a single instance in which a Union dispensary had succeeded; while Mr. Cane in 1854 "did not re-

* Evidence, 1562. † Ibid. 1563. ‡ Ibid. 142. ‖ Ibid. 287.
¶ Ibid. 2446. ** *Report* (1844), 9803.

member an instance where Boards of Guardians having agreed to provide drugs, had abandoned it, *after a trial.*"*

This pleasing variety—may it not be called, discrepancy?—in official statements, relieves the monotony of a public inquiry; and, as coming from gentlemen high in the civil service, who belong to the same department, is quite refreshing to ordinary blunderers.

The fact appears to be,—that, before recent changes in the local administration of the large towns of Birmingham, Bristol, Exeter, Leeds, Nottingham, and Norwich,—these could all boast of parochial dispensaries in active and successful operation.† Two, if not three, of them can still do the same.

We also learn from Mr. Cane's evidence that one metropolitan‡ and four country Unions had adopted this measure.

If, in any earlier or more recent instance, the separate provision of drugs has worked unsatisfactorily;—it would be only fair to ascertain whether such want of success might not be attributable to defects in other parts of the system, and especially to the absence of that scientific inspection, which has proved so beneficial in the dispensary organization of Ireland.

§ 27. The most eminent medical authorities have ever supported this reform.

The late Dr. Yelloly was probably the first and ablest public advocate of a separate provision of remedies, under medical supervision.‖

Sir B. C. Brodie also gave the following opinion before Lord Ashley's Committee :—" I think it very desirable that the fur-

---

* Evidence, 140.

† *Health and Sickness of Town Populations,* pp. 63, 64.

‡ The Stepney Union deserves notice, because the intelligent Chairman and another Guardian of that Union, gave valuable evidence on this subject before Lord Ashley's Committee (see Evid. 622, 715); and this accounts for their adoption of the reformed system.

‖ To him the public are indebted for collecting evidence on the subject from the heads of the medical departments of the Army, Navy, and Hon. East India Company's Service. Their statements are contained in his admirable *Letter to Lord John Russell.* Second Edition. London: Longman. 1837. pp. 19—20.

nishing of medicines should be made a distinct thing from the medical attendance."* He recommended that it should be placed on the same footing as in the Army and Navy, where "the medicines are furnished by the heads of the department, and the officers account for their use."†

The advice, so neatly given to a parochial Board, by one of the Metropolitan Cholera Inspectors, lately deceased, should be heard by every local authority in the kingdom:—

"I am not going to meddle," said Mr. C. R. Walsh, "with the amount of the salaries you give your medical officers. What that amount ought to be can, I believe, never be settled, while the manner of paying them, and the nature of what you exact from them, remain as they are. Pay what you and they may agree upon, for services rendered. You will soon arrive at a correct judgment on this point, when the nature of those services shall have been defined and simplified. But first and foremost, give them the medicines they require to use. Provide medicines and dispensers for them. Let there be no stint and no waste. To illustrate the absurdity of the present mode of uniting the contract for medicines and attendance, I beg your patient attention to a short argument by analogy. It is admitted that wine and cordials are sometimes useful remedies. Let us suppose them the only ones, and that they differed greatly, as they really do, in their fitness for particular cases, in their strength, and in their price. Now, try to make a contract with a publican, to supply your poor with wines and cordials at a fixed price per district, or per score or hundred of pauper population. That seems absurd enough. But now add this fresh element in the contract; suppose the publican to be made the judge of what wine, and what cordial, and how much of it, was good for each patient. What amount of faith in human disinterestedness would it require to make you believe that the publican decided fairly when to give Curaçoa or Champagne at 12s. a bottle, or gin at 2s. Now go on one step, and imagine that a publican did take your contract, in hopes

---

* Evidence (1844), 3530—1.

† This suggestion indicates a method of preventing certain evils which might result from Dr. Wallis's plan of village stations.

Mr. Keate in 1844 objected, and with reason, to small depôts of drugs, not in constant use and dispensed by the medical attendants themselves.—See *Health and Sickness of Town Populations*, p. 65.

Mr. Cane took the same ground in 1854.—Evidence 156.

of getting other custom. What a comfortable relation you and he and the sick poor would stand in to one another! Yet the difference between quinine at 16s. an ounce, and nitre, or oak-bark, at a few pence a pound, is greater than this; and besides it is not always easy to say which of the two is best fitted for the case. Fancy, how the difficulty is increased when the decision is hampered by the cost of the drug to the prescriber."*

§ 28. Successful precedents are now so numerous that the postponement of this reform can only be attributed to the powerful obstructiveness of official routine. In the army, previous to 1793, the regimental surgeons contracted for the supply of drugs to the sick soldiers, as the colonels, until 1853, contracted for the clothing of the regiments; and the same kind of abuses occurred in the physicking, as in the tailoring department, but with far less opportunity for detection.

In the navy, the old system continued until 1805. The separate provision of medicines has proved most beneficial, in all our war departments.

But the precedents most to our purpose are the charitable dispensaries of England; the public dispensaries of Ireland; and the universal practice among the civilized nations of Europe. These ought to decide the point against our Poor-Law peculiarity.

An important advantage, not often noticed, would result from abolishing drug-contracts. Physicians and surgeons of high scientific qualifications and most complete education, would, in that case, more readily undertake the parochial office, inferior as the rate of remuneration must always be.

In the Church, sons of Peers, and "first-class" men from the Universities, are constantly accepting curacies of 70*l.* or 80*l.* a year. Would they as willingly undertake those ill-requited duties, if the appointments involved contracts with parish vestries for the accessories of Divine service and the supply of Bibles, Prayer-books, and tracts, which they might nevertheless willingly contribute out of their own means?

* *Parish Maps,* &c., p. 6, *supra cit.*

§ 29. The practicability of establishing dispensaries in all populous districts was proved before Lord Ashley's Committee.

A calculation, then produced and never (that I know of,) invalidated, showed that the poor of four-fifths of the population of England might be supplied with medicines, &c., from public dispensaries, to be located in all towns which contain not less than 4000 inhabitants.* This might be done without the slightest additional trouble or inconvenience, either to the sick or to their doctors.

With regard however to the remaining fifth, residing in remote villages and strictly rural districts; it was admitted that, so long as country practitioners continue to supply their independent patients with medicines, it might be advisable for them, as medical officers, to do the same for the sick poor; although only in places of this description.

In these instances, a separate payment might be made for drugs, by the local authorities, according to the number of cases attended ; or, what would perhaps be better, a periodical supply of drugs, corresponding in kind and in amount with those given by the medical officer to the sick poor, might be returned to him from an appointed public dispensary.

Were the latter arrangement adopted, it would of course be necessary that an accurate record of the medicines consumed, taken by the dispenser from the case-books of the medical officer, should be at the command of duly qualified inspectors.

Dr. Wallis would not permit any medical officer to furnish medicines. Beside the establishment of depôts in villages, where it would probably be difficult to insure the conservation and correct preparation of the medicines,—he proposed that there should be at least one, sometimes more than one, dispensary in every district. This suggestion, evidently taken from the Irish system, would be wholly unnecessary in English districts, which

---

* See Evidence (1844), 9392, 9160—9161, reprinted in *Health and Sickness of Town Populations*, pp. 90—92.

are already much smaller than those in Ireland, and are in progress of further reduction.

There is no reason why two or more medical officers, residing near each other, or in the same market town, should not prescribe at the same public dispensary for the poor of their respective districts, living within convenient distance of such town. The number of dispensaries need not, therefore, nearly equal the number of districts.

§ 30. The cost of a public provision of medicines is now pretty accurately known, if only from the Reports of the Dispensary Commissioners of Ireland.

Calculated upon the cases of sickness relieved, the cost for each case averaged $8\frac{1}{4}d$. in 1853, and $5\frac{3}{10}d$. in 1854.

The rent of each dispensary building averages $9l.$ $6s.$ The cost of books, forms, stationery, printing and advertising,—of fuel, attendance, and incidental expenses,—averages $10l.$ $4s.$

Thus, *all* expenses, except the salaries of the medical officers and apothecaries,* average about $10\frac{3}{4}d.$ for each case of sickness. Dr. Wallis was therefore justified in estimating the average cost of drugs, on a large scale, at about $7d.$ per case.† We may add $5d.$ more for rent, and all other incidental expenses.

In the kind of dispensary suited for England, a thoroughly competent dispenser would be required, whose salary, on the whole, need not exceed $6d.$ per case.‡ This would bring the average cost of each case of sickness to $1s.$ $6d.$—which would fall, as it ought to do, upon the local rates.

The cost of dispensary establishments, and of medicines furnished to medical officers in rural districts, for the whole of England and Wales, would amount to $105,000l.$ per annum;—

---

* The duty of dispensing in Ireland generally falls upon the medical officer, but 40 out of the 720 dispensary districts are provided with apothecaries at an average salary of $43l.$

† Evidence, 1854, 2635.

‡ See *Dispensary Expenditure, Health and Sickness of Town Populations,* pp. 71 and 97—101.

assuming the correctness of the previous estimate of 1,400,000 cases of sickness among the poor who are not provided for in workhouses, hospitals, and charitable dispensaries, or by "self-supporting" associations.

If it be said that a more free provision of medical relief would tend to increase the number of cases, the reply is obvious;—all non-attended or imperfectly relieved sickness is a far greater expense to the public than the cost of its proper relief,—while an improved sanitary management of the people, such as is urged in these pages, would tend to reduce the public burdens in a vastly greater degree.

If, by wise measures of general policy, the ability and disposition of the working classes to provide medicines and dietetic remedies for themselves, were promoted, a still further reduction in the local charges would be effected.

VIII.—*As to the Medical Care of Workhouses.*

§ 31. Notwithstanding occasional instances of neglect, it may be safely affirmed that, on the whole, the treatment of the sick, in Union workhouses and other establishments under the control of the Poor-Law authorities, is adequately provided for, and carefully performed.

There seem to be no such reasons for suggesting organic changes in this department, as in that of attendance upon districts. The in-door paupers are a separate class, maintained wholly by the poor-rates, and subject, in every respect, to the authorities appointed by law to regulate the expenditure of those rates.

There may be, as there has been, serious sanitary mismanagement in some of these institutions. The inmates have been here and there sadly overcrowded.* Cleanliness has been

---

* The Workhouses planned in 1835 by the Poor-Law Commissioners were awful negations of the first principles of hygiéne. A rural workhouse, adopted by several of the Unions in Kent, on a plan devised by the eccentric Sir F. B. Head, allowed, on the average, only 117 cubic feet of breathing space to each

neglected. Drainage and ventilation have been, occasionally, very imperfect. Dietary tables have been not always wisely planned, nor judiciously applied to localities, climates and seasons, requiring very different ratios of nutriment and stimulation.

These and similar matters need the intervention of medical inspectors, to whom the surgeons also should be responsible for the due performance of preventive and curative duties;—and by whom they should be protected and supported in the fearless discharge of those duties.*

It is also important that a small and well-selected supply of medicines should be kept in every workhouse, under the charge of the master or other resident officers, for the sole use of the inmates; as has been recommended by the Inspectors of Prisons, for their inmates.

The poorer classes, residing in districts, should never be sent to workhouses for their medicines. The medical connexion between the *workhouse* and the *district* is one of those dangerous fetters which have hitherto bound the working classes to pauperism.

---

inmate of the dormitories. Even the larger and better-contrived Workhouses, supposing the rooms were ten feet high (although not even that height was insisted upon), allowed from 160 to 200 cubic feet per head for the ordinary dormitories; —less than 500, in the best wards, for "lying-in" patients;—and from 300 to 400 in the other sick wards.

About the same time, Motard and other foreign writers on State Medicine were recommending from 866 to 1040 cubic feet for each patient in hospital; and our own Prison Inspectors allowed 1000 for each prisoner!

It was a notion of certain Poor-Law sanitarians, that, by a sufficiently *rapid current* of fresh air, the smallest room might be rendered as wholesome as the largest room without proper ventilation:—a theory which, carried to the extreme then proposed, was not only absurd, but proved most pernicious to the unfortunate subjects of the experiment.

See also Dr. Maunsell's clever critique of Sir F. B. Head's plan, in his *Discourse on Political Medicine*, 1839, p. 44.

* Such flagrant cases as that of Dr. Semple, of Islington, surgeon to the parish infirmary, ought never to have been allowed in a civilized country. That gentleman was, only last year, driven from his post for reporting on the defective cubic space of the establishment, its want of classification, and the shocking state of its drainage and ventilation.

If therefore the medical provision for workhouses be left to Boards of Guardians, under proper inspection, there appears to be no sufficient reason for not defraying the salaries of their surgeons, as of their chaplains, wholly out of the local poor-fund.

I have estimated that the workhouse appointments, separated from the districts, would cost about 36,000*l.* per annum for the whole of England and Wales. Adding this estimate to that already made for dispensary establishments, there would be a total charge of about 141,000*l.* per annum upon the poor-rates of the several Unions. This would be in lieu of the existing charge made upon them for medical relief, which in 1853 was, we are told, half of 215,000*l.*;—and has since then increased.

On the whole, therefore, the adoption of the changes recommended in this Essay, would not materially increase the present cost of medical relief to the local rate-payers.

IX.—*As to the bearing of the Medical Charities of England upon the question of Poor-Law Medical Aid.*

§ 32. The munificent provision for the accommodation and treatment of disease and injury among the working classes, made in the hospitals and infirmaries of England, taken as a whole, is probably not surpassed in any country.

But until lately, it has so little affected the question at issue, that I need not have recurred to the subject,[*] had not these institutions been called upon, within the last few years, to aid in diminishing the Union supply of medical relief.

A barrister examined before the late Committee, showed how Boards of Guardians, taking advantage, as they were perfectly justified in doing, of a clause in a recent Act of Parliament,[†] made use of their hospital subscriptions, so as to appropriate an

---

[*] See the brief historical notice of English hospitals (p. 150);—and suggestions in the preceding Essay for their co-operation in a national registration of sickness.

[†] 14 and 15 Vic. 1851, c. 105, § 4.

undue share of the privileges mutually secured to the founders and supporters of those institutions.*

Governors of infirmaries may be said to have the remedy in their own hands, and perhaps they may use it, in rare instances; but those who know anything of the management and working of endowed or voluntary charities, can understand the great difficulty of resisting the pressure of legally-constituted representative bodies, and of checking the tendency of the present system to shift the burden of sickness among the poor from the public to charitably disposed individuals.†

These remarks apply, in a limited sense, to the *extern* department of our hospitals, but without reserve to all the charitable dispensaries of England.

§ 33. It would be going out of the way to dwell now upon certain radical defects in these voluntary arrangements for the relief of "out-patients;" but I have seen no reason to doubt the correctness of statements which were made on this head before the Select Committee of 1844,‡ and founded on Returns procured by the Provincial Association from forty large towns.

No judicious person, however, would propose to swamp or sap these dispensaries, merely to attain a nominal uniformity of system.

Nor, on the other hand, can any one doubt that sound measures of general hygiéne, and of special preventive visitation, would immensely diminish the demands made upon them,—perhaps render many of them wholly unnecessary.

So long as the duties of their honorary physicians and surgeons are confined to prescribing, at appointed times, for such as desire their advice, it is obvious that much valuable aid in the treatment of chronic cases can be rendered in this

---

* "The Board of Guardians subscribe and take from us [the Governors of the Infirmary] something which is, in fact, in aid of the general fund raised for the relief of the poor."—Kettle, Evidence (1854), 995.

† "If dispensaries are so constituted as to shift this burthen from the whole parish, and to impose it upon those only who are charitably disposed, they are insomuch objectionable."—The late Lord Clarendon.

‡ See Supplementary Note D.

way by an order of medical men who would not undertake the visitation of a district. And a very deserving class of poor, it is said, exists in most communities, to which it is found advisable to administer medical aid apart from a State provision. This class, indeed, would be very inconsiderable, if the State provision were not a "pauper" one. But however that might be, the benefit of charitable dispensaries ought to be confined to those objects and those methods of relief, for which they are essentially adapted. Such institutions can only be regarded as merciful auxiliaries in a good work. They cannot safely be relied on as substitutes for a national provision. Let them therefore never be pleaded as an excuse for neglecting a public duty!

As they now operate, they invite hostile criticism, if not public interference.

The entire want of unity of purpose and action among the several sources of medical aid in large towns, is extremely detrimental to the sick, while it inflicts needless expense on the community.

In the attempts, however heartless and supine, of the poor to obtain orders or tickets for medical aid, it has been shown that they suffer additional uncertainty, perplexity, and delay from the circumstance that the various provisions of aid are not only separate, but conflicting. Their interests are opposed.

Those poor "who, on the present theory, ought to be attended at the expense of the Union, are perpetually applying for assistance to charitable institutions; and the parish medical officers, who are required by their non-remunerative contracts to furnish medicines as well as attendance to the sick paupers, naturally feel disposed to acquiesce in the admission of these patients (chronic cases especially) at the dispensary or infirmary;"—which, in their turn, vainly endeavour "to limit their benefits to such as are not in the receipt of parochial relief."*

* In Supplementary Note D. will be found the published statements of the Governors of two provincial dispensaries on this point. That of the Huddersfield Dispensary applies to the whole class.

Thus, instead of anything like cordial co-operation, each medical-relief institution is constantly seeking to get rid of a portion of its liabilities, by throwing them upon the other; the poor being necessarily the victims of the struggle.

§ 34. Again, the labour of medical men practising among the poor is uselessly increased by the multiplicity of media through which their aid may be procured.*

A mere tyro in political economy knows that such waste of labour, and especially of skilled labour, creates an ultimate money loss to society.

The amount of professional exertion, which might be promptly and economically performed, in the same small district, at one time, by one responsible medico-sanitary visitor, is now imperfectly and casually distributed among several ill paid, or gratuitous and irresponsible, medical attendants; and, as a necessary result, many sick remain unvisited, and many precautions are neglected; disease extends, and lives are lost, or health permanently injured; all for want of what our Gallican friends call—Organization.†

It is said that·many of the existing dispensaries would readily co-operate with a national system; and thus save the cost of new establishments.

When the finances of charitable dispensaries are in a pre-

---

* The following description of the confusion existing in a provincial city, a few years since, may apply to many other places :—"Take, for instance, one of the thickly-inhabited lanes or courts of this city during any prevalent sickness. Some of the families succeed in obtaining orders for the attendance of the Union officers; others, with almost equal difficulty, procure recommendations to some of the medical charities, several physicians or surgeons of which may have patients in the same spot, at the same time. A few of the labourers and artisans belong to sick clubs, and are supposed to be attended by the medical contractors of their respective societies. Another portion of the residents receive gratuitous advice from private sources, or otherwise recklessly demand professional services, with the promise of remuneration, seldom if ever fulfilled. A still larger proportion, probably more than half the population, frequent the druggists' shops; diminishing their chances of recovery, and wasting their scanty resources upon improper remedies boldly administered by ignorant and unqualified persons."

† See Supplementary Note E.

carious condition, as is too commonly the case*—a condition from which they are rescued, if at all, by mere spasmodic efforts of bustling benevolence—they would not be likely to refuse a regulated contribution, from local authorities, for medicines supplied to each case of sickness attended by the district officers; even if a more methodical coalition were impracticable.

X.—*On the existing means of Directing and Inspecting medical duties among the Poor.*

§ 35. The real amount of benefit secured by subjecting medical officers to the control of Poor-Law Boards, and the necessity for a superior machinery for supervision, are questions which, as far as facts and arguments can decide them, have been already settled.

In the Third Essay, I remarked upon the very defective character of the customary medical returns and reports of pauper sickness, which are at the same time unnecessarily frequent and minute. We have briefly to consider the incompetence of the existing authorities to make any good use of important information, even were it afforded them.

Some evidence given in 1854, on this point, deserves notice.

Whilst the English Poor-Law Inspectors unanimously deprecated the appointment of *medical* authorities, they nevertheless admitted that there were no securities for the proper treatment of the sick, beyond the legal or nominal standard of qualification possessed by the medical officers† and the general trustworthiness of the Faculty; that there was no supervision of practice, except a cursory perusal by the Board of Guardians of the weekly sick lists presented to them, which led, in some instances, to further inquiry.

Mr. Austin exerted himself to defend an untenable position.

---

* Six or seven reports of Dispensaries for one year (1843) are quoted in the *Appendix to Report of Select Committee of* 1844 (p. 958), and show the desperate state to which their finances are liable to be reduced.

† Evidence, 126—7.

He thought that, although Boards of Guardians might not have any more scientific knowledge of the matter than himself, they are able " to detect, as they quickly do, that a case had remained under treatment too long."* If they thought it had, " they would require the attendance of the medical man before them." If, on the contrary, a rapid decease took place, without notorious neglect or mismanagement, the surgeon was of course released from further trouble and responsibility!

Notwithstanding the Inspector's ingenious and convincing proof of the competency of the Boards of Guardians to superintend the practice of their medical officers, those Boards do not seem to be equally confident of their own capacities.

It was a Guardian who proposed to the late Committee, that medical officers should be appointed by the Home Office, and responsible to it; and, at all events, "entirely independent of local influence."†

But, what is more to the purpose, the late Dr. Gavin, reporting to the General Board of Health in 1849, stated that—

" At an interview with the Board of Guardians of Bethnal Green, the chairman of the Board, who is a magistrate, expressed himself to the effect, that they were quite sick of having charge of the medical arrangements for the relief of the poor, and that they would be heartily glad to get rid of it. This statement was made deliberately, and appeared to be the unanimous feeling of the Board. Though expressed in consequence of the feeling of responsibility arising from the charge of the extraordinary arrangements imposed upon the Board by the prevalence of cholera, yet I know the opinion is the same with reference to *the ordinary superintendence of medical relief*."

Both of the Inspectors of the Poor Law Board, who were examined in 1854, felt themselves fully competent to direct inquiries into the conduct of medical officers. One of those gentlemen was, indeed, somewhat oblivious about the nature and

---

* Evidence, 306—8.
† Ibid. 1946—8.

Mr. Howman said, " *Under a different constitution of the Board of Guardians,* perhaps I might give them more power and more privileges."—Ibid. 2013.

results of the inquiries which he had held;* but the other was quite clear that he had been able to deal, without medical assistance, with every case he had been required to investigate.†

Throughout the whole country, complaints were said by Mr. Cane to be so rare, that the Poor-Law Board had found it quite sufficient to call in a superior physician or surgeon as assessor‡ in any case needing a scientific opinion. This had been done occasionally; but there was no necessity, he thought, for the constant employment of a medical man at the office of the Poor-Law Board. It would be a sinecure.‖

§ 36. Long ago, however, it was objected that medical opinions, procured for the nonce by the Poor-Law Board and Inspectors, at their own discretion, and selected in accordance with their personal preferences, are not calculated to satisfy the public or the profession.

But we have the means of meeting more directly the argument of the English Inspectors.

The Commissioner from Dublin was at hand to invalidate the self-complacent conclusions of his quondam colleagues. He had experienced the benefit of medical assistance.

He held, that to inquire and report upon complaints arising out of want of due attendance, was "a most important duty" for a *medical* inspector;¶ that the case-books and prescriptions of the medical officers constituted "a very important record"** to aid him in questions of alleged *mala praxis;* and he assured the Committee that the Poor-Law Board of Ireland had derived

---

* Evidence, 322. † Ibid. 341.
‡ Ibid. 34. See also Mr. Austin's case, 227.
‖ Ibid. 60. Yet it appears that, although complaints had very much diminished in number, there were no less than seven cases in 1853 in which the Poor-Law Board had required the resignation of a medical officer,—though not one in which they had formally dismissed the officer. It was rare indeed that a year had previously passed without a formal dismissal "of some medical officer or another" (Ibid. 43). Surely here was work for a medical authority.
¶ Ibid. 564. ** Ibid. 568.

"great advantage from the *medical* commissioner in the administration of the medical charities."*

When pressed, however, for his opinion as to the introduction of the Irish system of *medical* superintendence into England, he suggested that a Poor-Law Board, administering general outdoor relief on the English principle, would find immense difficulty in directing, at the same time, *a National Dispensary System*.† He was doubtless right.

This incompatibility of the two departments is the true reason for disconnecting extern medical relief from the Poor-Law administration, and therefore constitutes a sufficient objection to Dr. Wallis's proposal for a "Physician-in-chief" and medical "Curators" in connexion with the Poor-Law Board ;‡ a plan which was only another version of Sir T. N. Talfourd's and Mr. Guthrie's Medical Commissioner and Lord Shaftesbury's Medical Inspectors, and is thus fully open to the criticism already bestowed upon those older projects.

XI.—*As to the Sanitary Duties and Reports of the District Medical Officers.*

§ 37. Who would not rejoice to escape from the Stygian regions of pauperism and disease, "*superasque evadere ad auras,*" into the upper air and fresh breezes of Hygieia? And what weary traveller in this miry path has not been cheered and invigorated to proceed, when he first perceived that a machinery of rude device, and originally adapted for a mere *therapeia*, might be so improved in material and construction, as to become one of the most powerful agents in *prophylaxis*?

In the previous Essay (on Sanitary Inquiry) I endeavoured to

---

* Evidence, 588.   † Ibid. 576.

‡ Dr. Wallis may safely be left to settle with Mr. Guthrie whether the head of their Poor-Law medical department should be a physician or a surgeon. But one would like to hear the view taken by such men as Sir B. C. Brodie and Mr. Propert of Dr. Wallis's cool parallel between the respective grades in law—of barrister, attorney and law-stationer—with those in medicine—of physician, surgeon, and apothecary!!—See Dr Wallis's *New Design* &c., 1850 ; p. 29, note.

show that many momentous and perplexing questions in ætiology and prevention arise from time to time—questions both scientific and administrative—which can be solved only by a continuous, regular, and general collection of facts, to be reported by skilled and trained observers.

One of our chief *desiderata* is a Public Registration of Disease —a record which would apply equally to sporadic attacks and to epidemic visitations, and which would include all the local and physical circumstances connected with sickness.

The late Medical Council, appointed merely for a temporary purpose, have in their excellent Reports strongly urged the disadvantage of a system of inquiry and record which is not available in periods of immunity from unusual sickness, as well as in seasons of public alarm and excessive mortality.

The machinery for registration must be ready at hand and always at work. And such a machinery is already possessed by this nation.

The corps of district medical officers is, in most respects, and might become in all points, excellently qualified for forming the basis of a State Registration of Disease. That corps merely requires to be placed in its proper position, and to be re-organized in connexion with sanitary authorities.

At present, as I have before observed, the imperfect, though regular and laborious, records of sickness among the poor, are useless for the objects of scientific or philanthropic research.

The hard-worked and well-informed medical practitioner, toiling in a populous district, under a Board of Guardians, can think only with vexation of time and labour now wasted in mere pencraft, upon bundles of ruled paper, which serve no higher purpose than that of economical checks upon poor-rate expenditure.

How would his toil be lightened if he knew that his little spring of facts and observations ever ran on to swell the mighty river formed by four thousand such contributions; and that the benefits which medical science might confer upon his countrymen, would be increased, perhaps a hundred-fold, by the invaluable collection of those returns, their careful analysis and comparison, and their general publication; all which might be secured by that complete and effective organization to which he would then belong.

It is not my intention here to suggest those particular modifications and amendments in the periodical returns of the district medical officers, which would fit them for the purposes of a scientific registration of sickness, without diminishing their direct and immediate utility.

A few practical men, accustomed to parochial duty and to medical or sanitary inquiry, might soon devise suitable forms and schedules for these objects; and some valuable hints have been already offered on the subject.*

My design now is mainly to show that the poor being the chief and generally the earliest victims of epidemic invasions and of the neglect of sanitary precautions, their *medical* visitors are obviously the persons not only to notice, to collect, and to report on such facts, but practically to carry into effect all medical measures of prevention.

§ 38. To Mr. Chadwick belongs the credit of first pointing out the advantage which the public would derive from employing the medical attendants of districts in sanitary duties.†

This view was developed at greater length before Lord Ashley's Committee in 1844.‡ Mr. Liddle and others supported it with various facts and illustrations in 1848.‖ Mr. Simon, in most

---

* Mr. Liddle contributed a very good paper on this subject to the former *Journal of Public Health*, vol. i. p. 92. And the able Editor of the present Journal of that name has favoured me with a sight of some excellent suggestions on the same subject, which he offered in March last to the Epidemiological Society.

† "Were it practicable," said Mr. Chadwick in 1842, "to attach as numerous a body of paid officers to any local Boards of Health that could be established, it would scarcely be practicable to insure as certain and well-directed an examination of the residences of the labouring classes, as I conceive may be insured from the medical officers of the Unions."—*General Sanitary Report*, 1842, p. 343.

‡ Evidence (1844), 9361, &c.: also, *Health and Sickness of Town Populations*, p. 53, &c.

‖ *Journal of Public Health*, 1848, vol. i. pp. 92, 158.

apt and eloquent terms, urged it upon the civic authorities of London in 1849.*

We have already seen the manner in which the preventive and remedial services of medical officers were demanded in the cholera epidemic of 1848-9, how admirably they were performed, and how miserably they were requited.

With regard to more permanent sanitary functions, not depending on temporary emergencies, Mr. Kingsley's plain yet striking statement was as follows:—

"My own feeling is that the Medical Officer having been made a sanitary officer now, it becomes a question whether we can help looking on him as permanently such, because the Nuisances Removal Act makes him one of the public informers.

"There is no one thing which affects the condition of the medical officers of Unions now so much as the duties imposed upon them by that Act . . . In any improvements in the present medical relief, *that* connects itself with the pith and marrow of the whole matter . . . affecting the position of medical officer, and the question of his salary, because it imposes new and very onerous and very invidious duties upon him."†

The appointment, under any sanitary enactment, of "Inspectors of Nuisances,"—or, as they ought to be called in homely Saxon, "Searchers,"—could only relieve the Medical Officer of a small portion of those inquisitorial and preventive duties which he is the most competent person to perform. Besides, as the same clerical philanthropist observed with respect to mere nuisances, "they are known to the Medical Officer better than to any man;—it is he who must tell the Inspector in the long run."‡ A common searcher would often fail to detect them.

§ 39. But there are much higher functions of a preventive

---

* See Simon *On the Sanitary Condition of the City of London.* 1854, pp. 62—64.

† Evidence (1854), 1572.

‡ Ibid. 1578.

Mr. Leigh, also, the able Medical Registrar of Manchester, gave his opinion, that the district medical officers would make the best—the most practically useful—Health Inspectors.—Evidence, 2253.

nature* than those of a mere "public informer," which the district Medical Officer ought to perform.

He should become the sanitary adviser of the poor in their dwellings. Many removable causes of sickness within their own control would be pointed out during his beneficent visits. The miserable effects of alcoholic stimulation might be impressed on the minds of sufferers from intemperance, at times when no warnings or counsel save those of a *medical* visitor would be listened to.

The state of the apartments of the poor, their clothing and bedding, the choice and preparation of their food, the physical management of their children, their nursing in sickness,— would all come occasionally under his cognizance. He would often be the first to detect unwholesome occupations or trades in the neighbourhood, by their effects on those under his charge. In the execution of his ordinary duties, he might often be led to suspect the adulteration or impurity or decay of some article of food, or the deleterious quality of some pretended medicine or falsified drug taken by the poor;—and if the precise cause of mischief were beyond his means of detection, he would direct the attention of the superior Officer of Health, or the local administrative body, to the matter.

Injuries sustained in factories and other employments, for which the law provides a remedy, and which might never transpire but for his observation, would be reported by him to the authorities. His opinion would often decide a knotty question of sanitary improvement between the working man and his landlord. His information, not less than his mediation, would be of the highest value, both to the poor and to the local Boards of Health. He should always be *the* Vaccinator of the district, whoever else might assist in carrying that measure into effect.

---

* "The very responsible duties of active sanitary inspection, in conjunction with those of vigilant supervision of the health of the different districts, are thus devolved upon those who, by their local knowledge, and their professional avocations, can most efficiently discharge them; thus making a first, but most important step towards the formation of a health police."—*Times, Nov.* 1854.

Advice as to the removal and interment of the dead, and protection of the survivors, in zymotic disease, would also be his province in ordinary times.

I do not mean that he should perform those duties, which belong, as will hereafter be shown, to a Medical Superintendent or consulting Officer of Health, in a district of districts. But he would be, in a peculiar sense, the Missionary of Health in his own parish or district — instructing the working classes in personal and domestic hygiéne—and practically proving to the helpless and the debased, the disheartened and disaffected, that the State cares for them,—a fact of which, until of late, they have seen but little evidence.

I have no hesitation in affirming that a well-organized domiciliary visitation, to be performed by a medico-sanitary staff, whose duty and interest it would be to raise the standard of health in their respective districts, would be a much more effectual step than any yet adopted, towards diminishing the rate of sickness and mortality, and averting the consequences (as injurious to society at large, as to the individual) of neglected ailments, by attention to their causes and premonitory stages.

XII.—*As to the Qualifications, Number, Salaries, and Appointment of District Medico-Sanitary Officers.*

§ 40. It is not enough that the existing body of Union surgeons have proved their ready capability for a wider and higher sphere of duty, under the pressure and during the perils of recent pestilences.

The special qualifications needed for such an office as I have described in the preceding section, ought to be insured and tested in all future appointments. As vacancies occur in this corps, they should, as a general rule, be filled up by those only, whose theoretical knowledge of various branches of preventive medicine has been ascertained by such legally constituted examining bodies, as have been recommended in the Second

Essay; and who have also been practically trained for employment in the public service under officers already appointed.

An ordeal of this kind is as necessary for the Civil Medical Service* as it is for the Military or Naval; and it deserves consideration whether special, if not competitive,† examinations should not follow upon the general examination, and licence which forms the portal of the profession.

The AGE of those elected to district appointments is another important element in their qualification.

In Ireland, the Dispensary Commissioners have wisely raised the minimum of age to twenty-three years.‡ If, as I have before suggested, the age required for the licence, simply to practise, were twenty-three, an additional period of two years of study and experience would very properly be demanded of candidates for the full District Surgeoncy.

To render that further period of probation of the greatest public utility, it would be advisable to permit those young men who had acquired the State licence, to act officially, as unpaid deputies, or supernumeraries, in districts, until they had attained the age of twenty-five, and were elected to a vacancy in the higher charge.‖

§ 41. The *number* of officers needs to be augmented by a further diminution in the extent of the Visitation Districts, which require revision throughout the kingdom.

Their original faultiness, — namely, non-adaptation to the medical and sanitary wants of the people,—has been remedied, in some measure, by the failure of inconsiderate and mischievous arrangements; but, together with the establishment of public dispensaries, and liberation from poor-law control, many terri-

---

* Papers on the Re-organization of the Civil Service, Mr. Chadwick, p. 171.

† Competitive examinations are again noticed in the Sixth Essay.

‡ General Rules for Dispensary Districts—Ireland, Art. 16, II.—See *First Annual Report*, p. 46.

‖ Mr. Kingsley urged the importance of experience and *a knowledge of the locality* for several years, in taking charge of the general health of a district.—Evidence (1854), 1599. Hippocrates was of the same opinion.

torial changes of great practical utility might be made in medical districts, with reference to the sanitary and registration divisions of the country.

I have seen no reason to think that my original estimate* of 4000 medical districts is at all too large.

This would, in most places, allow two medical visitation districts to one registration district; and to each surgeon an average population of 4500. Preventive and remedial duties among the poor of such a population would be amply sufficient to occupy as large a portion of his time as the public could remunerate, even were his toils lightened by a deputy or supernumerary.

In large towns, where the inhabitants have abundant choice of medical advice, the office might be made independent of private practice, as suggested by Mr. Liddle, and under such an arrangement a larger population would be included.

But even in those instances the Bristol error† must be shunned; and throughout the greater part of England, it would be found most conducive to the public advantage to proceed in that course of reform which has been pursued for the last fifteen years;‡ and to divide the country among an increased number of medical officers who are engaged in private practice.

I repeat this, because Mr. Simon's evidence, before the Committee on the Adulteration of Food, would lead one to infer that an official scheme is preparing for a general separation of medical

---

* *Health and Sickness of Town Populations*, p. 73.

† See p. 229.

‡ The last official attempt to oppose this reform was made by the author of the *General Sanitary Report*, in 1842. "Whatever," said he, in that Report, p. 354, "may yet be required for placing the Union medical officers on a completely satisfactory footing, the combination of the services of several parish doctors in the service of fewer Union medical officers will be found to be advances in a beneficial direction." These "advances" have fortunately long ceased; and the principle for which Mr. Chadwick so long and so ardently contended has been proved inapplicable to a therapeutic office.

It is nevertheless perfectly true and extremely beneficial, when applied to the higher preventive grade of office, of which the next Essay treats.

attendance on the poor from that on other classes of society. He supposes that—

"Eventually there will be a set of public officers distributed through the country, *having no private practice*, but attending entirely to the sick poor and matters of public health."*

We need not go back to John Bellers, in 1715, for a conclusive objection to this project;† Mr. Ceely's admirable remarks in 1844, ought to determine the question:—

"I think that the union of private with public practice is desirable; first, that it is more satisfactory to the poor; secondly, that it is beneficial to them to have the advantage of the long and varied experience of established practitioners; thirdly, that it is beneficial to the rate-payers on the same grounds; it is equally beneficial to the rate-payers also to have the advantage of medical experience gained from an attendance on the poor, more particularly during the prevalence of epidemics, which generally attack the poor early, and in large numbers; and [the separation of the appointment from private practice] is more expensive (particularly in rural districts) if the districts are of the proper size."‡

The more wealthy classes ought not to be deprived of the advantages which belong to the patients of an order of practitioners so usefully qualified, and with such large opportunities of experience, as the district Medical Staff.

§ 42. When the vexed question of remuneration shall have been simplified by charging the cost of medicines and surgical apparatus upon a dispensary establishment, and by separating the workhouse appointments from the district office, it may easily be settled.

We see that in 1853 the district salaries alone amounted to about 180,000*l.*,|| including the cost of medicines. It should be raised at once to 200,000*l.*, exclusive of the dispensary provision; allowing, on the average, 50*l.* to each of the proposed 4000 districts, for attendance only, beside fees for midwifery and vaccination.

If all the preventive functions which have been stated to per-

* *First Report*, Minutes of Evidence, 866. † See p. 149.
‡ *Medical Relief Report* (1844), p. 604. || See p. 240.

tain theoretically to this appointment were committed to the officer, a salary of 50*l.*, or even 75*l.*, for a population of 4500, even with private practice, would be wholly inadequate. But it would be a considerable advance upon the present rate of remuneration,* and a step towards an endowment more worthy of so wealthy a nation.

The prospect of promotion to the higher post† of Superintending Officer of Health would be some compensation for a salary which, while paid out of public funds, will always be inferior to the deserts of the office.

But if the laws of England sufficiently encouraged and protected permanent endowments for the medico-sanitary care of parishes or districts, I hope and believe that there are landed proprietors, manufacturing and mining millionaires, and merchant princes, who would rejoice in being afforded such an opportunity of providing permanently and adequately for the welfare of the working people, by whose vigorous and willing toil their wealth increases, and on whose physical, moral, and social improvement their very safety depends.

The precise apportionment of salaries paid out of public funds to the respective districts, about which so much ink has been wasted, is too generally considered with reference merely to pauperism and to curative duties.

All such paltry calculations would be set aside under a sanitary rule.

A salary varying inversely with the density of population, as proposed by Dr. Wallis, involves another hygienic anomaly; though there is much to be said for it in rural districts.

On the whole, the suggestion‡ for which I was indebted to Dr. Farr is the most reasonable and generally applicable; namely, that the calculation should be based on the number of houses

---

* In 1853, 59*l.* was paid, on the average, for a population of 5700; the doctor having to defray the cost of medicines and appliances, which on the proposed arrangement would be borne by the public.

† See Fifth and Sixth Essays.   ‡ Evidence (1844), p. 598.

under a certain rental, say 10*l*., the salary being subject to a fixed rate of augmentation in thinly-populated districts.

§ 43. As to the fund from whence these salaries should be paid.

All the foregoing facts, arguments, and suggestions are utterly inconsistent with a system which would leave any portion of the district medical salary chargeable upon the rates of the locality.

The office would become one of State relations, and should be in no way dependent on the locality. The Rev. Mr. Oxenden had no idea of " paying medical men out of the parochial rates." "*I look upon this*," said he, "*as a national act.*"*

The Consolidated Fund at present bears more than 100,000*l*. of the annual medical expenditure of the unions.

I propose that, in lieu thereof, it should bear the whole 200,000*l*. to be paid to the medico-sanitary staff.

One very sufficient reason (not before mentioned) for the change is, that those districts in which a more than average ratio of destitution, a larger proportion of cottages, and a generally unhealthy condition would render the duties of this office the more arduous, and would therefore justify a higher remuneration, are, owing to those very conditions, the least able to defray the charge of the office. It would be quite enough for the rate-payers of such a locality to bear the cost of the *materiel*.

The transfer of the medical salaries to the consolidated fund, or to a separate rate levied uniformly on the whole country, would also remove the principal difficulty, which the Poor-Law Board has always felt, in issuing instructions for the equitable determination of these salaries.†

§ 44. The estimated cost of the medico-sanitary appointments would include a composition for surgical fees.‡

Midwifery, however, should continue a matter for separate

---

* Evidence, 1514.

† See note, p. 177. Other difficulties there mentioned would be removed by the General Dispensary Provision suggested in these pages, and by the facilities which that provision would afford to Insurance Societies for the supply of medicines to their sick members.

‡ See p. 178.

arrangement, because it is a distinct branch of medical practice, and because, as a matter of State policy, it would be undesirable to lead the wives of labourers to rely, as a matter of course, on public aid in natural and ordinary emergencies.

What the country most needs in this respect, is the provision of a thoroughly instructed class of midwives, as on the continent.* If the path to such employment were judiciously opened, many well-educated women in the middle classes would prepare themselves, by a proper course of study and hospital practice, for examination and licence by an obstetrical Board.†

§ 45. Supposing all the previous conditions fulfilled, there would be no plea whatever for leaving the power of appointment in the hands of Boards of Guardians.

The last General Order, which merely removes from those Boards the power of dismissal, is insufficient to secure the due independence of the medico-sanitary corps on poor-law control.

It may not be advisable to go so far in the centralizing direction as the clerical Guardian,‡ who proposed to leave the appointment to the Home Office.

Nor can we hope that the Parliament of England will admit the lofty principle of the Roman Civil Law. The remarkable edict, which serves as a motto for this Essay, committed the duty of selection to those who had already attained to the dignity of the Popular Medical Office, the Imperial sanction to the Collegiate act being alone required.

It was in Rome and its dependencies, that the poorest of the people, the inhabitants of the upper stories of the *Insulæ*, the

---

* The present fee of 10s. paid by Boards of Guardians to the Union Medical Officer is degrading and inadequate, yet a fee of only 7s. would remunerate a well-trained female midwife; whilst the difference between 7s. and 10s., on a multitude of cases, would much more than provide consultation fees of 2l. 2s. for medical men, called in to difficult and exceptional cases.

† Sir G. Cornewall Lewis, in 1844, made some valuable suggestions on this head, in which I beg mainly to concur. Evidence, 9822—9825.

‡ Evid. (1854), 1946.

Cænacularii, shared with the household of Cæsar the services of an honourable Iatrarchy. It was there that the baneful influence of local patronage and magisterial favour was prohibited, —*non patrocinio Præponentium, non gratiâ Judicantis.* It was there that the honest and circumspect choice of a learned body was judged to be the best safeguard for the public welfare.

These principles are still in operation in Belgium.*

But to look homewards: we may, at all events, be excused for requiring some gentle restraints to be placed upon the pranks and caprices of the representatives of rate-payers.

The power of appointment should at least be shared between local and superior courts. And it is most desirable to bring influences and motives of a high order to bear upon those who may exercise the primary duty of selection or recommendation in each locality.

Whether this object may not be attained in great measure by the constitution about to be suggested for Dispensary Committees and local Courts or Boards of Health, may be left to the judgment of the reader. And it is to one or both of these bodies, with the assent of the medical faculty of the neighbourhood, that it is proposed to leave the power of appointment.†

XIII.—*On the Constitution of Local Bodies for the Management of the proposed Public Dispensaries.*

§ 46. The Irish system makes these committees mere offsets of the Boards of Guardians. The nomination and addition of certain heavy rate-payers does not alter their peculiar character. Dr. Wallis's proposed introduction of the parochial clergy‡ (the magistrates are already *ex officio* Guardians) would be a decided improvement, but it might rouse the *odium theologicum* of the

---

* See Supplementary Note E.
† The organization by which the District Office should be connected with the Central Sanitary Council will be considered in the following Essays.
‡ This was originally proposed by Mr. Ceely in 1844. Evidence, 9400.

district, unless accompanied by some such compensation to the religious "denominations," as I am about to suggest in the formation of a new and superior kind of local sanitary courts.*

My own proposal† was, simply to combine the scientific and philanthropic elements with that of financial control.

As the cost of dispensaries would be charged upon the rates of the Union, the Guardians would, with the greatest propriety, nominate a certain proportion of the members of each Dispensary Committee, as in Ireland. But I propose that voluntary benefactions should be encouraged, by conferring on subscribers and donors of certain sums, the privilege of electing another portion of the Committee,‡ which should bear the same numerical ratio to the nominees of the Guardians as the total amount of income from voluntary sources might bear to the annual charge upon the poor-rates.

A certain injudicious method of combining voluntary contributions with a public tax for the support of dispensaries, once failed, as we have seen, in Ireland; but this fact does not, in the slightest degree, warrant the inference that every other method of combining these elements of income must be always and everywhere objectionable or unsuccessful. On the contrary, we have in England a remarkable group of examples of the success of such a combination, in our flourishing County Lunatic Asylums.

A third portion of the Dispensary Committee should consist of a limited and proportionate number of persons, well known in the neighbourhood for their general intelligence, scientific attainments, or philanthropic pursuits.

They should be selected by those local administrative bodies, which I propose to be constituted for the sanitary management of every part of the kingdom. They might either be members of such bodies, or other persons appointed by them.

* Fifth Essay, † Evidence (1854), 2036.
‡ A similar principle was recommended by the Parliamentary Committee on the Medical Charities of Ireland in 1843, and advocated in the debate of 1851 by Mr. Vesey and Mr. Sidney Herbert.—See p. 207.

A fourth portion of the Dispensary Committee should consist of one or two medical assessors, nominated by the medical faculty of a larger jurisdiction.*

§ 47. The Dispensary Committees ought to meet weekly, and oftener in times of pestilence.

Ordinarily, their duties would be to maintain a proper stock of medicines and remedial appliances at the institution, under regulations to be made by a central Council—to provide the surgeons of remote parishes or dependent rural districts with necessary drugs, unless a pecuniary allowance be made them for drugs consumed;—to appoint the Dispenser, and to inspect his entries and proceedings; to examine the register of patients, and to demand compensation for medicines, &c., supplied to persons who in the judgment of the Committee ought not to receive them gratuitously;† to employ nurses for the sick, under the direction of the Medical Officers; and to regulate the financial affairs of the institution.

In times of epidemic visitation, the Dispensary Committee would be the fittest authority to provide additional medical aid, if required by the district officers; and to form additional depôts, open day and night, for the prompt supply of remedies to the sufferers.

All poor persons,‡ having any ground of complaint against the district attendant, the dispenser, or the nurse, would make it to this Committee. It should be entered on their minutes; an explanation should be required from the person accused; and the statements of both parties should be referred, with the opinion of the Committee, to the Superior Sanitary Court, and to the Medical Inspector of the Circuit, for a decision, or for further inquiry.

---

* See First and Second Essays, pp. 43, 81.
† Strict demand would be made in a prescribed form, and enforced, if necessary, by legal process.
‡ Evidence, Dr. Wallis, 2830.

Conclusion.

§ 48. In concluding this Essay, I would briefly recall attention to circumstances which appear to have led to a strange misconception, current in England, with regard to the nature and objects of a public system of sanative care and regulation.

The notion prevails, and has long prevailed—that "medical relief," as we call it, is a commodity,—that it consists in a supply of "physic"—that it is an article to be procured, like food or clothing, for a specific necessity—and, therefore, that it may be provided, like any other comfort or convenience of life, by ordinary traffic, as between buyer and seller.

It has become the identical "*rem*" which, Pliny said, the Roman republicans "*non damnabant*," though, like our rulers, they rejected the "*artem*."*

The early condition of the Faculty in England may account for our traditional error. Coevally with a fearful ratio of mortality and sickness, and a brief average term of life, there was for centuries in this country a scarcity of fully educated physicians and surgeons far exceeding any deficiency in Italy, France, Germany, or Spain.

The people, therefore, had no help for it but to recognise and employ, as their medical advisers, apothecaries, who lived by the sale of their wares.

The healing art thus came to mean the sale and administration of medicines; and, conversely, the purchase of pills, potions, and plasters, became the provision of medical aid. Hence arose the "bills" of parish doctors, and then—parish contracts.

Hence, sensible people talked about an indiscriminate supply of medical "relief" producing pauperism; not, indeed, for the true reasons—that it involved an application to the overseer and a grant of "relief" in money or food, and that the doctor was one of the "Bumble" staff; but, forsooth, because it was a thing,

---

* Pliny, *Hist. Nat.* lib. xxix. c. 8.

(the "rem" again) which the independent poor ought to provide for themselves. Hence, also, accomplished writers like Sir J. P. K. Shuttleworth thought that charitable dispensaries pauperized the working classes, because medicines were in this way distributed without being paid for by the patients. Hence reasoners, as acute and logical as Sir G. C. Lewis, said:—

"Medical care is one of those things which each person provides for himself, according to his class in society. The highest class provide a better sort of medical attendance than the middle class; and the middle class better than the poorest class." *

Happily for the poor, and for society in general, his view of the case is not acted upon in the charitable institutions of England. The medical advice supplied to the poorest classes, in our great hospitals and dispensaries, comes, with occasional exceptions, from the same order of practitioners as that consulted by the highest classes of society.

Placing medical attendance in the light of a more correct analogy, one might as well urge that an inferior kind of moral and religious instruction, and a less amount of legal security against personal aggression, are the inevitable lot of the poor.† As well might the State profess to administer justice according to the means of the party seeking it. As well might education be limited to those who can afford to pay for it. At any rate, few statesmen would avow such principles, whatever may be our defects in practice on these points.

If it be in any case "the duty of the State to establish equal rights," as the learned Commissioner admitted,‡ it is pre-eminently so in matters of public salubrity, where the welfare of the whole community depends on the protection afforded to each individual. If, on the other hand, medical care be "one of those things which each person is to provide for himself according to his class in society," then it follows that the parochial provision is already too good, for no one doubts that the present

---

* Evidence (1844), 9834, p. 687.
† *Health and Sickness of Town Populations*, p. 32.   ‡ Ibid. *loc. cit.*

supply of medical advice to the pauper is very far superior to that which the independent labourer could procure by his own unaided efforts.

To sweep away these popular fallacies, and to revert to clear and just notions of the objects of a public sanative provision, we must get rid—first, of its Poor-Law connexion,—next, of the drug-supply by medical officers.

It will then be seen, that an efficient national establishment,—for visiting the sick, tending the wounded, soothing pain, and restoring health,—yet further, for preventing diseases by scientific expedients, and for instructing the people, at their houses, how to preserve health and prolong a useful life,—can no more degrade or pauperize the persons thus benefited, than enlarging their knowledge by public lectures, free libraries and museums,—training and disciplining their minds by endowed schools and colleges,—instilling the truths and morals of Christianity by pastoral visits and ministrations,—protecting them from personal injury by a police force and a magistracy,—or defending them by Counsel in courts of law, when threatened with the forfeiture of liberty or life.

Will any one have the boldness to affirm that the last-mentioned public provisions tend to lower the independence and self-reliance of the gratuitous recipients?

Neither, then, will medical attendance and sanitary advice have such an effect when freed from their pauperizing concomitants and associations.

The real cure, both for the perverted idea and for the practical evils to which it has led, is what in substance we recommended eleven years ago—namely, to connect medical duties among the poorer classes with the preventive visitation of districts,—to separate the drug-provision,—and to place the renovated office under professional supervision, co-operating with highly qualified Central and Local Councils of Health.

ESSAY V.

LOCAL SANITARY ADMINISTRATION.

"Speramus enim et cupimus futurum, ut id plurimorum bono fiat; atque ut medici nobiliores animos nonnihil erigant, neque toti sint in curarum sordibus; neque solum propter necessitatem honorentur, sed fiant demum Omnipotentiæ et Clementiæ Divinæ administri, in vitâ hominum prorogandâ et instaurandâ; presertim cùm hoc agatur per vias tutas et commodas, et civiles, licet intentatas."

BACON. *Hist. Vitæ et Mortis.*

ESSAY V.

CHAPTER FIRST.

Officers of Health; their Primary Design and Function.

§ 1. An Office, most beneficial in its design, yet anomalous in its relations both to the community and to the medical profession has existed for a short time in a few towns of England and Wales. In no other civilized country, nor at any former period of history—it may be safely affirmed—have similar appointments been made.

§ 2. The States of Ancient Greece and Asia Minor maintained famous physicians for public duties, at the public cost.

Such, say some, was Hippocrates at Athens. Such, also, was Democedes successively at Ægina, Athens, and Samos.[*]

Plato held that the Government of the commonwealth was not complete without the Æsculapian element; "for," added he, "is it not necessary to provide good physicians for the State, and must not these be, for the most part, such as have been conversant with the greatest number of healthy and sick people?"[†]

"It was quite common, in ancient times," says one of the most learned men of our day, "for the Asclepiadæ to be publicly consulted by cities and States respecting the general health of

---

[*] Herod. *Thalia,* 125—131.
[†] The original passage is prefixed to the Introductory Essay.

the inhabitants, and this, both for the prevention and cure of diseases."*

§ 3. The Romans under the Republic, on the contrary, scouted the healing art, refused to recognise its prophylactic office, expelled the Greek medical philosophers,† and reduced practitioners of medicine to a servile condition.

Under the first Cæsars, however, the profession was released from its degradation,‡ and a reaction followed, as extreme in the opposite direction. The embellishment of Naples, and the fortifications of Marseilles∥ bore witness to the enormous wealth, not less than to the munificence and public spirit of successful Roman physicians in the first and second centuries.

But another century had scarcely passed, when the people, disgusted with the venality and extortion of the private doctors—regulars and irregulars¶—and confused by the noisy pretensions of conflicting medical sects, were fain to take refuge in a municipal organization of the authorized faculty.

Antoninus Pius seems to have been the first to appoint physicians to towns, the number being regulated in each place by the population.** The elder Valentinian and Valens,†† at all events, confirmed with greater privileges the colleges of *Archiatri populares* in Rome, Constantinople, and other chief cities.‡‡

These officers do not appear to have been debarred from private practice, although the object of their public appointment —the care of the poor—for which they received yearly stipends, was made paramount.

They were not permitted by the civil law to receive specific remuneration, promised for cure during the alarm and peril of

---
* Adams's *Life of Hippocrates*, p. 13.
† Pliny, *Hist. Nat.* lib. xxix. c. 8.   See Supplementary Note F.
‡ Sueton. *Vit. Cæsar.* c. 42.
∥ Pliny, *Hist. Nat.* lib. xxix. c. 5.   ¶ Ibid.
** Sprengel, *Geschichte der Arzneik.* Theil ii. s. 218. Digest (Juris Civilis), lib. xxvii. tit. 1. De excusation. leg. vi. § 1.
†† *Cod. Theod. De Medicis et Professoribus*, lib. xiii. tit. 3, leg. 8, 9, 13.
‡‡ Frank *Med. Pol.* Band 6, s. 157.

sickness; but they might be retained, and their attendance secured under agreement by persons in good health.*

This was a measure of prevention, however imperfect; and the people were thus provided with the best medical care and sanitary advice which the age could afford.

§ 4. Some remains of the Roman Iatrarchy descended to the Mediæval Western Empire; and the towns of Italy, in the fifteenth century, are said to have had their *Medici condotti.*

Such, it seems, was the learned Veronese, Alexander Benedictus† (Benedetti), who, after distinguished services in the army, was appointed to the public charge of Padua.

Probably he held the same office as the learned Kaye (who advanced Gonvil Hall, Cambridge, into the College which now bears his name,) mentions in the following passage:‡—

"Wishīg for the better executiō hereof and ouersight of good and helthsome victalles, ther wer appointed certein Masters of Helth in euery citie and toune, as there is in Italie, whiche for the good order in all thynges, maye be in al places an example."

In the earlier part of the same century (1440) the office of *Meister Arzt*, or chief doctor, had been created by the Emperor Sigismund, in every imperial city, with a salary from the ecclesiastical revenues, and a solemn charge to the person appointed, to attend the poor gratuitously, and to earn his stipend by a zealous and faithful discharge of duty.‖ This enactment is,

* "Quos etiam ea patimur accipere, quæ sani offerunt pro obsequiis, non ea, quæ periclitantes pro salute promittunt." See the Edict of Valentinian and Valens, a part of which serves for a motto to the second part of Essay IV.

† Schroeckh's *Kirchen Geschichte,* Band xxx.

‡ "A Boke or Counseill against The Sweate, or Sweating Sicknesse, made by Jhon Caius, Doctour in Physicke," 1552.—See Hecker's *Epid. Sydenham Soc.,* 1844, p. 369.

‖ This curious Edict of Sigismund has been thus translated from its barbarous original.—"Generally, in every imperial city there shall be a *Meister Arzt,* who shall have a salary of 100 gulden. He may receive it out of some church endowment, as was ordained in the Council of Lyons. Let not, however, that church incur any damage on this account, but let it stand higher in estimation (*in der ordnung*). The *Meister Arzt* shall supply (?) medicines gratuitously, and shall earn his living zealously and faithfully. Nevertheless, if any [sick persons] require costly however, characterized by the same objurgatory tone towards the faculty, which has been noticed in the old English Statute of Henry the Eighth.*

Nuremberg appointed a *Stadt-arzt* in 1518,† and the office became general in the free towns of Germany before the end of the sixteenth century.‡

John Evvich, the *Medicus Ordinarius* of Bremen, published, in 1582, a singular book, entitled, *De officio fidelis et prudentis Magistratûs in tempore Pestilentiæ*. His notions about the constitution of sanitary authorities are sound, and his advice to the Government marked by much good sense and right feeling. His practical suggestions, also, are not underserving of notice, even in a more enlightened age. His plea for dedicating this work on preventive medicine to the civic authorities, was a sense of public duty as salaried adviser of the State.||

§ 5. The duties of the *Stadt-arzt*, or town doctor, were formerly partly of a prophylactic, partly of a therapeutic character.

The office, in some parts of Germany, is now merged in that of the District Physician (*Kreis-physicus*) and in others made subordinate to it.

As civilization has progressed, the duties have become more distinctly those of inspection and prevention,—yet always with definite relations to the duties of other medical office-bearers.

articles from the apothecary (*appentek*) they must pay for them. But the poor shall pay nothing. For on their account he is to receive his stipend.

"It is blessed to share God's gifts with the poor. But as for the high masters in physic (*meister in physica*) they practise fraudulently merely for gain. They attend on nobody unpaid. So they are going to hell.

"Some receive a stipend and enjoy it undeservedly; therefore, be it ordained, that no physician be hereafter allowed a stipend unless he swear to keep the rules formerly ordered by the Council."—Frank. *Med. Pol.* Band vi. § 173—5.

* 34 and 35 Hen. VIII. cap. 8. See Essay IV. p. 146.
† Niemann, *Med. Pol.* § 5.
‡ At Frankfort am Oder in 1503; at Brandenburgh in 1550; at Berlin in 1580. —Rönne and Simon, *Preussichen Medicinal Wesen*. Breslau, 1844, Th. i. s. 115.
|| "Quippe in quorum ditione, jam prope annos 18, medicinam faciendo, stipendio mihi imprimis observandæ Reipublicæ Bremensis consumsi, vitæque meæ terminum quodammodo fixi, ut a quibus plurimum acceperim beneficii, iisdem redderem quantum possum, officii."—p. 10.

A succinct and intelligible description of the modern appointments of *Kreis-* and *Stadt-physicus*, and indeed of the whole medical polity in the different States of Germany, is still a desideratum in the literature of Hygiéne.

At present, however, it is more to my purpose merely to mention, that in Prussia these officers were originally appointed by the local magistracy, subject to the approval of the State *collegium medicum* as to their qualifications.*

In 1809, the choice of town doctors and surgeons was committed to the Assembly of the City Delegates, subject to similar conditions. But the plan did not answer, and the permission was soon revoked; for its consequences convinced the Government that actual detriment to the public welfare might reasonably be apprehended from an arrangement which placed health officers, belonging entirely to the general polity† of the State, "in a position of dependence on the locality, incompatible with their efficiency."‡ It was also considered, that the variety of functions and correlations of such an appointment, rendered the city delegates unfit judges of the qualifications necessary for the office,‖ which was, properly speaking, a national, rather than a municipal affair; and it was said that the towns did not ask for the preventive *Stadt-physicus*, being already empowered to provide for their own medical wants.¶

The same consideration bore on the appointment of the district physician, *Kreis-physicus;* and in 1812, his election by district councils, *Kreis-stände*, was also superseded by the direct appointment of Government.

§ 6. Without exclusive reference to the regulations of any particular State, it may be observed, in general, that the *Kreisphysicus* has to superintend**—

---

* Rönne and Simon, vol. i. p. 116.
† "Polizei" has a much wider signification in Germany than "Police" in England.
‡ "Für ihre Wirksamkeit nicht zuträgliche Abhängigkeit."
‖ Royal decree, Jan. 30, 1810.—Rönne, p. 117.   ¶ Ibid. vol. i. p. 260.
** Niemann, s. 36—52. Rohatsch, *Handbuch für die Physikats Verwaltung*, 1846.

i. The general sanitary condition of his district;

ii. The medical treatment of the sick poor; in some States, attending personally; in others (where the *Kreis* is larger) inspecting the curative duties, the vaccination, &c. performed by the district surgeons—*Land-ärzte* and *Wund-ärzte;*

iii. Hospitals and houses of recovery, mineral baths, foundling and orphan institutions, poor-houses, prisons and houses of correction, schools and colleges, and police force, so far as relates to the *hygiène* of these establishments.

iv. During epidemics and epizöotics, the *Kreis-physicus* is to furnish instructions for health preservation, for attendance on the sick, and for general management; and to superintend their execution. In this department he is often aided by the surgeon —*Kreis-wundarzt,* and the veterinarian of the district—*Kreisthierarzt.* Although regarded as equal in official rank with the Magistrate or *Land-rath* of the *Kreis,* he is to receive all necessary directions from him, and to carry them into effect;

v. He is to promote and aid medico-legal inquiries of all kinds. With the co-operation of the district surgeon, he is to make examinations for inquests, and to attend on all sudden occurrences dangerous to the public safety;

vi. It is his special business to inspect and register medical men of all classes within his district, whether physicians, surgeons, apothecaries, or midwives, according to their respective qualifications and modes of practice. In some States he is to advance scientific medicine, by establishing a medical book-society, either in his whole district solely, or in conjunction with a neighbouring *Kreis-physicus;*

vii. He is to visit the shops of apothecaries, and to inspect their drugs and preparations;

viii. He is carefully to notice the produce and sale of all articles of food, as far as health-police is concerned;

ix. He is to report quarterly on the preceding matters; and, in addition, (*a*) on medical topography, including meteorological observations, notices of natural phenomena, and changes in the organic world ; (*b*) on agricultural statistics ;* (*c*) on the sickness or epidemic constitution of the period, with a summary of the cases attended by individual practitioners, and a particular notice of important events, such especially as affect medical police ; (*d*) on quackery, irregular or novel practice of all kinds, incompetency of practitioners, and contravention of medical laws ; (*e*) and, once yearly, on the census of population, with remarks on the returns of vital statistics (*tabellen biostatische*).

§ 7. Such is the provision made, and the example set, in Germany, for a local organization of sanitary officers.

Had I given even the fullest account of these appointments, it would be readily perceived that several matters of importance are omitted in the German schemes ; others are very partially dealt with ; while, on the other hand, a few of their regulations are unnecessary and unsuitable for England.

In France, the *officiers de santé*, instituted more than half a century ago, have merely served to suggest a name for the office. As to their duties and position, the precedent is worthless. They were, generally speaking, a class of inferior surgeons, of defective qualifications, and scarcely equal to the Bavarian *Land-ärzte*. Their preventive or public duties, if any, were very limited.

It appears that they received no fixed stipend from either the State or the commune. The office is now about to merge into an improved organization of salaried medical attendants for arrondissements and communes, connected with the *bureaux de bienfaisance,* and under the administration of public aid.

§ 8. Those who were actively engaged more than ten years ago in guiding legislation concerning the public health in England, had formed some strong, though perhaps not very definite opinions respecting the objects and advantages of a purely *preventive* medical office.

---

* " Im ersten Quartalberichte, wird über den dermaligen Wachsthum der Saatfelder Auskunft gegeben,—im Zweiten, über die Aussichten zur Getreideernte, und zum Gewinn an Gartenfrüchten,—im Dritten über den Ausfall der Ernte im Felde, in den Gärten und Weinbergen."—Niemann, p. 37.

Many valuable isolated suggestions were thrown out, without a complete view of the scope, design, functions, and relations of such an appointment. Mr. Chadwick's original propositions on the subject,* and the subsequent evidence of Dr. Southwood Smith to the same effect, supported by the independent opinions of a veteran philanthropist, Dr. Walker, of Huddersfield, have been already compared by me† with the earliest parliamentary project.

The conclusion, obviously, to be drawn from the whole argument was, that a paramount necessity existed for the appointment of a medico-sanitary officer, released from the engagements of private practice, for the superintendence of a district sufficiently extensive to embrace several medical relief districts; for the aid and supervision of the officers employed in administering such relief; for the examination of mortuary registries; for the detection of causes of disease among certain classes and occupations of the people, in certain localities and institutions; for inquiries into the quality and purity of the food and medicines supplied to the inhabitants; for investigating the causes of violent or sudden deaths; and for performing certain sanitary functions connected with interment of the dead.

The time had therefore arrived for legislation on the subject.

§ 9. The Duke of Newcastle's excellent Bill of 1845 contained a clause, which Sir B. Hall has just adopted word for word, as far as the duties of the office are concerned, in his Act for the Local Management of the Metropolis. In the Bill of 1845, however, the salary was to be determined by the Secretary of State.

During the second and ultimately successful attempt to carry a public health bill, by Lord Carlisle in 1848, this clause underwent several alterations. At one time it was even withdrawn; and, at last, a merely partial and permissive clause was inserted.

Each local Board might appoint a Medical Officer of Health. But two or more Boards might appoint the same person. His

---

* *General Sanitary Report,* 1842, p. 350 *et seq.*; *Supplementary Report on Interments,* pp. 139, &c.; *Health of Towns Commissioners' Report,* 1844, *loc. cit.*
† *Health and Sickness of Town Populations,* pp. 17, 20, 43, 73.

salary was to be paid out of the district-rates, and its amount determined by the local Board, or Boards. Both his appointment and dismissal were, however, subjected to the approval of the General Board, which was also authorized to direct his duties.

After three years' consideration of the subject, that Board proceeded in 1851 to prescribe these duties by a General Order, and to issue " Minutes" of instruction with reference to the appointment. These official documents, though needlessly prolix, prove that their framers knew well enough, that a sanitary superintendent, of high medical and scientific attainments, might be of incalculable benefit to the inhabitants of his district, by an energetic and independent discharge of those functions which had been clearly indicated in the directions referred to.

But these Minutes and Orders, no less than the history of their operations, also prove incontestably the existence of serious defects in the legal constitution and jurisdiction both of the office itself, and of the local authority, in which the power of making the appointment and determining its remuneration was unfortunately vested. It is not too much to say—that, had the framers and supporters of the Public Health Bill been sufficiently informed on the principles of medical police, or even had they listened to suggestions offered by others who had studied the question, a more effective provision would have been generally adopted.

§ 11. In a little tract, " On the Constitution of the Authorities about to be appointed under the Public Health Bill,"* I endeavoured to show that the true intent and object of such an appointment could scarcely be realized—unless the sphere of duty were so enlarged as to occupy the whole time and attention of the officer,—unless his functions were placed in official relation with those of the medical relief officers,—unless the appointment were removed from local influences, calculated to impair the independent discharge of its duties,—unless the salary were paid by the nation, and the appointment were controlled by the Government, —and unless every parish in the kingdom were included in some

* Those "Remarks" were first published in the *Journal of Public Health*, vol. i. 1848.

sànitary district. It became, therefore, a matter of much interest to me, to ascertain the results of the imperfect arrangements made under the Act on this point.

Accordingly, in July, 1854, I commenced a correspondence with all the provincial officers of health whose names I had been able to learn ;* and I circulated a series of questions among them. Twenty-two of the twenty-nine gentlemen thus addressed, favoured me with a body of very valuable and interesting information.

The whole affords a remarkable proof of the irregular, uncertain, and unsystematic character of English attempts at sanitary organization.

§ 12. Of the 182 towns, to which (as we learn from the Report of the original Board of Health)† the Public Health Act or local Acts incorporating that measure had been applied, it seems that only twenty-nine had appointed an Officer of Health —or less than one in six.

Such is the natural result of leaving the adoption of an indispensable measure to the option of bodies necessarily uninformed on so difficult and complicated a question as the prevention of disease ; and too generally unwilling to acknowledge their need of counsel and guidance by trained, experienced and scientific advisers.

The twenty-nine Officers of Health were thus distributed, according to the Registrar-General's division of England and Wales :—

	No. of Officers.
I. In the London division	1‡
II. South-Eastern	1
III. South-Midland	2
IV. Eastern	0
V. South-Western	0
VI. West-Midland	7
VII. North-Midland	3
VIII. North-Western	3
IX. Yorkshire	4
X. Northern	3
XI. Wales and Monmouthshire	5

* From Knight's *Parish Clerk's Almanac and Companion,* and from professional inquiries.

† *Report of the General Board of Health on the Administration of the Public Health Act,* &c., *from* 1848 *to* 1854, p. 14.

‡ Beside the officer for the City of London.

This little table shows that the office has been more frequently instituted in the north and west, than in the south and east of England.

§ 13. Of the twenty-two who favoured me with returns, three were appointed under Local Acts, seven by Town Councils, and twelve by local Boards under the Public Health Act.

The population of the district, committed to an Officer of Health, varied from nearly 400,000 in Liverpool, to less than 1400 in a little Welsh parish.

The sanitary district was co-terminous with a parochial Union in only two instances. It was, however, sometimes co-terminous with one or more districts for medical relief.*

The sanitary district of Liverpool appeared to contain fifteen medical relief districts,—that of Birmingham, eleven; Leicester, four; Swansea and Southampton, three; four other health-preserving areas contained a portion of two medical districts in each; while two contained exactly two medical districts in each; six seemed to be co-terminous with single medical districts, and five included only a part of such a district.

Thus, there existed a total absence of any thing like consent between medical and sanitary territorial divisions.

The perplexity which this defect must create in statistical observations and returns, as well as in practical operations, is manifest; and the confusion is increased by yet another division into Registration sub-districts, differing as to limits of area from both the former.

§ 14. It further appeared that seventeen of the twenty-nine were either themselves medical officers, or were connected by partnership with the medical officers of the Union containing the sanitary districts. Three, at least, were the sole medical officers in their sanitary districts; their healing and health-protecting spheres of action were co-extensive. In these, the actual con-

* The fact on this point is, however, not always clearly stated by my correspondents.

dition of the population, as regards mortality, sickness, and other causes, was more easily ascertained and reported, than in the others.

Most of those, who are not Union surgeons, complained of insufficient information respecting the diseases of the population.

Five are explicit as to their want of precise and regular intelligence from the medical officers, and urge the importance of some legally established systematic and direct communication.

Any proposals, on the part of Health Officers, to inspect the Union Medical Relief books—not authorized by the Boards of Guardians—would, of course, lead to some uneasiness between the two orders of officials. One Health Officer says,—

" it requires caution and tact to keep down feelings of jealousy, and to avoid the appearance of claiming supervision over the Union Medical Officers."

Medical charities do not exist in all these twenty-two places, and they co-operate with the Officer of Health only in two or three. Much valuable material is thus unemployed.

§ 15. In most instances, either the Inspectors of nuisances (as they are called), or the road surveyors, or the police, were said to notify to the Officer of Health any sources of impure air, or insalubrious emanations, which they may have observed.

But, reports of this kind were evidently much more promptly and regularly made in the larger towns. Some stated that an increased staff of Searchers for nuisances was exceedingly wanted. In three or four of the smallest towns, no assistance was afforded to the Health Officer in this arduous employment.

§ 16. The salaries of these officers differed still more remarkably than their areas of jurisdiction; but without any rational or uniform proportion to their duties.

In the only town where the directions of the General Board of Health have been fulfilled, by debarring the officer from private practice,—namely, at Liverpool—the salary was 750*l.*

In all other places, private practitioners were employed, and the salary varied from 150*l*.* to nothing.

Two places, with populations of 35,000 and 30,000, paid 150*l*. In one town, with 60,000 inhabitants, the salary was 100*l*.; in one of 24,000, 60*l*.; in one of 40,000, 50*l*.; another of 12,000, 30*l*., which, said the officer, was 20*l*. less than the salary of his colleague, the Scavenger! In other towns the salary is 25*l*., 20*l*., 15*l*., 10*l*. In four places, the office is performed gratuitously. In two, there is no fixed salary. From eleven out of twenty-nine, no return is made on this point.

On looking over these returns, one can scarcely fail to be strongly impressed with the disinterested and courageous zeal manifested by those medical men, who, before accepting the post of officer of health, had placed themselves in front of the sanitary movement; sometimes even refusing any stipend for their official appointment, lest their motives should be suspected; and everywhere promoting and guiding improvements which tend to cut off the only source of profitable employment at present open to them in this country.

§ 17. The amount of duty appertaining to this office varied as strangely as the other particulars. Some of the health officers seemed to consider it a very trifling affair; rather a sort of recreation in the intervals of practice. These gentlemen were evidently sanitary amateurs. The services of one "have never been required, the town being remarkably clean and healthy," in fact, a "model" for all other communities. I need not say this is but a small place.

The multifarious instructions of the General Board, with reference to the duties of the appointment, were evidently considered in most places as shadowing forth an imaginary standard of perfection, not intended to be literally and immediately acted

---

* The sharp-witted Americans pay their health-officers more liberally. The annual salary of this officer, in the city of Buffalo, is 900 dollars,—for a population probably less than half of that of either of the English towns which pay their health-officers 150*l*.—*Medical Press*, Sept. 6, 1854.

upon. The reports, where required, were usually made according to the directions of the General Board, in places under the Public Health Act. In those under local acts, the frequency and form of reports vary. In one of the latter, a periodical return of all cases of zymotic disease, on a printed form, was requested of every resident private practitioner. The plan had not been in operation long enough to determine its success. Probabilities are surely against it.

The reports appear to be printed for local use in but few places. Two or three of these documents, which have been sent to me, are highly creditable to their authors, and calculated to be of essential service in their respective localities. The only ground for regret is, that they should mostly refer to very limited areas.

§ 18. In Liverpool only, I repeat, was the Officer of Health debarred from private practice.

Ten, perhaps eleven, other officers expressed opinions, more or less decided, against the combination of this appointment with private professional engagements. Eight or nine considered that the ordinary duties of a practitioner were compatible with the office; but four of these admitted that their opinions were grounded merely on the smallness of their districts, the inconsiderable amount of their public duty, or the limited extent of their own practice. Of those who approved of the directions of the General Board on this point, some adduced very forcible reasons, based on their own experience, in favour of the principle. The following are a few extracts from their communications:—

(No. 4.) " In general practice, the many claims upon one's time and attention often clash with public duties; and again, the course of studies which sanitary improvements render necessary, are far out of the track of ordinary medical knowledge and requirements."

" The whole time of the Officer of Health should be devoted to the duties of his office, and where one district is too poor to pay, he should be appointed for a portion of a county. Legislation should not leave this to the option of the local authorities, but should render it compulsory."

"Co-operation with other medical men is imperfect, owing to my being myself a private practitioner."

(No. 5.) "I find the two occupations of a public officer and a private practitioner continually clash, sometimes much to my disadvantage."

"I cannot efficiently perform either my practice, or always attend to my official duties."

"The Officer of Health ought certainly to be independent of practice and of local authority. He cannot otherwise be really useful, nor carry out sanitary principles. He should be fairly paid, and if the town is not large enough to occupy all his time, several towns or unions ought to be grouped together; his whole time should be given up to the public. The duties of an officer of health are very important and onerous, and require special devotion."

(No. 6.) "No one who takes this appointment ought to continue in private practice. I have injured myself considerably in endeavouring to make this town healthy. I have been obliged to expose some members of the local Board, whose property was in a disgraceful state, and have been frequently brought into collision with some of my best patients."

"The Government ought to *appoint*, and *pay* adequately."

(No. 16.) "Unless the salary of Health Officer be paid by Government, independently of the local Board,—the inhabitants of such a town as this (population, 14,000) would object to pay a proper remuneration to an efficient medical officer, who ought not to receive less than 500*l.* a-year, if compelled to relinquish all private practice, and if capable of filling the office. Unless such an appointment is independent of local authority, it is perfectly useless."

(No. 20.) "The Officer of Health should also be Superintendent of the Medical Relief, and consultant to the Union Medical Officers; his salary should be such as to render private practice unnecessary."

(No. 23.) "The conscientious discharge of the officer's duties must necessarily involve trouble, and frequently expense to landlords, many of whom—in agricultural districts especially—will not see the necessity for such efforts. A local Officer of Health is unwilling to oppose facts to the prejudices and supposed interests of those from whom he probably derives his livelihood. He is thus tempted to overlook decided causes of malaria, to the injury of those who have no claim upon him. The Officer of Health ought therefore to be a Medical Commissioner appointed by the General Board to visit several districts, and to act independently of the local Boards, which should be compelled to afford him all the aid he requires."

§ 19. Several of these gentlemen concurred in complaining that their authority was injuriously limited and wholly inadequate. Not shrinking from greater responsibility, they urged that powers more clearly defined, and more summary, should be placed in their hands, especially in anticipation, and during the prevalence of epidemics.*

§ 20. The results of this inquiry are surely sufficient to convince any unprejudiced person that the 40th clause of the Public Health Act, and the orders of the late General Board thereupon, have singularly failed of their object.

Comparing these results, again, with that sketch of the proper position and duties of a superintending Officer of Health, which has been suggested in the introductory Essay;—can any one doubt, for a moment, which of the two is calculated to prove the more efficient and publicly-useful arrangement?

We may be told, however, that owing to the powers unfortunately conferred on Councils and Boards representing certain occupiers and ratepayers in towns, it has become almost impracticable to re-constitute the local machinery on correct principles, simultaneously, in every place.

I shall endeavour to show that this objection is by no means insuperable; and, even if it were, the superior plan might be carried into effect in all districts where such an officer has *not* been appointed; and every local Board might be empowered to merge its own arrangements in a general organization of health officers at the national expense.

§ 21. It has been remarked, that in very small sanitary districts the combination of the medical-relief office with the disease-prevention office, has been found to work advantageously, as regards authentic information on the causes and amount of public sickness; and it has been asked whether the officers employed in such an improved administration of medical-

* If every municipality could place its health officer in the same independent and commanding position as the borough of Liverpool, the 40th clause of the Public Health Act (under which, by the bye, Dr. Duncan was not appointed) might, perhaps, work well. It cannot be expected to do so under actual circumstances.

relief as is recommended in the Fourth Essay, might not also in some places become the sole health officers of their respective districts?* For instance, might it be left to the option of local Boards superior in constitution to those at present in operation, *either* to nominate ONE superintending officer of health, in definite relation with the district medical officers, and as a referee on all questions and measures of prevention, *or* to constitute each medical-relief officer the sanitary superintendent of his own district?

In reply to these questions, it is to be observed: *first*—that, whichever plan were adopted by any local authority, the Officer of Health should undoubtedly be debarred from private practice, and salaried either out of the consolidated fund or by means of an equalized national rate: And, *secondly*—that there are ample grounds, confirmed by experience and reflection, for deciding in favour of the universal adoption of the former plans.

The following reasons for the separate establishment of the higher sanitary post have already been noticed,—the special and undivided attention requisite for success in statistical, scientific, and forensic investigations; the peculiar and exceptional nature of certain preventive functions, and their more satisfactory performance by one in the rank of consultant; the great advantage to be derived by the public from the Medical Superintendent's exercise of such functions in an extensive sanitary jurisdiction, and from his collation of results in different districts; and lastly, the substantial benefit to be conferred on the poorer classes, and the useful aid to be afforded to their medical attendants, by providing a second opinion in obscure cases, within an accessible distance, free of cost,† and above all suspicion of professional rivalry.

* At one time I thought that this might be managed, and that such preventive duties as were incompatible with a local appointment, might be vested in a circuit-inspector appointed by the Crown.—[*Remarks on Constitution of Authorities*, &c., p. 10, 1848.] But maturer reflection has convinced me that the number of inspectors required on such a system would be so great, that the still higher duties of extensive comparison and communication with the Central Council would be too minutely divided.

† Travelling expenses would of course be allowed, as to coroners.

§ 22. Such being the conclusions, almost inevitable, from the premises and considerations here submitted; it becomes a matter for deep concern to find that, in the Act of the last Session for the better local management of the Metropolis, the 132nd clause ignores the entire result of administrative experience with reference to these appointments.

Every parish "vestry" (for vestries are not defunct, as some might have hoped) and every district parochial Board is to appoint "one or more" medical practitioners, to be called "Medical Officers of Health."

Even supposing that the subsequent (139th) clause may empower the Supreme Metropolitan Board, with the consent of the vestries, to constitute a larger area than is comprised in one parish or district, for the action of one Officer of Health,—it remains to be seen whether this provision will lead to combinations of districts, under fewer sanitary officers.

Such doubts, therefore, as the following, force themselves upon one's mind.

Why should "one or more" of these officers be appointed in each parish or district, without the slightest recognition of the existing corps of sanitary officers, *i. e.*, the medical attendants of the poor? Are the latter to be discharged from their preventive responsibilities? Or, as "doctors differ," are they to get up lively discussions with the new officers of health on those controverted points of management which continually arise in every locality?

Without any pre-determined co-operation between these two classes of officers, how are the proposed sanitary superintendents to arrive at a knowledge of all the numerous facts relating to prevalent sickness?

What security has been taken for something like correspondence between the areas in which palliative functions are now executed, and those in which preventive duties are to be performed? or, rather, has not this crude enactment almost annihilated the hope of a speedy adjustment of these diverse and conflicting jurisdictions?

If the Health Office is to be purely preventive and superintending, why "one or more" in *each* parochial district?

Why "practitioners" at all? Why not—as has been so strongly recommended by the highest sanitary authorities—physicians and surgeons restricted from practice?

What precaution is taken in the metropolis, against those anomalies and mistakes, of which the provincial Officers of Health so justly complain?

What approach to security for the free and conscientious discharge of the highest order of professional duties, is afforded by irresponsibly committing the appointment, the determination of salary, and the right of dismissal, to a body representing every kind of influence which is adverse to sanitary control?

Ought a class of officers, whose independence is of the greatest public importance, to be reduced to a position of moral thraldom, from which even the medical officers of districts have just been rescued? Is an office of exalted object and design to become a matter for taunt and scoff among those who delight to show how professional opinions may be bought in favour of any and every abuse?

What would have been the result of committing the choice of Judges of County Courts to local elective bodies?

Why does the Lord Chancellor appoint, and the Treasury pay, these district Judges, but to secure their absolute freedom from local bias, and their impartial administration of justice?

Are not the majesty of the law and the liberty of the subject vindicated alike by this exercise of prerogative, and by the permanence of the judicial appointment? Why, then, are opposite principles to be applied to the superior offices of State Medicine, in which an equal amount of independence of thought and action are necessary?

Could no members of his "Medical Council" have instructed Sir Benjamin Hall as to the principles on which these appointments must be based, if they are to secure positive and reliable protection to the community?

§ 23. Let not these speculations and questions be thought needless or irrelevant.

Recent events in the metropolis indicate the probable application of a modified "Tender System" to the new sanitary appointments, after its abolition in the therapeutic office. If the salaries are to be cut down, at each successive vacancy, to the point at which it is understood that men of skill and science will compete for the office,—why not apply the same principle to the presidency and other appointments of the General Board of Health?

Why, at all events, is the stipend of the Chairman of the Metropolitan Board of Works fixed at a sum, which, however suitable for a barrister of good standing, is considered extravagant by a majority of that Board; whilst the pay of the Metropolitan Officers of Health is to depend on the opinions—perhaps the prejudices—of those, who, for the most part, are unavoidably ignorant of the science upon which the duties and responsibilities of those officers are based?

The last defect in this enactment which need be noticed in this place, is the entire absence of any provision for securing the proper qualification of the officer. The Act requires no examination by competent authorities, no period of professional standing, no length or amount of public service, no testimonials or evidence of character.

In a subsequent chapter of this Essay, I hope to offer some practical suggestions on the appointment and organization of future Officers of Health. It is enough here to have shown the impediments which have already been raised to the adoption of correct measures, and to remind my readers of the very appropriate remarks of Inspector Sutherland on this subject:—

"So-called sanitary improvements carried out in the absence of the necessary knowledge of the effects of those local conditions which they are intended to remedy, may be in any case, as they have been in many cases, mere empiricism and waste of money. And this can only be avoided by making use of the assistance of qualified Officers of Health."*

* *Report,* 1855, p. 65.

CHAPTER SECOND.

A. LOCAL BOARDS AS THEY HAVE BEEN AND ARE.

§ 1. IN some countries, powers of deliberation and advice only have been conferred upon scientific councils and officers.* In others, ill-defined powers of legislation and action have been committed only to unskilled and incompetent municipal bodies. And it is difficult to say which of the two errors has caused the greatest amount of failure in sanitary improvements.

In England, however, the latter system of public administration has chiefly prevailed; and—as, in the preceding Essay, a consideration of the duties and relations of the Medical Relief Office led to questions respecting the competency of the local Boards at present directing that department of State Medicine—so, the subject of this Essay involves an examination of the grounds on which Boards of Guardians, Town Councils, and other municipal or district corporate bodies, are assumed by the legislature to be qualified for discharging the sanitary duties and responsibilities now committed to them.

§ 2. It becomes necessary, in the first place, to consider published evidence respecting the exercise of preventive and palliative functions by BOARDS OF GUARDIANS, especially in epidemic visitations. This was a point eschewed by the Parliamentary Committee on Medical Relief in 1854. The Right Honourable Chairman seemed anxiously to deprecate any criticism of the sanitary proceedings of these Boards.

The truth, however, more than once came out. A medical officer manfully affirmed:—

"I have myself constantly experienced the difficulty of carrying out sanitary regulations under the control of a Board of Guardians, when

* See supplementary Note G.

several members of that Board are themselves the owners of property, which becomes taxed by sanitary changes at my suggestion."*

§ 3. Other corroborative testimony from private sources can be adduced on this head, but I prefer availing myself of official documents, as less likely to be called in question.

The senior medical superintending Inspector of the General Board of Health, remarked† with regard to the execution of precautionary measures in some places, previous to and during the visitation of cholera in 1848, that—

"To all intents and purposes, no one fact of sanitary science might ever have been ascertained, so far as the local authorities were concerned; and as might have been expected, the most disastrous consequences have, in these instances, ensued."

And, concerning remedial measures,—

"with a few exceptions, the General Regulations, as to medical aid, dispensaries and houses of refuge, were certainly not exercised in such a manner as to fulful the intentions of the Board."

Again ;—

"At a period when a properly constituted local Board of Health would probably have carried out relief measures on the widest and most liberal scale to save life, the money aspect of the measures in certain instances appears to have occupied the largest share of attention. At a time when the self-sustaining heads of families were being cut off in all directions, the question appears to have been in these cases, not how the largest saving of productive human life could be effected, but what was the smallest increase of rates which the parish could escape with? The kind of inquiries, which are natural to parochial bodies, occupied the chief place in their consideration; and thence, the medical assistance provided has sometimes been very inadequate. I have walked through affected districts, and seen the people in terror running about in all directions, seeking for medical aid where none was to be found. I have entered houses, and seen the sick and the dying lying without help. In a whole district of the metropolis the people were falling before the ravages of the epidemic, apparently without the knowledge that the legislature had made any provision for their relief. In one town, the medical staff was broken up and dismissed in the midst of a wasting pestilence, on account of some paltry

* Evid. (1854), 3287.   † App. A.—*Report on Cholera,* 1850, pp. 136, 137.

pecuniary consideration, and numbers of families were thrown into mourning in consequence; *the decisions of one meeting on matters of instant and vital importance having been upset by another meeting called by a cabal for the purpose.* I know one case, in which, on the very eve of one of the most disastrous outbursts of cholera I have ever witnessed, the medical staff was dismissed, and the dispensaries closed, and where hundreds died without being able to obtain a single dose of medicine.

"Similar difficulties arose in the exercise of the power of providing houses of refuge by the parochial authorities. . . . .

"On the part of some Boards there was often a great unwillingness to open refuges; and on the part of the people there was often as great an unwillingness to enter those which had been provided. I cannot help thinking that the workhouse idea influenced both parties. Indeed, I have known a portion of a workhouse set apart for a refuge for persons who abhorred the very name of the place."

Mr. Grainger, another of the principal Inspectors, reported:—

"The most serious, or rather, as it ought from its results to be called, the most fatal, mistake which pervaded the whole of these remedial measures from first to last, was this:—The guardians—herein departing diametrically from the injunction of the General Board, that cases should be sought out—in all their arrangements acted upon the principle that the poor, when attacked, should apply to the medical officer, who thus, instead of discovering cases in their first incipient stage, waited for an application; a delay which led, as I am prepared to show, to the most fatal consequences. The evidence collected from all parts of the metropolis points but to one conclusion: the patients who suffered from cholera, and who were treated under the system of the guardians, were, in the great majority of cases, seen for the first time by the medical officers when in complete or incipient collapse: when, consequently, the aid of medicine was almost as nothing; when, whatever mode of treatment was adopted, from forty to fifty per cent. of those attacked would perish. So generally, or rather universally, was this the case, that on reflection, I cannot recall the instance of a single parish or union in London where, so far as the proceedings of the local authorities were concerned, apart from the Board of Health, any plan was adopted for seeking out persons affected with the premonitory, first, and curable stage of cholera. That partial steps were taken— that the medical officers overtaxed their powers in the effort to supply assistance to the multitudinous sufferers—that they again and again visited the afflicted localities, is true: but, large as were the numbers relieved by their meritorious exertions, still larger numbers were overlooked, many of whom subsequently fell into collapse, and swelled the weekly tables of mortality."*

After such disclosures, through their superintending Inspectors, the General Board of Health was perfectly justified in passing the following decisive judgment upon the Union Boards, to which Parliament had so unwisely committed the local administration of sanitary measures.†

"It is a matter of deep regret to us, that during the entire prevalence of the epidemic we have, in many instances, been wholly unable to carry into effect the beneficent intentions of the Legislature, in consequence of the inappropriate and inadequate machinery provided by the Act for its local administration; and this regret is increased by a consideration of the extent to which suffering and loss of life have been prevented in the towns in which we have succeeded in inducing the local authorities to exercise, in an efficient manner, the powers intrusted to them for the prevention of disease.

. . . .

"The provision intended by the Legislature was one for the common protection against impending dangers to *all* classes, against which the individual means of private persons were inadequate.

"But the common functions of the Poor-Law Guardians relate exclusively to one class, the destitute or the pauper class only.

"Notwithstanding the scope of the Act, and explanatory notifications, the first and common impression of the Guardians of the poor was, to confine the measures of prevention to the destitute, and administer it according to their settled practice as respects the relief of paupers, which is, to do nothing except on application, and then only upon proof given of the urgency of the case."

§ 4. I have been the more particular in citing these Reports, lest it should be pretended that the Government and Parliament had not ample notice and warning of the incompetency of these Boards, before the last visitation of cholera.

It might perhaps have been supposed, that, however indifferently the Boards of Guardians acted in 1848, the experience they then acquired, and the censures since passed on them by the Board of Health, would have produced some change of intention, exaltation of motive, and amendment in practice. Yet, in 1854, the

* *Report on Cholera*, 1850, p. 138.   † Ibid. p. 137.

same indisputable testimony proved the fallacy of any such expectations, and established the correctness of former observations.

Although Dr. Milroy's report from the provinces is not yet published—(no reason is assigned for its being withheld), there is abundant evidence from the metropolis to show—that, owing to the inefficiency of the parochial Boards, the epidemic was in many places allowed to take its own course; and that much aggravation of suffering, much actual loss of life, resulted.

§ 5. *With regard to precautionary measures.*—Searchers for nuisances were not appointed in sufficient number, nor for a sufficient period, nor from a sufficiently instructed and energetic class of persons.*

In Chelsea, Dr. Greenhow reports :†

"Nothing really had been done by the authorities to prepare for the epidemic, and the condition of the inferior class of property has been gradually retrograding in a sanitary point of view."

In two populous districts, Deptford and Greenwich, inspected by Dr. Glover, there were *no* such searchers, even when cholera was at the worst.‡

"Taking all the parishes (of the metropolis) together," says the chief reporter, "in which the epidemic was most fatal, it appears that in not one of them was the preventive machinery, sanitary and medical, organized in accordance with the minute of instruction, although some parishes had done more than others."

As to Houses of Refuge.—Although the attention of Boards of Guardians had been specially directed to this most valuable means of checking the spread of pestilence, Dr. Sutherland states:

"I do not know of a single instance of any metropolitan parish having had a place of refuge, *except the workhouse,*|| in readiness before the epidemic broke out. In only one or two instances was a place of refuge provided after the disease appeared, and in only one parish, so

* Dr. Sutherland's Report, p. 49.   † Ibid. p. 50.   ‡ Ibid. p. 51.

|| Dr. Glover reports :—" In a few cases people were removed to workhouses, but the working classes very naturally refused to avail themselves of such a provision for their safety."

Dr. Greenhow says :—"One woman told me, that rather than become a pauper she would drown both herself and her children."

far as I have been able to ascertain, was the accommodation so provided made use of."

As to Medical House-to-House Visitation.—The expediency of forcing medical attendance upon afflicted or threatened districts was suggested to the Medical Poor-Relief Committee in 1844.* The first definite scheme in England for this kind of visitation, was recommended by Dr. Sutherland to the General Board of Health in December 1848, and was applied with some success to Dumfries and other towns. Much good was effected by that measure, carried out only partially in the metropolis, in 1849; and the results would have been more decisive, says Dr. Sutherland, but for "the remissness of the local authorities."†

The General Board of Health, in anticipation of the last outbreak, had sent instructions on the subject to all the unions and parishes in the kingdom. "Every means of conveying practical information to these Boards had been adopted." Yet with what effect? Absolutely less was done than in 1849.

"With one or two exceptions of more healthy parishes, none of the metropolitan parishes had made arrangements for putting into operation the instructions of the General Board on this point. In a few places, after great exertions on the part of the Inspectors, and repeated recommendations on the part of the President of the General Board, a few Visitors were appointed, but in most instances, nothing effectual had been done, and some of the parish authorities eventually did nothing."‡

* See *Health and Sickness of Town Populations*, p. 53, with Sir G. Cornewall Lewis's remarks on my evidence, in the foot note.

† Dr Sutherland's Report, p. 56.

‡ Ibid. Dr. Hassall gives the following account of the medical relief measures in operation in Lambeth on the 4th September, when he first inspected the parish, during the height of the epidemic.

There were no day or night dispensaries.
There were no houses of refuge.
There were no house-to-house visitors.
The accommodation for cholera cases consisted of two wards in the workhouse.
The medical relief for the whole parish, with its 140,000 inhabitants, consisted of nine medical officers and two assistants.
Dr. Hassall, with the approval of the President of the General Board of Health, recommended that eight dispensaries should be opened; and that nine visitors

As to Measures for Medical Relief.—Here, also, the arrangements adopted by the different Boards were said to be destitute of anything like uniformity and adequacy.*

The efforts of the Guardians seem to have been generally directed to one end—namely, how best to evade or resist the directions of the Central Board; while in one parish—

"from the first there was an openly expressed determination not to be in any way interfered with by the Board. The inspector was treated with discourtesy, and the district medical officers and their recommendations were regarded with contempt."†

One is really wearied with the repeated statements to the same effect, which occur in page after page of this Report. They may be summed up in Dr. Sutherland's concluding observations:—

"The result of the whole inquiry, as regards the administration of the sanitary and medical relief measures by the Boards of Guardians, is that, generally speaking, they were inefficient in character and extent, except in some of the larger and more healthy parishes, where they were least wanted. The experience in this respect is essentially the same as that obtained during the cholera of 1849, and it demonstrates that some more suitable local authorities, with adequate powers for carrying out permanent sanitary works and measures, and for providing the working classes with adequate medical relief, during seasons of pestilence, are absolutely necessary for the metropolis."

§ 6. In investigating the causes of defective sanitary administration by Boards of Guardians, it is necessary to consider the composition of these bodies, the design and scope of their institution, and the fact of their responsibilities being shared in many places with corporations and local Boards of Health.

They are composed of rate-payers, and cramped in every way by rate-paying notions. Their "imperfect and inefficient measures," and their "delay in adopting more active proceedings," preparatory to and during the invasion of epidemics, appear to

should be appointed, to act under the superintendence of the district surgeons, but the Lambeth Guardians declined to accede to these suggestions.

The parish was therefore left without any adequate protection against the epidemic.—Ibid. p. 57.
* Ibid. pp. 58—62. † Ibid. pp. 59, 60.

have arisen partly, says Dr. Sutherland, " from a mistaken sense of duty to the rate-payers," and partly from the fact, that the members of these Boards are " themselves occasionally large owners of cottage and other property,"* or else engaged in noxious trades, and interested in the perpetuation of particular nuisances.†

It is a remarkable fact that such men generally contrive to get elected on the local Boards; they " often attend most diligently all meetings, and thus acquire an influence which overpowers that of the better disposed,"‡ who may, nevertheless, constitute the majority.

§ 7. The design and scope of the original institution of Union and parochial Boards were well contrasted, by the General Board in 1849, with the responsibilities now imposed on them, and were shown to be a cause of their inefficiency and incompetency.

This view of the case is also confirmed most strongly by the Inspectors, in 1854.‖ The late Mr. Walsh pointed out, as the result of his experience, the utter unfitness of the Guardians of the *poor* to be the Guardians of the *people*, in a matter so important as the public health. As guardians of paupers against starvation, and guardians of the rates against all except paupers, " their functions are instinctively *exclusive*, not *inclusive*."¶

Again, the classes principally attacked by pestilence are not those under the protection of the Guardians.

The chief epidemic causes of disease require " a totally different body to deal with them." Guardians have no power to direct the larger structural improvements; and but little inclination to enforce those smaller measures which would require them " to interfere with each other's interests, or to place themselves in antagonism with other local authorities."**

§ 8. The replies of my recent correspondents on this subject deserve notice.

All those Officers of Health, *who are also Union Surgeons*,

---

* *Report* (1854), p. 62.   † Ibid. p. 36. Stepney Union.   ‡ Ibid. p. 62.
‖ Ibid. pp. 63—65.   ¶ Ibid. p. 64.   ** Ibid. p. 63.

report that the Boards of Guardians are "auxiliary" in sanitary measures. On the other hand, the majority of those who are *not* in office under Boards of Guardians (although, of course, as local practitioners not independent of their influence) report that these Boards are "indifferent" or "obstructive."

Those who appear to enter the most heartily and intelligently into the sanitary movement, speak the most plainly on this point.

In one large town, the parochial Board refused to act during the cholera visitation of 1849, until compelled by the General Board of Health; and even then took legal advice as to whether they were bound to obey. For two or three years, the Officer of Health had considerable difficulty with them: and in 1854, again, when cholera was carrying off numbers daily, the Guardians were doing their utmost to thwart the laudable efforts of the sanitary superintendent.

Another gentleman mentions a joint committee of the Board of Guardians and Board of Health, which separated without coming to any arrangement to meet the threatening advent of cholera, owing *to the jealousies existing between the two bodies.* He adds—

"The Board of Guardians will most probably refuse to recognise me in any way, deeming me an enthusiast wishing unnecessarily to alarm the public, and to spend large sums of money. They say, it is a got-up case! Such are the feelings of Boards of Guardians throughout the country, and also of many members of the Boards of Health."

A third Officer of Health, however, reports favourably of a joint committee appointed by the two local Boards.

A fourth states—

"There has been some collision between the local Board of Health and the Board of Guardians, arising mainly from the petty jealousies of their respective officials; and from the very circumstance of two Boards existing in the same place, and possessing common powers in sanitary matters."

§ 9. Nevertheless, with all this evidence against the hygienic administration of poor-law Guardians, there is much to be said in their behalf, if the Government and Parliament are resolved not to create new local authorities. They have certainly some claims for consideration, not possessed by other local bodies. Their jurisdictions include the whole of England and Wales; and they are in possession of important machinery for action.

Their superiority to town councils, in these respects, was very fairly put by Mr. Hawksley, in his evidence before the Select Committee on Sir B. Hall's Bills.

"The Town Councils do not come into communication constantly with the poor, or rather the working classes, for whose benefit, I apprehend, this Bill is principally promoted. .... The medical officers of the Boards of Guardians constantly visit the poorer classes, and altogether they are, in my opinion, much fitter bodies for the initiation of proceedings of this kind than Town Councils; and inasmuch as these councils do not exist everywhere, and as the Boards of Guardians, as nearly as possible, do exist everywhere, and as it is desirable to have one simple form of proceeding, and one well-known body all over the kingdom, to carry out purposes of this kind, I think it very much better that Boards of Guardians should have the powers than the Town Councils."*

The presence of the magistrates, also, as *ex-officio* members of the Union Boards, is some little compensation for the disturbing influence of annual elections upon their deliberations.

§ 10. In the second place, we have to consider LOCAL BOARDS OF HEALTH, created by recent Acts of Parliament.

Some of these are known only by that name, and are entirely new corporations. Others existed previously, as Town Councils, Commissions of Sewers, Town Improvement Commissions under local Acts, and bodies empowered for more limited objects, as highway management, lighting, watching, and cleansing.

Looking at the practical results of the authorization of Municipal Councils, and other town Boards, it would appear—that, with a few gratifying exceptions, they are not more nicely and judiciously adapted for the sanitary protection of the inhabitants than Boards of Guardians.

To show the manner in which they proceed to carry into effect

* *Report of Committee on Sir B. Hall's Bill*, p. 61.

the objects of their institution, it may suffice to refer to three places.

i. From a hospital surgeon of great repute, residing in the smallest of the three towns, I received the following account, in 1854, and can vouch for its accuracy.

"I can't say much in favour of our Local Board, which was expressly elected by those inhabitants most desirous of doing nothing. . . . . They have not yet got a plan of the parish on the scale and under the direction of the General Board, so that none of their measures have received the sanction of that Board . . . . The Local Board has evaded the law (imposing the control of the General Board) by contracting for the necessary works by fragments, for sums below the amount specified by the Act as needing the sanction of the General Board.

"I have very little doubt that much of the money laid out under the direction of our Board is thrown away; and, as a matter of course, our economic gentry will prove, eventually, to have conducted business in an extravagant way.

"The supply of water is both bad and insufficient, and none can be had, but from the distant hills, at an expense that will never be incurred. Hence one can entertain no hope of grand sanitary measures here at present. Wells are dug and pumps put down for the reception and diffusion of surface water; and hence, few (houses) are now otherwise than very short, or entirely destitute of water."

ii. In the city of Worcester, justly distinguished for its intelligence and public spirit, the weighty matters, for which the Local Board (the Town Council) was empowered, were absolutely at a stand for some months in 1852; the majority declining to transact any business relating to the public health, because they could not persuade the General Board, highly to its credit,—to sanction their dismissal of a very able and efficient officer.

iii. In Gloucester, once called the "fair city," we are told that the Local Board (there also the Town Council) frittered away more than 10,000*l.* of the citizens' money, or 10*s.* per head on the population, during its first three years of power, without even commencing a permanent sanitary work. No provision was made for a proper supply of water, the want of which was severely felt during the late visitation of cholera. The general sewerage was then planned and finished, before any arrangements were made for the water-supply; and, by a regulation of the Local Board, no houses could communicate with the main sewers until supplied with water. So that, more than half the householders were paying sewer-rates for a year and upwards, without the possibility of their availing themselves of the sewers. And these, moreover, are completed on the principle of allowing all their valuable contents to run to waste in the Severn. Thus, owing to the increased and increasing defilement of that fine river—the water of which in its natural state is admirably adapted for town supply—the inhabitants of Gloucester have been induced to expend a very large sum of money in procuring a harder and less generally useful kind of water, from a more distant source in the oolitic strata of the Cotswold hills.

§ 11. Without producing any more specimens of practical mismanagement, I proceed to notice the defective composition of these Local Boards. As might be supposed, the Officers of Health, with whom I have communicated, are somewhat reserved on this point. One of these gentlemen, indeed, does not hesitate to confess his opinion that the inadequacy and inefficiency of local arrangements are "due to the obstruction of unwilling members of the Local Boards," and that representatives of borough rate-payers are "ill informed and re-actionary."

In smaller towns, in fact, the two Boards are composed of the same class of persons, the same individuals often sitting at both.

In one such town, a surgeon—well known for his invaluable labours in a particular department of sanitary research—writes thus:

"The Union Board and the Town Board of Health have never yet clashed in their views or duties; the latter is and has been notoriously bent, from its first institution, on spending as little of the public money as possible. Hence, the two Boards perfectly agree! No medical officer of health here, nor any likely to be. This would be a gross piece of extravagance!"

§ 12. If the Union Boards are distinctively characterized by the predominance of the rate-paying interest,—we see in Town

Councils not only that, but other elements obstructive to sanitary progress.

Investments, trades and occupations, which are either insalubrious in their very essence, or are conducted in a manner prejudicial to the public health, are largely represented in these corporations. Above all, there exists in undiminished vigour the element of political party strife,—which Lord Carlisle was enthusiastic enough to hope to allay, by giving the town councils something better to think and talk about.

Now, when to these deteriorating influences is added the continued operation of depressing physical causes—a thick, smoky, and fœtid atmosphere, a crowding of inhabitants and a site of low elevation (as is the case in most of our large towns),—who can wonder if the individual perception should be obscured, the moral sense perverted, and the corporate conscience deadened?

It is generally observed that cultivated intelligence, professional knowledge, scientific research, philanthropic zeal, are rare constituents, almost always in the minority; while the claims of labour, the safety of the helpless, and the welfare of the unrepresented masses—women and children, I mean especially,—are considerations which are understood to carry but little weight in the decisions of these corporate bodies. Such an estimate of town councils is pretty generally made by thoughtful persons. An eminent solicitor and parliamentary agent, examined before the Committee on Sir B. Hall's Bills, says:—

"There are not, perhaps, ten municipal corporations in the kingdom in which you will find the gentlemen of the place or the leading and most intelligent inhabitants of the place, taking their part in that body and conducting its discussions. ... It is not an atmosphere in which it is found that such persons can stay.

"The experience of town councils does not present to us, in point of station, in point of intelligence, and in point of the power of the management of business, any pattern which it is safe to copy and apply universally to the management of all the local affairs of the kingdom."*

* *Report on Sir B. Hall's Bills.* Evid. 978, 980.

Mr. Baxter remarks, with regard to meetings of rate-payers:—

"You will never, for local purposes, practically get the more quiet and sensible

§ 13. It would not be uninstructive to compare the present administrative bodies with the Boards of Health, temporarily appointed in many towns by the Privy Council, during the cholera visitation of 1831-2. The general superiority of the earlier authorities may not be known to the younger portion of sanitary reformers; but if any one doubts it, let me suggest to him to visit a few of the principal provincial towns, and—having obtained for each place a list of the persons who acted in 1832, and another list of those composing the Local Board now in power in the same place,—let him lay the two before any old observant and reflective inhabitant, with this question,—"Which of these lists contains the best men of their day in this place, the most educated, judicious, liberal, and generally respected?"

Then let him inquire how the former selection was made; and I am much mistaken, if, at the close of his tour of inquiry, he will not have formed some clearer notions with regard to the relative merits of the past and present methods of appointing Local Boards of Health.

§ 14. The preceding observations are intended to apply, principally, to Municipal Corporations. But, in a very few of the more modern towns, a new description of Local Board has recently been created, under the name of "Improvement Commissioners."

It is said that the composition of these local commissions is generally far superior to that of the reformed Town Councils. Men of high intelligence, character, position, and public estimation, are found to seek and not unfrequently to obtain seats on these Boards. And it is no mean recommendation to such a body, when the right of voting at the election of its members is not confined to male burgesses, as in municipal corporations, but is extended to female occupiers and owners of property.

people to attend the meetings. The noise, and tumult, and jargon that go on at those meetings drive them away, and they will not go there."—Ibid. 991.

"You get, in point of fact, the votes of those who are, perhaps, least qualified to conduct the business; and particularly if anything becomes a party question, there is so much disturbance created by it, that all quiet people retire at once from interference in it.—Ibid. 992.

In these matters of local management, so deeply affecting domestic comfort, good order, and personal health, women have undoubtedly the greatest stake, and are probably the most competent judges.

§ 15. The needless limitation of the areas of jurisdiction, under the old Town Councils and the new Local Boards, is another weighty objection to their being constituted the sole sanitary managers of districts.

The only intelligible pretext for confining such jurisdictions to towns is, that vast public works, as aqueducts and reservoirs, main sewers and gasometers, are needed only for densely-peopled localities. It does not however follow, that the owners and occupiers of property so circumstanced should be isolated from the rest of the community, in order to effect their objects of water-supply, town-lighting, paving, and sewerage. Their rights and interests may be equally protected, and their responsibilities better enforced, by other and safer means.

Even as regards great structural works, much disadvantage and ultimate loss has arisen from the restriction of plans and designs to thickly inhabited areas. Moreover, it will be recollected that these architectural and engineering improvements are, after all, but a small portion of the details of sanitary management. With regard to all other arrangements, no less indispensable, for preventing disease, personal injury, and degeneracy of race, there seems to be no pretext whatever for limiting sanitary jurisdictions to aggregated populations of a given density.

As it is not for the benefit of the governed that the operation of laws for the public health should be confined to populous areas, so neither is it for the advantage of the local governing bodies, that they should be elected or selected solely from the inhabitants of such areas. Perhaps I may add, without giving offence, that the corporation of a borough sometimes needs ventilation as much as its streets and houses; and that the addition of a "country" element would not necessarily impair or debase it.*

§. 16. When, therefore, Town Councils and Commissions claim the undivided powers of health-protection and disease-palliation, within their own legal limits of jurisdiction, they should be unflinchingly met by asserting the broad principle—that measures of sanitary police, in order to be effectual, must be of universal application.

If the arrangements of every Local Board of Health were thoroughly and satisfactorily completed, they would benefit only 2,100,000† of the population of England and Wales—excluding the Metropolis. If every borough in the kingdom were under such a Local Board, the population provided for would amount to little more than a fourth of the whole.‡ Even if to these were added all the small market-towns, only half of the population would be thus protected.

But, why should there be any limit to the numbers benefited by a Public Health enactment, short of the frontiers and shores of the kingdom?

Seeing that the public provisions for collecting vital statistics —for medico-forensic inquiries—for vaccination—and for medical relief to the sick poor (not to specify other national arrangements for public order and safety),—apply to every parish, and most of them to every family, in the country,—why are general measures of health-preservation to be limited to *towns?* nay, even to those towns in which a stated proportion of the ratepayers happen to be sufficiently judicious and moderate in their

---

* It is worth notice, that the ancient limits of "Counties of Cities" were, in some instances, far more extensive than the modern boundaries of the same parliamentary boroughs. Among the records in the Town Clerk's Office, I have seen a map of Gloucester, which shows that the city jurisdiction, in the sixteenth century, included villages situated four and five miles beyond the present narrow boundary.

† See *Report* (1854) *of the General Board of Health*, p. 14.

‡ See Census. Dr. Farr has lately remarked that the municipal organization extends only to about 200 of all the towns that were enumerated at the Census. Minutes of Evidence (1586). *Report of Sir B. Hall's Committee.*

notions of "self-government," to apply for central aid and direction, in carrying into effect these most necessary reforms?

The more accurately and scientifically we investigate the causes of disease, the more clearly will it appear, that the artificial distinctions of town and country have but little to do with the administration of preventive medicine, except to limit and obstruct the execution of comprehensive measures.

§ 17. Further, the present narrow system tends directly to exclude large portions of the population most needing legal protection.

One remarkable instance of this tendency occurred under my own observation.

In 1848, I drew up a Report to the Registrar-General on the mortality of Gloucester; in which, by comparing the deaths, the ages at death, and the apparent causes of disease in the *city proper*, with those in the *suburbs*, it appeared that the latter were by far the more unhealthy, and therefore the more urgently in need of vigorous measures of sanitary reform. The superintending Inspector (Mr. Cresy, C.E.) confirmed this distinction, and accordingly recommended that a considerable district of country, extending in some directions two miles from the centre of the city, should be included within the jurisdiction of the Local Board. Nevertheless political questions arose, the influence of the Town Council prevailed, and the "Provisional Order" applied only to the Parliamentary borough.*

The result was thus described, in 1852, by a resident gentleman, of high intelligence, and belonging to no profession.

"The jurisdiction of the Local Board, I am sorry to say, does not extend beyond the boundaries fixed by the Municipal Act, which practically excludes one-third" (more now) "of the population from any control. Upon this serious obstruction to sanitary improvement, my attention has long been fixed. I counted 700 houses on one side of the city, whose only natural drainage is Sudbrook, all beyond control;

---

* A subsequent attempt to extend the sanitary jurisdiction has been defeated by another "party" manœuvre.

and, owing to the direction of the prevailing winds, the town has the full benefit of all the effluvia which their refuse creates."*

The suburban residents looked in vain to the managing authorities of the outlying districts for redress ; for, as the same impartial observer said,—

" The Board of Guardians does not co-operate with either the Local or the General Board, but (I believe) offers all the obstruction in its power."

§ 18. The error of commencing sanitary legislation by circumscribing sanitary jurisdictions, has led to the adoption of a canon of administration wholly unreasonable and indefensible; namely, that all districts, in which it cannot be proved that an excessive number of persons die annually, shall be exempted from the operation of sanitary law.

Observe the difficulties into which the movement party has brought itself by this concession. The first question of the objectors is—What do you mean by an excess of mortality? All above an annual *twenty-three* in a thousand of the population, the average of English mortality, according to Sir B. Hall's Bill. All above an annual *seventeen* in the thousand—the "natural rate" of mortality—pleaded the first vital statist in England. All above *twenty-seven* in a thousand, replied an ingenious casuist, whose object apparently was to defeat any efficient Public Health Bill. All above *twenty-five* in a thousand concludes Parliament, because that number splits the difference between Sir Benjamin Hall and Mr. Toulmin Smith.

The excess of mortality being thus summarily, if not satis-

---

* Sir Benjamin Hall, in introducing his Public Health Bills, is supposed to have selected Gloucester, as an illustration for the necessity for more comprehensive legislation. During a certain period previous to his Parliamentary Statement, the mortality of the city proper was reported to have sunk to 21 in 1000, the mortality of the suburbs to have risen to 39 in 1000. Subsequent and more minute calculation has proved that this extraordinary difference was somewhat overrated; but the fact remains, that the city mortality had diminished, and the suburban mortality had increased, since my Report in 1848, thus corroborating my conclusions. No wonder, then, that Sir B. Hall proposed to attach such outlying districts to places where the Act was already in operation.

factorily, settled—the fatal effects of the want of a preventive law having been correctly calculated—the required number of lives having been prematurely sacrificed to the regulated neglect, —the preventive law may then, and not till then, be enforced. One is irresistibly reminded of the stolen steed and the order to fasten the stable-door.

All this, be it observed, is based on the assumption, that a certain annual ratio of deaths, in any spot, is *the* test of its insalubrity. But we live in the nineteenth century, and under the glorious privileges of local self-government—freedom and science to boot—who could wish for more?

To argue further on such a point would seem to be a mere waste of time. Yet I must be allowed, by way of illustration, to ask—What would have been thought of a proposition to restrict the application of the new Poor-Law to parishes in which the rates exceeded so many shillings in the pound? Or, of a Bill to abolish the constabulary force in every county or district, in which less than an average number of crimes were committed annually?

§ 19. Before proceeding to details of suggestion, I must not omit to remark upon the measures, which have so lately received the sanction of Parliament,—the one for the better Local Management of the Metropolis,—the other,* an amended "Nuisance Removal and Diseases Prevention Act" for the whole of England. Both these enactments have created new local administrative bodies.

Those for the metropolis are either parochial Vestries or Boards of parochial districts—thirty-eight in number—all of them external to the boundaries of the old city, and, together with that, including the whole of the extensive territory now covered by modern London.

* Another small Act for the Prevention of Diseases (cap. 116, 1855) embodies a few special regulations, relating chiefly to medical duties in times of epidemic, endemic, and contagious disease, which would have more properly emanated from a Council of Health having plenary authority.

From and by these Boards and the authorities of the City, a Metropolitan Board of Works is elected, consisting of forty-five members. Each of the vestries of the six largest parishes elects two members of the Metropolitan Board; other vestries and districts send, each, one representative; four smaller districts are paired, for the purpose of electing two members.

Considerable ingenuity is shown in this formula for constructing a single administrative body by a triple process of selection from the rate-payers. The pressure of the democratic principle is doubtless diminished by each stage of the operation; but the result is a concentrated essence of parish vestries. And it remains to be seen whether the nobler or baser elements of the raw material will predominate in the extract.

§ 20. In whatever degree the new Metropolitan Board threatens to trench upon the domain of the Imperial Legislature, it may, nevertheless, insure a certain amount of uniformity and consistency in the government of this petty State.

The superior Board is empowered to exercise certain superintending functions,—such as the supervision of great structural works and main sewers. Important alterations in streets and lines of road, as well as corrections of parochial boundaries, where the ancient divisions are found to be inconvenient, may be directed by this Board.

Other powers of local management are committed to the Vestries and district Boards, which will absorb and consolidate many of those conflicting jurisdictions, for which London was so famous, with regard to paving, lighting, watching, and cleansing. They will execute the powers of surveyors of highways. They will control footways, courts, cellar-dwellings, and slaughter-houses. They are to be the local authorities for carrying into effect the Nuisances Removal Act. They are to appoint scavengers, "inspectors" of nuisances, and, as we have seen, medical officers of health.

Nevertheless, the provision and control of baths and washhouses, the interment of the dead, the supervision of markets, and the administration of charitable trusts, remain under former management.

The medical visitation of districts, also, whether in ordinary times or during epidemics, is not mentioned in the Act; so that this and all other duties of prevention and palliation of disease, which appertain to Boards of Guardians, will also remain in the same unsettled and unsatisfactory position.

§ 21. The conclusion, therefore, to which I am led by an examination of this Act, is—that the greater anomalies and difficulties of the sanitary question are not met by it.

For, *as to limits of jurisdiction :*—Comparing the Schedules of parishes and districts appended to this Act with the thirty-six Registration districts of the metropolis,—there seems, at first sight, to be some attempt to identify, or at least to approximate, the two systems of distribution ; but, on a closer inspection, it will be found that the discrepancies are neither few nor trifling. And unless the Registrar-General should see fit to alter the limits of his districts, the areas for sanitary and statistical returns will remain at variance with the areas of local management.

Again, *as to the constitution of these Boards :*—We have seen how miserably the old Vestries provided for the public safety in perilous emergencies. But it would be difficult to show that any real security has been taken by Parliament for a more liberal and judicious management of sanitary affairs by these new Vestries.

It will scarcely be affirmed that the " qualification" is raised. For, although the aspirant to municipal distinction must now be assessed upon a rental of 40*l.* a year*—said to be the average rental of the metropolis,—this is positively the only guarantee provided for a superior class of local directors.

But if moral worth, intellectual cultivation, freedom from sordid views, and zeal for the welfare of the masses, are desirable qualifications for those engaged in local administration,—if such

---

* The qualification in all provincial boroughs, fixed by the Municipal Reform Act, and for local Boards of Health, by the Act of 1848, is 30*l.* Considering the difference of house rent between London and other towns, the provincial qualification is perhaps relatively higher.

'qualifications do not specifically belong to occupiers rated at 40*l*. (Heaven forbid they should!)—if the large and probably increasing proportion of persons of condition and intelligence, who are not "occupiers" at all, in a legal sense, (such as refined and highly-educated residents in furnished houses, and well-informed artisans in lodgings,) are decidedly more likely to possess the higher endowments I have mentioned;—on what grounds, let me ask, is a mere rate-paying qualification adopted?

Are dealers in all sorts of food, drugs, and chemicals, or owners of obnoxious stores and manufactories of various kinds, more likely to assist cordially in abolishing the causes of disease, because they rent premises of 40*l*. and upwards, than those who have no opportunity or temptation to profit at the expense of their neighbours' health and comfort? Does a forty-pound house "make the man, and want of it the fellow?" If such odious and fallacious distinctions are not utterly opposed to the diffusion of knowledge, to the prevalence of Christianity, and to the progress of social improvement, they are at all events revolutionary, because they tend to create discontent among the working classes, who are thus stigmatized as unworthy to deliberate on matters more seriously affecting their welfare than that of any other class in society.

Lastly—*As to various preventive and remedial measures:*— Several most important duties of this nature, as we have seen, are still shared by other bodies; so that, until further legislation takes place, we must expect to hear of the same miserable results of irresponsibility and apathy as were so recently exposed by the Inspectors of the General Board of Health.

§ 22. The "Nuisances Removal and Diseases Prevention Act" of 1855, has also authorized new local administrative bodies of various descriptions, as follows:—

(1) Local Boards of Health under the Act of 1848;
(2) Town Councils;
(3) Bodies of Trustees and Town Improvement Commissioners;
(4) Highway Boards;

(5) new local authorities, to be called "Nuisances Removal Committees," and to be annually appointed by Vestries;
(6) Boards for lighting and watching;
(7) and, as a *dernier ressort*,* Boards of Guardians.

The surveyors of highways are to be added to the three last named authorities. Each description of Board named in this singular category is deemed less worthy of confidence and less capable of administration than that preceding it; but the "wooden spoon" in the list of sanitary honours is reserved for the poor-law Guardians, who, it seems, do not feel particularly complimented by the distinction. And when we consider the extremely remote connexion with affairs of public health which some of the more favoured bodies can claim, such a slight to Boards of Guardians is surely undeserved. Practically however, in most instances, the latter Boards will be unaffected by the change, and will continue to exercise their sanitary functions over the greater part of England, and their remedial duties over the whole, until they are superseded by more comprehensive legislation..

When so many local bodies were specified, one does not readily see why the Burial Boards, of which there are at least fifty-eight in the kingdom, were not included. Surely, the interment of the dead has as much to do with the public health, as repair of the highways, or watching and lighting the streets.

§ 23. Doubtless, by fixing upon one of these numerous little authorities to execute the Act in every place, the legislature has done something to prevent that unseemly evasion of responsibility, which prevailed when not even the lawyers employed could determine which of the local Boards was to act in a given case. But, on the other hand, by directing the performance of the same duties by different Boards in different places, a new element of confusion is introduced; and we are left to wonder that the legislator, who was bold enough to create an authority which may

---

* Mr. Lewis, a solicitor, examined before Sir B. Hall's Committee, said,—"The gentlemen with whom I am acting, think that the Boards of Guardians, being gentlemen of great respectability, instead of being the *last* upon the list, should be the *second*."—(409.)

some day prove a dangerous rival to the Imperial Parliament in the metropolis of the kingdom, did not venture his constructive hand upon a new order of local Boards of superior constitution, identical in kind, and embracing the whole population in their united jurisdictions.

This Act, moreover, leaves medical relief and other palliative measures during pestilence in the present incompetent hands.

It is true that this and other important omissions,* especially the absence of any provision compelling local Boards to perform the duties specified in the Act, may be attributed to that neutralizing process which every promising Bill must be expected to undergo before it can escape from the double parliamentary ordeal as an Act. The measure is in all respects so small and imperfect an affair that it can be only temporary; but it was probably thought necessary to do something to appease troublesome reformers until another session.

§ 24. The absurd outcry against what is commonly termed "centralization," but more correctly, responsibility; and in favour of what is called "local self-government," meaning irresponsibility,—an outcry which has been of late so unwisely and unfairly abetted by some whose commanding position might have enabled them to allay the misapprehension and remove the prejudice,—may, for a short time, make an undue impression upon the temporizing, the ill-informed, and the infirm of purpose.

But the worth and intelligence of the country will not be long deluded by mere words and names. If a really popular influence, that is, a representation of the vital interests of all who have souls and bodies to be cared for, can be best secured by means of a constitutional Government—a central power, resting upon the confidence and support of a nation—why should we fear the establishment of such a power?

At all events, we must cease to expect more of local Boards than they are calculated to fulfil. Much of importance, if judi-

---

* Some of these changes for the worse are well exposed in a vigorous article on Sir B. Hall's Bill, in the *Saturday Review* of Dec. 29, 1855.

ciously constituted, they might effect; but the experiment recently made in England has been singularly unfortunate. As an able writer* has pithily said,—" Boards have been so created that they could not do what they might, and might not do what they could."

§ 25. From the dilemma into which we have been brought by an inconsiderate, a too confiding, legislation, we can now only escape by comprehensive and decisive measures.

"Government direction will not remedy the evil of local incompetency. Unless the constitution of the corporate bodies should be so modified as to work harmoniously with the Central Board and its Inspectors, we must look for a perpetual struggle between the motive power of the State and the obstructive resistance of the municipalities, in which the latter will generally come off victorious."†

The preceding sentence has been in print more than seven years, during which period malignant epidemic cholera has twice invaded this country. Have not my predictions, with regard to the struggle between the local and central administrative bodies, been literally fulfilled in each of these visitations? Will it not also be found that " rights and powers, once conferred on representative bodies, are not easily recalled, however miserably executed?"

Further legislative interference is now, however, generally admitted to be inevitable, and another Parliamentary Session will hardly pass without a new Public Health Bill.

The question, therefore, with regard to local Boards, is not whether some change shall be made, but what that change should be, and how it should be carried into effect.

B. Local Boards as they might be.

§ 26. The primary requisite for a Sanitary Code of laws—as was urged in 1848—is the employment of a uniform administrative machinery, applicable to every part of the country, whether town or rural parish. The next principle—to be deduced from the preceding evidence—is no longer to delegate common

* *Fraser's Magazine*, Aug. 1854, p. 23.   † *Remarks, supra cit.* p. 6.

or mixed functions to two or more local boards, in the same place, yet with different areas of jurisdiction.

After all that has passed, the Guardians of the poor will scarcely be allowed to remain the sole local authorities, as regards measures of prevention and palliation, in places which are not included in the jurisdiction of existing Local Boards of Health, Town Councils, and other bodies of this kind.

Still less probable is it that the latter bodies will be authorized to supersede Boards of Guardians in the direction of medico-sanitary duties (medical relief—vaccination—registration) within the narrow bounds of their circumscribed jurisdictions. Nor yet can we reasonably expect that "joint committees" will adequately meet the difficulties of the case, so long as the respective areas of administration of the two bodies are so widely different.

The third main conclusion, as to future legislation, is, that NEW local administrative bodies ought to be formed, with larger jurisdictions than those of any existing bodies,* and constituted, in great measure, of delegates from all those corporate authorities which the Legislature has already empowered and cannot easily set aside. By this means alone, as it seems to me, can Boards of Guardians be equitably and reasonably dealt with. If a considerable portion of each new Sanitary Court were to consist of delegates from the Board or Boards of Guardians within its sphere, few objections, and these not insuperable, would be raised to the transfer of all palliative functions, now performed by the existing parochial authorities, to the new and superior body, or to committees of that body.

§ 27. Nevertheless, the difficulties created by existing territorial divisions and jurisdictions, are not to be summarily disposed of.† In theory, as has been repeatedly urged, "areas for

* This is not intended to apply to the metropolis,—perhaps not to three or four other first-class towns.

† "The inconveniences and perplexities which the variety of ecclesiastical, military and civil, fiscal and judicial, ancient and modern, municipal and parliamentary, subdivisions of the country occasion, have been sensibly felt by us, as they were brought under our notice in the enumeration of the population. It is not within our province to reduce all these to simplicity and harmony, but we

the management of the Public Health should be co-terminous with those adopted for statistical returns." And practically, could the established divisions of England and Wales, for enumerating the population and for registering births, deaths, and marriages, be revised and corrected with reference to sanitary considerations, the identification of the two systems of distribution would in this country become easy and obvious. But, it must not be forgotten that the Registration districts were, without any sufficient reason, based on the Poor-Law division of the country into "Unions," which are too often inconvenient in form, and unscientific in arrangement.

Indeed, as Unions were not originally planned with any reference to the public health, but, in general, either simply for fiscal purposes, or to meet the views of landed proprietors, there could be no pretext, save that of use and custom (and these but of short duration), for applying them to statistical and sanitary objects.

§ 28. Aware of the objections which may fairly be urged against almost every attempt to re-distribute the population, and conscious that I have neither the materials nor the opportunity to enable me to meet all such objections by a perfect scheme, I am nevertheless disposed to submit the following suggestions,— which would, of course, apply only beyond the limits of the metropolis.

i. That each sanitary district should contain, on the average, 60,000 to 80,000 inhabitants;* that is, more than double the extent of the existing Registration districts.

ii. That towns and cities containing more than 60,000 inhabitants, should constitute sanitary districts of themselves, and

---

call attention to their existence, and venture humbly to suggest, that the task of taking any future census, the comparison of statistical facts of every kind, and probably all administrative arrangements, would be greatly facilitated by the adoption of a uniform system of territorial divisions in Great Britain."—Census (1851). *Report*, 8vo ed. p. 25.

* In Prussia, in 1852, each *Kreis*—287 in number—was said to contain an average population of 56,000.—See a Statistical Account in the *Med. Times and Gaz.*, April 30, 1853. In Austria, the size of the *Kreis* is more variable, containing from 30,000 to 120,000 inhabitants.

should include no more of the surrounding country than would be indicated by the natural features of the locality or required for the sanitary purposes of the population.

iii. That, in other districts, of mixed town and country population, a conveniently situated county or market-town be selected for the meeting-place of the Local Court, and confer its name on the district.

iv. That the boundaries of the several districts, following generally the limits of parishes or townships, be so determined, that each cluster of population might be included in that district, the capital town of which is most easy of access; subject nevertheless, in some cases, to considerations of physical topography.

v. That every sanitary district be an exact aggregate of a number of medical-visitation districts—the boundaries of the latter being corrected for the purpose if necessary.

If a revision of the Registration districts should be refused, the only course would be, to make use of them as they are, with all their imperfections, combining two or more of them in one superior district.*

§ 29. Let me next suggest an amended constitution for the local administrative bodies, on the principles already indicated. In each of the proposed sanitary districts, it is presumed that one such body should be instituted, and that it should consist of:—

1stly. A definite proportion of the Guardians of the several parishes contained within the boundaries of the new district, to be selected by the Board or Boards of which such Guardians are already members:

2ndly. Representatives of any or every local Board of Health, Town Council, or other similar body, the jurisdictions of which may be contained within the new district; the total number of

---

* "The Registration District," says Dr. Farr, "is the basis of the Census, and of the registration of births, deaths, causes of death, and marriages, which supply ready means of determining the state of the public health."

He would therefore make the Registration District "the area for the operation of the Public Health Act." So would I, on condition that the Registration Districts be revised and amended.

these representatives not to exceed the number of the selected Guardians ; a scheme for such representation to be submitted, in the first place, by a Government Inspector, to the several bodies concerned, and their objections, if any, to be respectfully received and fairly considered ; and the ultimate decision to remain with the Home Office or the Central Board :

3rdly. A limited number of the magistrates, resident and acting within the district, to be selected at Quarter Sessions, or at a general meeting of magistrates.

The three preceding elements of the new Court should, at their first meeting, proceed to add to their number, as follows :—

4thly. A limited number—not exceeding that of the selected magistrates—of the parochial clergy, chosen in consideration of their known zeal and success in promoting the moral and social welfare of their parishioners :

And, 5thly, the same proportion of other specially qualified scientific and philanthropic residents,—such as civil engineers, professors of the natural and exact sciences, and instructors of youth, or (if required by a majority or even a large minority of the Court) ministers of various religious societies.

§ 30. A medical Council or Faculty* should be chosen by the registered practitioners resident in each sanitary district, for the promotion of scientific research, for the consideration of questions belonging to the duties of the profession, and especially for the aid and counsel of the District Court of Health, which should be required to refer certain matters for their opinion.

The relation of this local faculty to the District Court, would be analogous to that which the late medical council of the metropolis bore to the General Board of Health ; and the public would derive a greater amount of benefit from the separate session of the medical element than from introducing it into the proposed District Court.

§ 31. With regard to the duties of the proposed local administrative bodies, little need be said.

* See Introductory Essay, p. 43 ; and Essay II. p. 81.

The Public Health Act, the "Nuisances Removal and Diseases Prevention" Acts, and various other measures already enacted by, or laid before, Parliament, will be found to indicate many of the sanitary regulations which would have to be enforced by the local authority. Other provisions, again, which the English Legislature has not yet attempted, scarcely even contemplated, for the public health, and which are pointed out in the Introductory Essay, would be carried into effect by these Courts.

In ordinary circumstances, and when a resort to compulsory legal process might not be required, their mode of action would be through skilful and properly qualified officers. The number, titles, and functions of such officers have been already suggested.*

In most places, some alteration of the existing "medical relief" districts would be found desirable. The sanitary jurisdiction should contain a number of these, amply sufficient for the needs of the poorer population, and they should be called " visitation districts." This revision would be one of the first duties of the Sanitary Court; and the localization of dispensaries would be determined, at the same time, with the aid and approval of the circuit inspector.

After the preliminary arrangements for dispensary establishments were completed, the Sanitary Court would appoint its quotum of members for each dispensary committee; and, as being the superior body, would call upon the Boards of Guardians, the subscribers to the dispensaries,† and the medical faculty, to elect the other quota; and thus complete the formation of these committees.

Large structural works would, of course, apply only to the more closely aggregated portions of population; and these portions (where the sanitary district did not consist wholly of a town) would alone be charged with the cost of such works.

* See Introductory Essay, pp. 50—52. † Essay IV. p. 244.

ESSAY VI.

ON CERTAIN DEPARTMENTS OF HEALTH POLICE, IN
THEIR RELATIONS WITH LOCAL SANITARY
ADMINISTRATION.

" Porro, si cui novum videatur quod dico, sciat, non hîc novam quidem, sed tamen prorsus utilem necessariamque politiæ partem moliri."

. . . .

" Cùmque in aliis omnibus Reipublicæ partibus prudenter aliquot præfecti sunt, qui earum curam gerunt, ut Ædiles structuris, Tribuni militiæ, Scholarchæ ludo literario, seplasiarum Inspectores pharmacis; præterea quando in omnibus rebus semper præstat ordo ataxiæ, sitque Deus ipse ordinis autor et propugnator; spero cordatos homines facile concessuros, ut hanc novitatem Respublicæ admittant.

" JOHANNES EVVICH,
Reipublicæ Bremensis Medicus Ordinarius," MDLXXXII.

ESSAY VI.

CHAPTER FIRST.

THE REGISTRATION OF BIRTHS AND DEATHS.

§ 1. AT the termination of the Third Essay, I mentioned three classes of officers—now performing duties connected with the public health in England—who might in combination, and under an improved organization, act far more efficiently and usefully than they do at present.

Two of these classes have already been under consideration —namely, Medical Officers of Visitation districts, and Health Officers of Sanitary districts.

The third class, on which I proceed to make a few remarks, consists of the Registrars and Superintendent Registrars of Births, Deaths, and Marriages.

§ 2. The very obvious connexion in every locality between the medical care of the poorer classes and a scientific record of births and deaths, induced certain official authorities, soon after the passing of the English Registration Act, to point out the probable advantages that might be expected from committing the duties of Registrar in every sub-district to the Union Surgeons.

But the extreme dissatisfaction with which the poor-law arrangements were at that time justly viewed by the mass of medical practitioners, and the peculiar manner in which the proposal was put forth,* prevented in some degree a calm con-

---

* A circular was issued from the Poor-Law Commission Office in 1836, to the Clerks of the several Boards of Guardians, announcing that, in consequence of the

sideration of the very rational principle on which it was founded. Yet it had a certain effect, for we were informed by the Registrar-General, that (416 + 111*) 527 members of the medical profession had accepted office as registrars of sub-districts; that is, nearly a fourth part of the total number (2190) of Registrars.

By 1853, however, the number of *Medical* Registrars must have greatly decreased, for at the close of the year there were only 340† Registrars of Births and Deaths, either physicians, surgeons, or apothecaries; that is, not one in six of the whole number.

Probably, this diminution may show that there is something in the present position and relations of the office not agreeable or suitable to medical men. And it is of no small importance to endeavour to discover the real objection, in order that, if it be removable, the combination of the medico-sanitary office with that of registering births and deaths in the same sub-district may be promoted.

§ 3. The appointment of Registrar is, now, too frequently held by persons of inferior education, unprepared and indisposed to appreciate the importance of accuracy in recording the physical events and circumstances attending upon every commencement and termination of human life.

My recent correspondence with "Officers of Health" elicited some very important facts respecting the application of the registration machinery to local sanitary management.

It appears that in some towns the Registrars supplied copies of their entries to the Health Officer, weekly in the largest places, and either monthly or quarterly in others. The Registrars were paid for this information by the local Board of Health, in at least

---

registration enactment, Registrars would be wanted immediately, and suggesting that the paid officers of the Unions, especially the Medical Officers, would be the fittest persons to hold those appointments.—See a review of this document, *Med. Gaz.* vol. xviii. p. 879.

* *First Annual Report of Registrar-General,* p. 4, 8vo, 1839.

† Forty-nine of these 340 were also Registrars of Marriages, together with twenty-one who were *only* Registrars of Marriages, making seventy of this class.

four of the twenty-two towns, and those the largest. In three or four others, the Registrars furnished facts gratuitously. In two, objections were made by the Registrars to grant this aid. In another small place, it was said—" the Registrar-General does not sanction the singling out a small parish for mortality returns from the rest of the district." And it is manifest that all pretext for such an application to the Registrar-General would be removed by identifying the areas of statistical inquiry with those of sanitary management. Generally the Officers of Health report—that the Registration machinery is available, and, except in the cases above-mentioned, those officers or their deputies make their own extracts from the registers.

As to the quality of the information thus obtained, some observations have been already made in this work (pp. 103, 104). It may suffice here to repeat, that in several places the statements respecting the causes of death have been not only imperfect and unsatisfactory, but supplied (in disobedience to the Registrar-General's orders) by unqualified persons.

§ 4. The certification of the physical circumstances of deaths, (as before said) by regularly qualified medical men, should be imperatively demanded in all cases under equitable arrangements.

If, moreover, a scientific and sanitary character were conferred on the office of Registrar, the leading facts of each disease, or at all events the signs, if any, of injury or morbid change,—the duration of the case, and the apparent predisposing and proximate causes of the event, would be correctly described; and by employing the district surgeons as registrars, the public would possess a tolerably sure guarantee, not only for an accurate mortuary registration, but for a trustworthy physiological record of births.

But, notwithstanding the advantages to the community and to scie ce of such an amendment in the registration machinery, any attempt to enforce universally the appointment of medical registrars is to be deprecated; and the precise arrangement in each sanitary district might be very reasonably left to the joint deliberation of the proposed sanitary Court and Medical Faculty.

Whether or not the district medical officers should, as vacancies occur, become the Registrars of births and deaths,—it is unquestionably desirable that the two systems of territorial division should be made to correspond. If, as suggested in the fourth Essay, the number of visitation districts were increased from 3040 to 4000; and if it should be deemed unadvisable (though why, I know not) to increase the number (2190) of Registration sub-districts to the same amount; it might be neither inexpedient nor impracticable to direct such a revision of local jurisdictions as would in most cases form *one* Registration sub-district, out of *two* medical districts. It cannot be too often urged that areas for returns of vital statistics should correspond with those instituted for sanitary care.

§ 5. But there are yet stronger and perhaps unanswerable reasons for concluding that so much of the office of Superintendent Registrar, as relates to births and deaths, should in future vacancies be committed to physicians or surgeons of a certain standing.

The Officer of Health would obviously be the fittest person to hold that appointment; whilst the performance of merely civil marriages, and the collective registration of all marriages, might be left to the Clerks of Unions, or other non-medical persons, now holding the office of Superintendent Registrar. But, as it would be preferable to keep the whole arrangements for Registration under one system of local management, the marriage department of Registration might, with still greater propriety, be committed to the Clerk or Secretary of the proposed Sanitary Court: and this officer would generally belong to the legal profession.

In 1853, it appears that only four of the 624 Superintendent Registrars were medical men. Yet, beyond all question, medical supervision would render the registration of births and deaths, by whomsoever performed, far more serviceable in a legal or forensic point of view; for it could hardly fail of securing more precise attention on the part of the Registrars to the causes and conditions of mortality.*

Dr. Southwood Smith's opinion on this point, given in 1843,† is too valuable to be omitted:—

"Nor will it be regarded," said he, "as the least important part of the service capable of being rendered by such an instructed body of men [superior Officers of Health] to whom the present local registrars might act as auxiliaries, that they would soon give to the registration that degree of accuracy and completeness which would fit it in a perfect manner for every use, civil and legislative, to which a perfect registration is capable of being applied."

Conversely also, the Officer of Health, in the execution of his high functions of advice and prevention, and aided by such an official co-operation, would have at his command certified statements of the fact and cause of every death occurring within his jurisdiction. He would thus be enabled immediately to direct the attention of the local administrative authority to any circumstances connected with locality or occupation, which might appear to him on investigation likely to have caused the deaths.

These various considerations show that many substantial advantages would arise from the establishment of a close and well-defined connexion between the Registration department and the civil medical service.

---

* Dr. Greenhill, who has bestowed much careful attention on the Registration of Births and Deaths, and who is therefore particularly qualified to give an opinion on the subject, thus writes to me:—"A *Medical* Registrar would be especially useful in avoiding mistakes in copying the medical certificates of death. At present many monstrous words and ridiculous errors occur from the illegibility of the certificate, which a *Medical* Registrar would be able to avoid. A *Medical Superintendent* Registrar would be useful in detecting the errors of the *non*-medical Registrar, when he collates the certified copy of the register with the original before it goes to London. *Both* would be useful in asking now and then for additional information or explanation from the medical practitioner who gave the certificate."

† *Health of Towns Commission Report,* loc. cit.

CHAPTER SECOND.

MEDICAL EVIDENCE IN FORENSIC INQUIRIES.

§ 1. So many matters of sanitary police claim to be dealt with, under a national organization of medical service, and special legislation upon some of those matters is now so urgently called for, that I may be expected to treat of, at least, the more prominent among them; and, without confining myself to system, I shall now consider some of them, in the order which seems naturally to suggest itself.

The preceding remarks on the advantages of medical assistance, in the Registration of Deaths, lead almost inevitably to a consideration of our legal provisions for Forensic Inquiry; the main object of both these departments being to ensure a correct determination of the causes of mortality.

Judicial investigations concerning suspicious deaths, are conducted in England on principles widely differing from those in operation on the Continent; and the comparison is not to our advantage. A Coroner's Inquest, as we all know, is demanded* whenever a death has taken place in an apparently unnatural manner; or where some suspicion of foul play has been aroused, or some rumour to that effect has prevailed; or where the fatal event has obviously resulted from some horrible accident, startling the neighbourhood or the nation into a spasmodic effort to ascertain the precise cause.

A remarkable feature of the English Inquest is, that the law does not require the presence and aid of a scientific person, specially instructed and practised in forensic medicine—an

---

* "The Coroner, upon information, shall go to the place where any be slain, or suddenly dead or wounded, and shall forthwith, &c."—Old Statute *De Officio Coronatoris*, 4 Edw. I. stat. 2.

expert, as the French call him—to enlighten the researches of the Coroner and Jury.

§ 2. The Medical Witnesses Act (6 and 7 Wm. IV. c. 89) empowers the Coroner to call for the attendance of any legally-qualified medical practitioner, and secures his remuneration out of the poor-rates. The guinea fee is to be doubled when a post-mortem examination, with or without chemical analysis, is deemed necessary by the majority of the jury; but every practitioner is liable to a penalty of five pounds for declining to undertake this peculiar and disagreeable duty, however incompetent he may feel himself for it.

No attempt, be it observed, has ever been made by the Legislature to ensure the competency of medical evidence on the many abstruse questions which come before these Courts. It is entirely at the option of this petty judge and jury to summon any professional or scientific witnesses; and the State has provided no official persons of learning and skill to whom the Court may resort in emergencies.

We have been told of the invaluable protection afforded to the public by this ancient institution; but, when all the froth of so empty a boast has subsided, the plain fact remains, that a very large proportion of Coroners' Inquests leave the cause of death wholly unexplained. Hence our medico-legal investigations have sunk to a very low ebb in the estimation of the better informed, both at home and abroad. Such common verdicts as "Died by the visitation of God," and "Died from natural causes," however true in the abstract, generally amount to simple avowals, that the Coroner and Jury are alike unable to solve the difficulties, and at the same time unwilling to refer them to more competent authorities.

§ 3. It is no discredit to a practitioner engaged in the toilsome routine of ordinary medical duties, if he should feel himself at a loss when called upon for a decisive opinion in some obscure case of poisoning, infanticide, or legitimacy. His scanty opportunities for the study of these points, and for post-mortem examinations, cannot suffice to qualify him for answering the delicate and important questions which he must answer before a jury can find a proper verdict.

One of our leading periodicals* lately exposed in a single number two cases, which even of themselves ought to leave no doubt, that some very different method of determining the cause of death should be provided by the State.

i. A well-known baronet was lately found dead in his bed. A coroner's order was issued for examination. The abdomen and thorax only were opened. Nothing peculiar was noticed, except some "fat outside of the heart," which was supposed to be sufficient to account for death. The head was not opened, because " the position and appearance of the corpse did not indicate any mischief in the brain"!

ii. An old man, in a parish of Surrey, died after lying down in pain. An order was issued to Mr. C., to make a *post-mortem* inspection. On his arrival at the house, forty-eight hours after death, he found that the body had been already opened, the viscera cut and detached, and the pericardium and large vessels about the heart not to be found. It appears that a Mr. Y. thought that he ought to have had the order, and so revenged himself by anticipating Mr. C., opening the body early in the morning, and causing the missing parts to be buried! His behaviour at the inquest, if reported correctly, was as unbecoming as his prior conduct was disgraceful.

Such cases could not have occurred in France or Germany; and the mere possibility of their occurrence here is a stain upon our national institutions.

§ 4. The custom of indiscriminately summoning medical practitioners of all sorts, and of all degrees of pathological knowledge and forensic skill, has sadly depreciated the value of medical evidence in courts of justice. Public confidence in the profession has been shaken; and the appearance of a "doctor" in the witness-box is but too often a signal for sport among gentlemen of the long robe.

It is really disheartening when one sees that even those who are supposed to be specially qualified for forensic examinations by their peculiar pursuits and exceptional position, not unfre-

---

* *Medical Times and Gaz.*, Feb. 3, 1855.

quently expose their incompetence as much as their less distinguished brethren. Would any impartial reader of the very fair and courteous cross-examination to which the physicians retained by the Crown, in the case of the insane murderer, Luigi Buranelli,* were subjected, conclude that one of those gentlemen had any clear notion of his assumed difference between an *illusion* and a *delusion?* And should the momentous decision between life and death be allowed to depend, as it did in this case, on so shadowy a distinction?

There is nothing, apparently, that the Bar delights in more than a request, made with a mischievously bland smile, that the medical witness would be so kind as to " define insanity." The unhappy witness, flattering himself that he can take an original and safe step in a path where hundreds have stumbled before him, generally falls into the trap. A question of fact in a particular case, which his professional experience might enable him correctly to determine, thus becomes a question of theory; and he is soon lost in a maze of logical refinements and contradictions, to the triumph of the "learned gentleman," and the hopeless perplexity of the jury.

§ 5. The results—ludicrous or lamentable—of our system of medical jurisprudence being patent to every one, it would be deemed most unreasonable to tax the community with the cost of more frequent inquests of such doubtful utility.† Yet it is

* See the " Case of Luigi Buranelli," by Dr. Forbes Winslow, London, 1855.

† " Not many years ago, the following incident occurred at the London Hospital, and occasioned much interest. A Coroner and Jury sat upon the body of an unfortunate person who had died suddenly, and connected with whose death there did not chance to be any circumstances known of a nature to make either suicide or murder suspected. Satisfied with this negative evidence the Coroner refused to order a *post-mortem*, and despite the doubts expressed by the medical witnesses, a verdict of death from natural causes was recorded, the hypothesis of an apoplectic fit having been adopted. After the inquest, as a matter of pathological interest, an autopsy was made, and in the stomach was found a large quantity of oxalic acid."

" One would have expected that a man who had once in his life been placed in a ridiculous position of President over the farcical inquiry just alluded to would have taken good care in future to avoid like errors."

" A few days ago, at the same Hospital, an inquest had been held, in which the certain that a large proportion of sudden deaths escape any legal investigation whatever.

Dr. A. B. Granville, who has paid much attention to the subject, asserts, that not half of the number of sudden deaths in the metropolis are subjected to inquiry.* If even a tenth part were exempted, how much crime might pass undetected and unpunished!

These extraordinary imperfections of the English methods of medico-legal research have led some to advocate a combination of technical knowledge with the judicial function in the appointment of MEDICAL CORONERS.

There may be instances† of the successful working of such a combination; but it ought, in my opinion, to be looked upon as merely an exceptional and temporary arrangement for supplying a fundamental defect in the national system. It is at best but a very inadequate compensation for the want of an appointed scientific referee in each locality.

The Coroner is, in theory, both magistrate and judge. He ought therefore to be versed in the technicalities of law. He ought to possess the faculty of weighing evidence, and to be trained in the art of "summing up" for a jury. These are

house-surgeon had given evidence. At its conclusion, one of the officials (not the Coroner himself) addressed the house-surgeon to this effect:—'Here is another man here, sir, brought in dead, having spit blood, perhaps you will be good enough to save us the trouble by deposing to his death also.' This being declined, the proper medical officer was summoned and the due forms gone through. He deposed to the fact of the man having been brought in dead, but as to the cause of death, stated that he could give no opinion unless an autopsy was first performed. This the Coroner refused to order, and under his direction a verdict of death from natural causes was returned by the Jury."

" We instance this on account of its absurdity, not on account of its supposed rarity. We fear, from information which reaches us from time to time, that proceedings such as it exhibits are but too frequently allowed to disgrace our Coroners' Courts and to defeat the ends of public inquiry."—*Medical Times and Gaz.*, p. 167, Aug. 18, 1855.

* Ibid. Feb. 17, 1855. See also a corroborative statement by Mr. Amyott, of Diss (Norfolk), ibid. March 3, 1855.

† The most remarkable instance of distinguished service in this office is afforded by the able Coroner for Middlesex, to whom also the profession is indebted for the Medical Witnesses Act.

qualifications belonging to the *legal* profession as specially, as the delivery of scientific, ætiological, or pathological opinions belong to the *medicql*. The supposition that lawyers have been unfairly thrust into medico-sanitary employment in this country, does not justify a retaliation on the part of the medical profession in the sphere of forensic medicine. The boundary line between the two vocations is plain enough, and the public interests will be best served by neither party overstepping it.

§ 6. It would be out of place here to enter upon a discussion which will soon force itself upon public attention—namely, whether the office of Coroner, and the form and constitution of his court, are judiciously adapted for their professed object;—whether a separate system of forensic inquiry (the jurisdiction of which is imperfectly defined) is necessary for that object;—and if so, whether the long-established though much-abused methods of electing and paying Coroners, do not cry out for a sweeping reform; whether also, a deliberative assembly, consisting of some score of small traders and village (or street) gossips, picked up in haste by the parish beadle, and meeting in an alehouse, represents adequately the impressive dignity and stern independence of Justice; and whether the results are calculated to satisfy the public mind in any of the perplexities arising out of such appalling events as are thus investigated.

These questions cannot be thrust aside, but they would be more properly considered by others and elsewhere.

Enough, probably, has been said to show—that, owing partly to a frequent defect in registering the causes of death, and partly to the absence of skilled evidence in medico-legal inquiries, the public has really no adequate or valid security for the detection of secret crime; and it is too probable that such crime is on the increase.*

* We are told by Dr. A. B. Granville that fifteen per cent. of the children born alive in England in the five years before 1852 died before reaching one year of age; while nearly five per cent. perished within thirty days of birth: also, that during a recent "strike" at Preston, the deaths of children under one year of age amounted to thirty-three per cent. of the general mortality, and of infants under a month to eight per cent. !

§ 7. Now according to previous suggestions, the medical superintendent of every sanitary jurisdiction—our Officer of Health—would, in virtue of his position, be entitled to information of the most valuable kind, respecting the latter stages and terminations of life, from the medical visitors and the Registrars of the several sub-districts under his inspection. It is also presumed that he would be well versed in questions of medical jurisprudence, and accustomed to give evidence upon them. He should therefore be required either to examine or to be present at the examination of every corpse subjected to an inquest; and to give all the information in his power respecting the cause of death to the Police Magistrate, or the Coroner and Jury.

Thus, three hundred selected Physicians or Surgeons, specially prepared for the embarrassments inseparable from these inquiries, would be at the service of the country, occupying posts of dignity and responsibility in places convenient of access to the entire population.

§ 8. It will be observed that these suggestions, respecting the forensic duties of the Officers of Health, contain no mention of minute chemical and microscopical analyses; for instance, in cases where poisoning is probable, and cannot be detected by the simpler methods of investigation. I am not prepared to affirm, that most of the proposed sanitary districts in England could be at once provided with resident scientific analysts, according to the programme in my introductory Essay. And it may well be doubted whether the medical superintendent of the Sanitary district would, as a general rule, be the proper ultimate referee in the cases supposed.

Medical men, even the more highly educated, are for the most part unprepared for the peculiar difficulties of an examination involving a delicate and protracted analysis of the viscera, their contents, adjacent structures, and other matters concerned.

It may also be assumed, that, although the proposed Medical Officer of Health would in general be better qualified for such an undertaking than other medical residents within his jurisdiction, he might not possess either that tact in chemical manipulation, which can only be acquired by continual practice, or the complicated apparatus which is needed for very refined examinations.

Again, neither this officer, nor the Circuit Inspectors hereafter to be proposed, would be advantageously employed in special and tedious researches, which would seriously interfere with their numerous and regular administrative duties; and which, after all, require merely a high degree of knowledge and skill in qualitative and quantitative analysis, or in practical toxicology.* On weighing these *consideranda*, it will I think appear, that—without interfering with the right of any local court to appoint an expert resident chemical analyst, subject to the approval of a central scientific Council—it would be a more judicious course, as regards the country generally, for such a Council to appoint three or four first-rate men in this department, *e. g.*, one or two in London, one in the north, and one in the west of England, who might be called in by the Officer of Health, with the sanction of the Coroner, in extraordinary cases.

This subject is, however, closely connected with another department of sanitary police, on which I now proceed to make a few observations.

* Dr. R. M. Glover, in a useful and suggestive paper on Sanitary Police, mentions the obvious objections to committing these analyses to an Inspector of Health in an extensive district with regular routine duties.—" The examiner (says Dr. Glover) has often to subject all the internal organs of the body to a careful analysis, and to search for the poison in the very tissues themselves. The labour of the inquiry is increased by the circumstance that arsenic has been found in somany of the re-agents which have to be employed. Before proceeding to the analysis itself, he has to satisfy himself of the purity of the materials which he employs;—and, in a word, a week or fortnight's labour may be expended before he can certify either the presence or the absence of the poison."—*Lancet*, March 25, 1854.

CHAPTER THIRD.

The Adulteration of Food, Drinks, and Medicines.

§ 1. In this matter, as in many others, Germany and France are far in advance of England, as to both legislation and practical administration; though the activity of current inquiries may lead us to hope that our national inferiority in this respect may be of but short duration.

The recent stir upon this question is in a great degree attributable to the spirited undertaking of the editor of the *Lancet*. The extraordinary disclosures of his Analytical Sanitary Commissioner,* Dr. Arthur Hassall, have most beneficially rivetted public attention upon a monstrous and growing evil, and established the fact, that impurity and falsification of articles of daily consumption—whether of nutriment, condiment, refreshment, or medicine—have prevailed in the metropolis to an extent which, but for incontrovertible evidence, would have been deemed incredible.

A most striking proof of the fidelity of these researches is, that, although their results, with the names of the sellers of adulterated and damaged articles, were published in a journal of wide circulation, legal proceedings were in no case taken against the courageous publisher.

* For a brief account of the origin of this "Commission" and of the valuable labours of Dr. O'Shaughnessy, Mr. F. H. Henry, M. Chevallier, Dr. Thomson, Dr. Normandy, Mr. Mitchell, and Dr. Letheby, see *Lancet*, Aug. 4, 1855.
But it is impossible to escape the conclusion that Dr. Arthur Hassall has been the chief scientific worker; and that to him belongs the principal share of the honour of the investigation and its successful results. The secret of Dr. Hassall's success has been very properly attributed to the fact,—" that in addition to chemical analysis, he has used the MICROSCOPE in his inquiries, and his merit not only consists in the able manner in which he has employed the instrument, but in his being the first to use it practically and to such an extent for this purpose."—*Dublin Review*, p. 63, Oct. 1855.

The public health has not suffered more severely from these prevalent abominations than the national character from their exposure. But the very vigour of this exposure is the redeeming feature of the case; the pledge of future reformation. These truly are not the days for the concealment of fraud, abuse and mismanagement, in either public or private concerns.

The *laissez faire* principle of local management meets with its death-blow, when corruption, falsehood, and dishonesty become the rule in the commonest transactions of society. How remarkable the ingenuity which has been perverted to the invention of some of these adulterations! How unpardonable the neglect which has permitted the regular debasement of the first necessaries of life!

§ 2. To attempt any description of the varied facts of the case, would extend these remarks far beyond their object and intended limits. Let those who do not object to be in turn amused, astounded, disgusted and appalled, read the First Report (recently published) of the Select Committee of the House of Commons in 1855, on the adulteration of Food, Drinks, and Medicines. No records of crime are more deeply and personally interesting to every inhabitant of this country; and if many such "blue-books" were published, a certain class of novels might sell for waste paper.

This important Parliamentary Inquiry is immediately due neither to Government nor to the metropolis. A great provincial town, as is not uncommon in public movements, took the lead in its promotion.

Mr. Postgate, the Lecturer on Anatomy in Sydenham College, Birmingham, and Mr. Scholefield, the member for that borough, commenced the provincial agitation. And on the motion of the latter gentleman, a Committee of Inquiry was granted by the House of Commons,—in this case, we may hope, not without the effect of hastening comprehensive legislation on the subject.

§ 3. The particular measures proposed for detecting and preventing these falsifications show, as might be expected, very little unity of purpose among the reformers; whilst nothing, as yet, is known of the views of the Committee or of Government.

One thing is certain, that the old official adage, *Quieta non movere*, is not to apply in the present instance.

The Birmingham Lecturer would empower Town Councils and County Magistrates to appoint public analyzers all over the kingdom.

The man of science would have all the investigations conducted by a Central Board, local agents being employed merely in collecting and forwarding the suspected articles to London for investigation. It was also suggested that the Excise Inspectors might be made use of, especially in the ports and larger manufacturing towns.*

The man of administration† wisely recollected, that we may in time possess a Board of Health "constituted according to its title"; that local Boards of Health, or something like them, might in all places direct inquiry and prosecution; that Officers of Health competent to conduct (at least all ordinary) investigations must be appointed; and that medical officers of districts already exist, who would everywhere be competent to act as primary detectors. He also showed, that not only the analytical chemist was required, but the pathological observer as well, who from particular symptoms would recognise the agency of certain deleterious *ingesta*.‡

The publication of popular treatises to facilitate detection, and the publication of the names of offenders, by way of prevention, were urged as useful auxiliary measures;|| and all agreed in the necessity for signal punishment by fine and imprisonment.

§ 4. One main root of the social evil was untouched by the Parliamentary Inquiry. No one showed that the preparation of the most necessary articles of food has been gradually banished from the cottage and the kitchen to the shop and the contractor. All of course are "ladies," who scorn the pickling and preserving arts in which their grandmothers excelled.

* Evidence, 182.   † Ibid. 806, 820, 795, 858.   ‡ Ibid. 844. || Ibid. p. 29.

And what is of still greater importance,—the wives of labourers and artisans, instead of baking, brewing and cooking, as in former times, and thus themselves supplying the coarse but wholesome food on which their lusty children thrived and their stalwart husbands toiled, are now too often employed from break of day till night, in the factory, the work-room, and the field. In addition, therefore, to all the other social and moral evils which are incident to the withdrawal of woman from her natural sphere of duty, she is now no longer able to protect her family from the impositions of the unscrupulous trader, by the home-manufacture of food.

Again, laws have been enacted from time to time, some of which tend avowedly to discourage the domestic preparation of articles of food, and to throw the helpless consumer into the power of the protected manufacturer: while other enactments promote the use of the most deleterious and fatal substances.

By removing restrictions upon the importation and distillation of spirits, and thus encouraging their unlimited consumption by the operatives of large towns, those "Gin Palaces" have arisen, which decimate the population and afford the speculator every facility for rendering the alcoholic poison still more destructive by the addition of powerful drugs.

By taxing malt, and thus checking the practice of brewing in private families; by abolishing the duty on the sale of beer, and thus multiplying the number of public-houses,—legislation has directly promoted the adulteration of our national beverage, and fostered that intemperance which at once marks and disgraces our national character. But these deplorable results must also be attributed in no small degree to the domestic desolation arising from the state of the dwellings of the poor, and from the removal of their wives and daughters from household cares and duties to compete with men in the great industrial struggle of the age.

Here then we see at least some of the reasons why the purity of bread, beer, and other necessaries of home-growth and home-manufacture can now only be secured by an expensive machinery of legal interference, administrative *espionnage*, and scientific inspection.

The real cure for many of these evils cannot be applied to the present generation. Much may nevertheless be done by an improved system of domiciliary visitation and instruction.* But we must look chiefly to the institution of sound and rational methods of EDUCATION, in which females may be practically taught how to perform home duties, and how to select and economize food, rather than to "define a cube" or to give the scientific name (genus and species) of the plant from which india-rubber is produced.†

§ 5. In connexion with the unchecked sale of pernicious medicines, I would notice a monstrous and mischievous absurdity maintained by law in this country. I allude to the Government stamp on *Patent Medicines*, the nature and composition of which are wholly unknown to the authority which thus warrants and promotes their sale. If a revenue must be derived from the sale of medicines, to which there seems to be no greater objection than to any other indirect mode of taxation, it may be reasonably asked—why the duty should not be levied upon all drugs, after their quality and properties have been tested, and their purity and genuineness certified by competent scientific examiners?

A very small tax, paid by importers or drug-brokers or manufacturers for such examination and verification, would, I believe, raise a larger revenue than the Government now obtains from aiding and abetting the consumption of all sorts of secret abominations.

§ 6. With regard to immediate legislation, the practical conclusions from the Parliamentary Inquiry seem to be obvious. Fraudulent admixtures, as well as spontaneous changes from

---
* See Note p. 115.
† I have myself heard these absurd questions put at a public examination of a parochial school.

disease or decomposition in organic matters, require for their detection profound knowledge and skill in the highest department of chemistry, and great analytical and microscopical experience.

It would be vain to look to Municipal Boards, as judges of the qualifications of those who are required for such delicate investigations. Besides, these bodies, containing (often in great proportion) tradesmen liable to the operation of such a law, could hardly be expected to provide for a vigorous and searching inquiry into abuses, the prevention of which might diminish their profits. But the position of public scientific analyzers might be, and ought to be, rendered as independent of local and political influence, as that of Judges in our Courts of Law.

Without any exclusive legislation on this subject, it is plain that the machinery suggested in these Essays provides for every administrative deficiency.

The Medical Visitors of districts would observe the effects of deleterious adulterations, and report them.

An improved class of "Searchers for Nuisances," beside the Excise Officers, would assist in discovering the sources of the suspected supply.

The Officers of Health would be the scientific agents of detection or instruments of proof, in ordinary cases; while Chemical Analysts, if such were appointed in any of the proposed sanitary jurisdictions, might relieve the Officers of Health of the special duty in those places. Elsewhere,—and in obscure and doubtful cases generally,—the eminent Chemists, whom I have before suggested to be appointed by the Central Council, for appeal in difficult toxicological inquiries, would complete the security which the public, and especially the working classes, ought to enjoy.

Full power of enforcing penalties, and adopting any other suitable preventive measures, should be vested in the Central and Local Sanitary Boards.

CHAPTER FOURTH.

Public Vaccination.

A.—*Historical.*

§ 1. The various proceedings of the Legislature for the promotion of Public Vaccination in this country, during the last half-century, may be arranged chronologically into three stages.

The first commenced in 1809, with the establishment of the National Vaccine Institution, which conferred upon the then novel and dubious practice the countenance and support of Government. And, at that time, its objects were more extensive and its operations more active than at a later period. It professed to do something for science, by carefully investigating alleged " opposing facts and incident anomalies," and thus determining the degree and extent of the protective influence of Vaccination.* But its main designs were administrative and practical. A central office in the metropolis, at which Vaccination was performed on a very extensive scale, under the immediate superintendence of a board of eminent physicians and surgeons ;—a depôt, from which vaccine lymph was promptly and gratuitously supplied, on application, to all parts of the empire, where also an authentic form of the vaccine disease was preserved, and where an approved method of vaccination professed to be taught ;—an institution of this kind could hardly fail of producing very important and beneficial effects in promoting the general adoption of this sanitary measure.

* For some valuable remarks and suggestions on the subject of this chapter, I am indebted to Mr. Ceely, whose original researches and scientific labours in this department of preventive medicine are too well known and appreciated to need any commendation from me. His opinions on public vaccination, in which I beg leave generally to concur, have been already laid before the Government.

§ 2. These objects, or most of them, were originally carried into effect by several classes of Public Vaccinators, "Stationary, Extraordinary, and Corresponding." The only salaried, and therefore the only legally responsible, officers were the "Stationary" Vaccinators of London, originally twelve in number, and at the present time sixteen. They were located in metropolitan and suburban districts, and required to vaccinate gratuitously all applicants, to keep up a succession of cases, and from them to furnish the central depôt with regular supplies of lymph. The other classes of vaccinators need not now be described. No notice is taken either of the "Extraordinary" or of the "Corresponding" Officers in recent programmes of the establishment.

The duties of the Board of Management gradually diminished, until they consisted merely in the preparation of an annual report to the Secretary of State. Of these reports it is impossible to speak satisfactorily, and the general opinion of scientific men respecting them, may be given in the words of an able professional critique on the Report for 1828.

"When we consider the mass of information which must necessarily be possessed by the Vaccine Board, we acknowledge that we cannot but look upon their reports generally, and the present one in particular, as wonderfully meagre and unsatisfactory. There are many questions connected with the subject which are of the highest pathological interest and of the most urgent practical importance; yet these are seldom referred to in the reports, which are for the most part limited to a few general assertions with regard to the 'protective influence' and 'wider diffusion' of vaccination, with an occasional, unwilling, and qualified admission that cases are 'very often' reported, in which small-pox has occurred after cow-pox. But from a Board, comprising the highest medical authorities in the country, expressly established for the purpose of constantly watching over the progress of vaccination, and annually presenting to Parliament a Report, by which they and the public at large might be enabled to form a judgment upon a subject which is more or less interesting to every member of the community, we expect something more than this. We expect some account of the grounds on which the general conclusions have been furnished; and we expect that the great questions which at the time press upon the attention of professional men, and cause anxiety in the public mind, should be met and candidly discussed.

"It is remarkable, however, that the Vaccine Board, instead of leading public opinion, follow in the wake; and it scarcely ever happens that they allude to the difficulties which surround any portion of the subject, until they have long excited the notice and been elucidated by the investigations of private practitioners. We do not look upon this as the fault of the individual members of the Board, but of its original and primary constitution. Men at the summit of professional eminence, and overwhelmed with business, cannot give to the subject the time and attention it requires; nor, on the other hand, can they whose connexion with the Board is but of a temporary nature, be supposed capable of entering, with much prospect of advantage to themselves or others, upon investigations, their immediate interest in which must terminate before they have become fairly acquainted with the subject—yet of these dissimilar and inefficient parts is the National Vaccine Board composed."*

§ 3. The Board originally consisted of eight members, a director, a registrar, and a secretary. The number of *ex-officio* members was from time to time reduced at the suggestion of the Secretary of State, and in 1832 was fixed at three, the present number.

Whether from discontent with "the meagre and unsatisfactory" annual reports, or from some suspicion of the sinecurism of the Board, or from general motives of economy, a select Parliamentary Committee was appointed in 1833—"To inquire into and report on the expediency of continuing the National Vaccine Institution." The Report of this Committee displays a thorough investigation of the subject. It is replete with historical information and many interesting practical details, well deserving attention even at the present time. The following were its chief recommendations:—

That the Board should for the future, consist of two Physicians and one Surgeon; all members of the profession to be eligible, and the appointments to be made by the Secretary of State:—that the Board should appoint an Inspector, to super-

* *London Medical Gazette*, vol. i. p. 507.

intend the vaccinations and attend to the distribution of lymph; and a Registrar to conduct the correspondence, and, in case of the Inspector's illness or absence, to officiate in his place:—that, as the duties of the Board would for the future be rather honorary than troublesome, the members, before their appointment, should signify their consent to superintend the executive officers, and to make the annual reports, gratuitously;—and that the annual charges should be reduced from 2321*l*., as in 1832, to 1605*l*.

The House of Commons, however, still sanctioned the salary of 100*l*. per annum to each member of the Board, and the appointment of the *ex-officio* authorities who now form it, acquiesced in the proposed limitation of its duties, and confirmed the recommendation of the Committee respecting the other officers.

§ 4. From that time, the essential duties of the National Vaccine Establishment have consisted in collecting, carefully registering, and promptly distributing gratuitous supplies of vaccine lymph to all parts of the empire, by means of one Inspector and Vaccinator, sixteen stationary Vaccinators, and a Registrar. Its objects are therefore to promote efficient vaccination, by directing its careful and scientific performance at the London stations, and by an extensive circulation of the lymph thus obtained.*

With reference to the necessities of the public, the defects of the National Institution were,—that its stations and officers were confined to the metropolis, that it was constituted without any definite administrative authority, and that the Board of Management consisted of gentlemen in high professional position, who might happen to be practically acquainted with the details of the subject, but who were not selected on that account.

* The Small-Pox Hospital and the London Vaccine Institution, or Jennerian Society, although supplying lymph very extensively, are not here mentioned as State establishments, because their incomes were derived entirely from private contributions.

§ 5. What, then, at that time, was the state of the provinces with regard to public vaccination? As regards a permanent supply of lymph, they were chiefly dependent on the London institutions. As regards executive arrangements, they were wholly dependent on the philanthropy and intelligence of old parochial managers. But, whatever amount of apathy and stolidity these might have often evinced, their more ready perception of danger, when small-pox threatened their own families and immediate neighbourhoods, led them, in many places, to arrange periodically with the parish doctor for the vaccination of the poor.

Thus, before the enactment of the new poor law, the churchwardens and overseers of probably more than half the parishes in the kingdom were in the habit of directing a general vaccination of poor children, either annually, or on the threatening of a small-pox epidemic.

But, after the reform of the Poor Laws, parochial vaccinations became less and less frequent; and the subject, in its local bearings and interests met with but little attention from the Boards of Guardians. Small-pox became far more prevalent and fatal. The deaths from this loathsome disease, in 1838, amounted to more than 16,000 in England and Wales, and to 3800 in London alone, or more than four times its average rate of mortality.

The effect of vaccination, as a permanent safeguard against small-pox, became to be more and more doubted by the people. Medical observers noticed some modification in the normal character of the vaccine vesicle and in its accompanying constitutional disturbance as described by Jenner.* It was generally believed that re-vaccinations took effect more frequently, and it was therefore thought that they had become more necessary.

§ 6. The anxieties of the nation and the Legislature were roused; and the admitted necessity for State intervention led to the second stage of public vaccination—namely, the enactment in 1840 of a law for its extension (generally known as Lord

* See Mr. Estlin's opinions. See Supplementary note H.

Ellenborough's Act), which applied to England, Wales, and Ireland, but not to Scotland.

The principal provisions of the Acts of 1840-41, have been thus described by the Epidemiological Society:—

"i. Boards of Guardians are authorized and required to contract with their medical officers or other practitioners, for the gratuitous vaccination of all persons resident in their respective unions or parishes, the expense being defrayed out of the poor-rates.

"ii. A copy of the contract so made is required to be transmitted to the Poor-Law Board, who have the power, within the period of fourteen days of the receipt of the contract, to annul the same if they see fit.

"iii. The Poor-Law Board are empowered and required to issue regulations which are binding on the Guardians.

"iv. The public vaccinators, appointed as above, are required from time to time to report the number of persons vaccinated by them. The practice is, that the books of the vaccinators are laid before the Guardians at each of their meetings, which are held weekly or fortnightly.

"v. Inoculation with variolous matter is declared to be an offence punishable by imprisonment for any term not exceeding one month.

"vi. Vaccination as performed under this Act, is declared not to constitute parochial relief or alms."*

§ 7. I have already shown (Essay IV.) the extreme inconsistency, on grounds of political economy, of committing a measure of sanitary police like public vaccination to authorities constituted merely for the control and relief of pauperism. But, the remarks on this subject, contained in the last memorial on Vaccination by the Epidemiological Society, are so much to the point, that I shall probably be excused for quoting them here at length:—

"It is manifest, in the first place, that the vaccination of the people, which is a measure undertaken by the State for the security of the public, has nothing in it of the character of alms, and does not fall properly under a department of Government, whose sole function is the distribution of alms; while it is equally obvious that it does fall naturally under a department charged with the maintenance of the

* *Report on Vaccination by Epid. Soc.*, 1853, p. 10.

public health. Had there been such a department in existence when vaccination was first made a matter of public concern, there can be no doubt that the duty would have been placed in their hands; and it is not only proper, but highly politic, that it should be transferred to them. Vaccination, like many other great and beneficial discoveries, has had, and still has, prejudices to encounter, and it is of the last importance that it should be presented for public acceptance in the manner most calculated to soften and subdue these prejudices. But to stamp it with pauperism, or give it even the semblance of an act of Poor-law relief, is not to soften and subdue, but to aggravate and add to prejudice; and this has unquestionably been the result (as has been repeatedly noticed indeed by the Poor-Law Board), and it has operated to retard the cause of vaccination."*

Such objections have occurred not only to medical investigators. The late chief of the Poor-Law Board, during a discussion on the Amendment Bill of 1854, is reported to have confessed, that—"for himself, he entertained doubts whether it was the wise course to place vaccination in connexion with the poor-laws in any way."†

Nevertheless, had the management of this protective provision by the local Boards been successful, and had its objects been satisfactorily carried out,—merely theoretical objections, however forcible, would hardly have established the necessity for a change of administration. It is true, that the Central Poor-Law Board made repeated efforts,‡ and displayed the utmost anxiety to carry into effect the beneficent designs of Parliament; but the inadequate arrangements made in most Unions, the repulsive character of a poor-law sanitary provision, and the pitiful semblance of remuneration paid by contract for the performance and record of public vaccination (not to mention other previously existing obstacles), checked the operation of this unpopular measure, and led to renewed discussion and agitation.

§ 8. The careful investigation and interesting report made by the Vaccination Committee of the Epidemiological Society,

---

* *Report*, 1855, p. 4. † Parliamentary Debate, July 18, 1854.
‡ Especially by a general appeal to the Boards of Guardians in 1844, and again in 1847.—See *Rep. cit.* p. 14.

threw fresh light upon the question; and their urgent recommendation of a law to compel vaccination universally under penalty, induced Parliament to try the experiment. But it is most remarkable, that—with all the evidence so clearly laid before the Government and Legislature by the Vaccination Committee itself, and by other well-informed persons, proving the utter inadequacy of the existing administrative machinery—the remedy adopted was to force the same imperfect system of vaccination upon an unwilling people, by means of the same inappropriate local organization.

Regardless of warnings from medical men whose opinions were entitled to respect, those members of the legislature who interfered in this matter, backed by a few heedless and inconsistent medical associations, recklessly pushed on their ill-considered and obnoxious measure, and succeeded in carrying it.

§ 9. Thus commenced the third stage of legislative intervention. It may be as well to recapitulate the main provisions of Lord Lyttelton's Act in 1853.

The Guardians of the poor were empowered to divide Unions into vaccination districts and to appoint a place in each district where the medical officer or practitioner "contracted with" should attend to vaccinate, &c. &c. (Cl. i.)

Every child born after August 1, 1853, was to be taken to the district vaccinator within three months, or under certain circumstances within four months, unless previously vaccinated and certified by some duly qualified practitioner; and to be taken for inspection on the eighth day after the operation. (Cl. ii. and iii.)*

Registrars of Births were to give notice of the requirement of vaccination, and, on failure of the parent or guardian, to comply a penalty of 20s. was to be enforced. (Cl. ix.)

A certificate of unfitness for vaccination (to be renewed every two months), and a certificate of insusceptibility to the disorder, protect from the penalty. (Cl. v.)

All who vaccinate, whether public or private practitioners, are directed to give certificates of successful vaccination to the parents and to the Registrar of Births; but no remuneration is awarded for this duty, nor is any provision made to insure its performance.* (Cl. iv.) The

* See note at the end of this chapter.

contractor for vaccination is to receive 1*s*. 6*d*. for each case within two miles of his residence, and 2*s*. 6*d*. if beyond that distance. (Cl. vi.)

The Registrar-General provides Books, Forms, and Regulations for carrying into effect the provisions of the Act. (Cl. xi.)

With all these positive directions for the performance of public vaccination,—all this apparent determination on the part of the Legislature that every child in the kingdom should be protected against the small-pox, and all the assistance so readily afforded by the Registration department,—the defects of this enactment soon became as obvious to ordinary observers, as they had been from the first to those who had studied the working of public arrangements for vaccination in this and other countries.

§ 10. It is needless to dwell upon those faults in the Act, and errors in its administration, which have been already noticed by the Epidemiological Society; but I may briefly mention the following—namely, the absence of a retrospective clause for the vaccination of all born before the date of the Act, or afterwards immigrating into this country; the want of some superintending officer or officers charged with the execution of the Act; and the entire absence of any provision for scientific inspection of the vaccinated cases, and for impartial and unimpeachable testimony as to their results. The " successful" character of the operation is now declared by the operators themselves; and one can readily understand how those who are scrupulously conscientious recoil from the disagreeable necessity of securing their payment by attesting the success of their own performances; and how, on the other hand, the certificates of the unscrupulous can afford no security to the community.

In the words of the Epidemiological Society, " administrative science, zeal, and activity are not brought to bear on public vaccination." No adequate inducement is afforded to the public vaccinators to insure the permanent success of their inoculations by a careful selection of the purest lymph and by studious attention to the several details on which Jenner believed the complete protection of the *variola vaccina* to depend.

§ 11. It thus appears that the second and third stages of legislative action were based on a principle, and took a direction, differing *in toto* from those which characterized the first stage.

We have seen that the earliest national attempt was limited to the establishment of a central office, partly for scientific purposes, and partly to secure an uninterrupted and general supply of unexceptionable lymph. The Acts of 1840 and 1853, on the other hand, provided only for the local performance of vaccination under non-professional superintendence; not recognising the existence of the National Establishment of 1809, and its necessary connexion with any properly organized system of public vaccination. The institution of similar centres of vaccine arrangements in populous districts has hitherto been wholly neglected by Parliament; unless it were erroneously supposed, that the object and design of such centres would be attained by the appointment of numerous petty "stations," one or more to each medical-relief district, as directed in the last enactment.

§ 12. On one point, indeed, which I now proceed to notice, the Legislature followed the advice of a scientific body—namely, in fixing the age of three or four months as the extreme limit for vaccination. But was this a wise decision? The opinion of a majority, I believe, of practical vaccinators throughout the kingdom, is adverse to a compulsory requirement of the measure at so early a period of infancy. And, judging from the reports of the Registrars, the general feeling of the people seems to be no less decidedly against it. The Epidemiological Society justify their "three months" clause, on the ground of the large proportion of small-pox mortality which happens in infancy; but even admitting that eleven per cent., as it is said,* of the total deaths from small-pox occur under the age of four months, it by no means follows that those early deaths would be prevented, or even materially diminished, by the fulfilment of such a requirement, were that possible.

By the laws of certain Continental States, wherein the deaths

* See Dr. Seaton's letter in the *Association Journal*, April 7, 1854.

from small-pox have been so remarkably diminished under a State-system of vaccination, the limit enforced is, practically, not less than *one* year, for the public vaccinations are ordered only annually. Thus the fears of the Epidemiological Society's Committee, that any extension of the period for vaccination would augment the ratio of infantile mortality, are not warranted by reference to the regulations of those countries in which vaccination is, on their own showing, most successful.

There can be no doubt that in this country the unpopularity of the compulsory Act has been greatly increased by the "three months" clause, which is continually evaded, and openly resisted throughout the winter months. The people are, in fact, justified in apprehending greater peril to the lives of their children from their exposure at that tender age in "stations," during the colder half of the year,* than from the remote contingency of small-pox, increased as that risk might be by deferring the operation until the following spring.

The effect of certain meteorological conditions upon the development of the vaccine vesicle, was well shown by Dr. Howison, of Edinburgh, in 1831; and most practical vaccinators will coincide in his conclusions—

"That diminished temperature and tempestuous weather diminish the appearances and properties of the vesicle; that increased temperature and dry weather again restore it to its perfect state; and that vaccination succeeds much better, and is more effectual as a preventive

---

* Mr. Martin, of Pulborough, a practitioner well known and universally respected, wrote thus sensibly on the subject:—"I am not myself a public vaccinator; but I saw infants brought out in the hardest weather of last winter, to meet the appointments of the practitioner, and with coughs and colds upon them; and I venture to predict that the mortality ascribed to the neglect of early vaccination, as stated by Dr. Seaton, will be very quickly transferred to some one of the heads of bronchial, or peripneumonic, or dysenteric, or others of the inflammatory diseases of children." . . . .

"I have other and strong objections against such early vaccination, where no danger of small-pox is imminent. I know that the poor little skinny arms of ill-clothed and ill-nurtured children can seldom (especially in cold weather) be readily infected, and if infected, can seldom be made to exhibit all the satisfactory characters of a successful vaccine."—*Association Journal*, April, 21, 1854.

against small-pox, when performed during the summer than during the winter months."*

§ 13. The idea of compulsory vaccination, in the minds of many, has been vague and inaccurate. Compulsion was called for by those who had no very clear notion of the extent or limitation of the term. In many European States, which were cited by the Epidemiological Society as precedents for a compulsory enactment, and in which is reported the lowest mortality from small-pox, the compulsion is only indirect,—that is, it is made essential to admission into schools and asylums, or a necessary qualification for citizenship, or apprenticeship, or domestic service, or relief from the public funds.

Direct compulsion by fine is the law, apparently, in only four of the States mentioned in that elaborate and valuable Report. In two of the four (Hanover and Bavaria), the vaccination is annual, and is performed at the most favourable period of the year. The majority of infants, therefore, are not vaccinated until they are more than a year old. In Prussia, there is no liability of fine for non-vaccination under a year. And in Sweden, where the mortality from small-pox appears to be at the lowest rate of any in this group, the compulsory measure applies only to children more than two years old; and even then, reprimand is tried for a time, and the fine only resorted to as an ultimatum.

The successful results of vaccination in some States, as Belgium, where no compulsion of any kind is resorted to, deserve some consideration.

§ 14. The plain practical inference from these facts is, that if the principle of compulsion is to be maintained in England, the parents of all children under one or even two years old, should be exempted from penalty and left to the influence of persuasion and encouragement. The arrangements for public vaccination should be made acceptable and attractive, and its efficiency should be considered more than its numerical relation to births.

* *London Medical Gazette*, vol. viii. p. 522, and vol. ix. p. 546.

The promoters of compulsory vaccination triumphantly appeal to the fact that in the year following that enactment, the practice had so remarkably increased, that the vaccinations exceeded the births of the year by more than a tenth part. A temporary impulse of this kind, however, proves nothing. The Epidemiological Society show that the surplus consisted of arrears. Although a crowd of applicants may have been forced into vaccination,—in many instances performed hastily, perhaps imperfectly and at an improper time (as it concerned the individual),—the effect as regards small-pox has yet to be tested.

§ 15. Some idea may be formed of the unpopularity of the Act and of its unsatisfactory working, from the Notes of the Registrars appended to the Quarterly Returns of the Registrar-General for the last two years, and especially of those made during the prevalence of small-pox in the year 1854-5. Passing over numerous statements relating to the extent and mortality of that epidemic, and the prevailing indifference, prejudice, and even hostility of the people to its substitute,—their distrust also of the sources from whence lymph is procured by the public vaccinators,—there is a considerable amount of very direct evidence with regard to the operation of the Act itself. The following remarks hastily extracted from four consecutive Quarterly Returns may suffice for my purpose:—

No. 22 (p. 41). BOLTON, *Eastern.*—" Several medical practitioners in my district refuse to supply duplicate certificates of successful vaccination ; and the Act of Parliament is evaded in other respects, no steps being taken to enforce its observance."

No. 23 (p. 36). BRIGHTON, *St. Peters.*—" The Act is imperfect, and is negligently carried out by the parents and some medical practitioners."

— (p. 37). MITFORD, *East Dereham.*—" I am sorry to state that the new Vaccination Act appears to be a total failure in my district, for although I have registered 224 births within the last thirteen months, only eighty-one children appear to have been vaccinated."

— (p. 38). LISKEARD, *Serrin.*—"Much more sickness among young children than I have ever known, and in many cases the parents attribute it entirely to too early vaccination. They insist that their other children who were vaccinated at six or eight months never suffered such bad effects."

— (p. 38). WELLS, *Glastonbury*.—" The Vaccination Act works very badly, few successful cases being returned in proportion to the number of children registered, say one in five."

No. 24 (p. 36). ST. MARTIN'S IN THE FIELDS, *Charing Cross*.— " The Vaccination Extension Act is almost inoperative; very few medical men in any district send duplicate certificates, and my Successful Vaccination Register in more than two-fifths consists of blanks."

— ST. GILES' IN THE FIELDS, *North*.—" It is impossible to work it in its present form."

— (p. 38). CAMBRIDGE, *Great St. Andrew*—" Vaccination is much neglected, and some surgeons refuse to send certificates, on the ground that they receive no remuneration, and that the Act does not render their service compulsory."

— ERPINGHAM, *Cromer*.—" It appears that the Act cannot be fully carried out in its present form."

— MITFORD, *East Dereham*.—" There is still an aversion to the Compulsory Vaccination Act, and I think people endeavour to avoid having the births of their children registered, to prevent their receiving the notice requiring vaccination, and this is common in other districts besides mine."

— REDRUTH, *Camborne*.—" I feel bound to call attention to the great neglect of the Vaccination Act, which is almost a dead letter. I have delivered 539 notices to the parents of children born, and have only received about 140 certificates of successful vaccination."

— (p. 40). PENKRIDGE, *Brewood*.—" The Vaccination Act is almost a dead letter in my district, as of all the children registered I do not receive certificates of the successful vaccination of more than one in six."

— (p. 41). HORNCASTLE, *Horncastle*.—" The working of the Vaccination Act is very unsatisfactory: I do not obtain more than one-third of the certificates of cases actually registered."

No. 25 (p. 24). DARTFORD, *Bexley*.—" Not more than one-third of the children born are vaccinated by the public vaccinator, and the other surgeons refuse to give certificates of successful vaccination. It cannot therefore be ascertained what proportion of the children born are vaccinated.

— (p. 25). OXFORD, *Oxford*.—" I am informed that at this time most of the medical profession have no sufficient supply of matter. The Act is now perfectly useless."

B.—*Suggestive.*

§ 16. Enough probably has now been adduced to prove the defective and impracticable character of the Compulsory Act. The general opinion of those who have considered the subject may be inferred from the many propositions recently made for fresh legislation.

To some of those suggestions I would now call attention. That which has been the most warmly pressed by medical practitioners is to throw open public vaccination to the whole profession, leaving parents, in every case, to select the operator. Such a change, however, would merely lead to the substitution of another set of difficulties for that in existence. It would render anything like superintendence or inspection next to impossible. It would separate the performance of vaccination from that of other prophylactic duties committed to district medical officers, and it would render all arrangements for the maintenance of a local succession and supply of vaccine lymph more hopeless even than at present.

§ 17. The Bill which originated last year with the Epidemiological Society, and is endorsed with Mr. Brady's name for the current Session of Parliament, suggests many extraordinary changes, which it would have been important to examine in detail, had not another Bill, prepared by the Board of Health and introduced by the heads of the Public-Health and Poor-Law Boards, made its appearance just as these sheets were passing through the press. It may, however, be advisable to notice cursorily both these measures; for even if Mr. Brady should withdraw his, some of its details may again be pressed by the Epidemiological Society. To avoid repetition, I shall generally designate Mr. Brady's Bill as No. 1, and the official Bill as No. 2.

i. The former proposed to place public vaccination under the control of the General Board of Health, and under the immediate direction of a Medical Superintendent of public vaccinations, to be appointed by the Board and paid by the Treasury (Cl. 2).

This officer is intended to supersede the Registrar-General in the duty of preparing forms and issuing regulations (Cl. 22).

Constituted as the General Board of Health now is, one does not exactly see what would be gained by the proposed change. The Registrar-General is provided with a medical counsellor of no less ability, and of longer administrative experience, than the gentleman who happily now assists the President of the so-called Board of Health. Moreover, the latter Board has no local machinery at its command; and the inability of any central authority—however highly qualified for general superintendence—to supersede the action of 600 local Boards, is practically acknowledged in Bill No. 2. For the Board of Health proposes to leave all local arrangements respecting "contracts" and districts, in the hands of the several Boards of Guardians, which it thus recognises as *the* local sanitary authorities of England;—a foregone conclusion, surely, —an admitted fallacy,—a conventionalism of no long standing, and soon, we may hope, to be for ever abandoned.

The Bill, No. 2, however, distributes the central duties among three Government departments. Boards of Guardians on this scheme, will have to serve three masters; for the Registrar-General is still to prepare forms and to frame regulations (Cl. 25); while the appointments and districts are to be revised, and special regulations in small-pox epidemics are to be issued by the General Board of Health, which is also to be empowered to inspect (by its officers) the books, records, and duties of the vaccinators (Cl. 6, 7, 9, 22, 26). Lastly, to the Poor-Law Board, thus relieved of many troublesome responsibilities, is left the sole duty of compelling the Boards of Guardians to obey both the other central authorities (Cl. 26).

Surely we have seen too much of the evils of divided responsibility to expect much advantage from such a settlement of the question. Unless some project be forthcoming for consolidating the sanitary functions of certain Government departments, neither vaccination nor any other preventive measures stand a chance of being efficiently dealt with.

Nothing is more clearly proved by these propositions than (*first*) the necessity for instituting competent sanitary authorities, central and local, and (*secondly*) the impropriety of legislating upon details until these have been created or re-constituted.

ii. According to Bill No. 1, Medical Inspectors were to be appointed* at the instance of the proposed Medical Superintendent of Public Vaccinations; and the Board of Health has also indicated its own Inspectors (Cl. 33) for the purpose of inquiry into the execution of the Act.

Admitting, to the fullest extent, the importance of a permanent organization of Inspectors, under a real Council of Health, I do not see what particular service to the cause of public vaccination is likely to result from that description and amount of inspection, which the General Board of Health would be empowered to provide, and which could only be exercised in very large circuits. *Local* supervision is, indeed, an essential feature of any project of national vaccination, and we shall soon see how that object might be satisfactorily accomplished.

iii. It is well that the General Board of Health declines the patronage which the Epidemiological Society would confer upon it, by committing to it the appointment of all future vaccinators. Granting the expediency of a limited Government control in this and other matters, I see no reason to anticipate any substantial or permanent improvement in local administration from so complete an abolition of all local responsibility.

iv. It is proposed in Bill No. 1, that at least one convenient place or station for the performance of vaccination, and its subsequent inspection, shall be appointed in each sub-registrar's

---

* The proposal of the Epidemiological Society is precisely analogous to the defective proposition made by Lord Shaftesbury in 1848 (see Essay IV. p. 197). His design was truly laudable; but while the superintendence of the medical care of the poor was the ostensible object, "the other sanitary duties of every kind" proposed to be committed to those medical inspectors, were, in fact, matters of more serious concern to the State. So now, if the object be—as it surely ought to be—the thorough sanitary inspection of circuits, under which both medical relief and vaccination, with many other matters of national importance, would take their proper place,—let it be boldly avowed.

district; whilst the Bill No. 2 leaves the appointment of this place in each vaccination district to the Board of Guardians, subject to the approbation of the General Board of Health.

One object, apparently, of the former of these proposals is, to promote something like identity of districts, or correspondence of arrangements in the registration and the vaccination systems; but, gladly as we might hail any recognition of a principle so often urged in these pages—namely, that the areas of all local administrations should be co-extensive,—it is surely desirable, in the first place, to require a general revision of the registration districts, or at least some investigation into their local fitness for the purposes of vaccination. And since 'registration, as well as vaccination and other preventive duties, ought invariably (if possible) to be performed in areas corresponding with the districts for medical visitation—or, as it is now called, medical relief,—it is important to notice that both the new vaccination Bills are open to criticism for treating their particular subject as if it were independent of any other public provision; although No. 2 would doubtless tend indirectly to confirm the very natural and obvious connexion between public vaccination and the medical care of districts.

If, as the Epidemiological Society and Mr. Brady doubtless think, and as I believe, the medical relief department is in improper hands, that evil will not be remedied by separating vaccination, and thus adding another to our already too numerous schemes of local jurisdiction. Nothing further on this point is required than a general revision of the medical relief districts for vaccination arrangements,* and their identification, as far as possible, with the registration divisions.

* I am tempted here to question the utility of establishing some thousands of stations or "places" in England and Wales. If a station be intended merely as a rendezvous for adults and children who are to be vaccinated or inspected, the object is too insignificant for notice by Parliament. *Nec deus intersit nisi dignus vindice nodus.* It may be safely left to the local sanitary administrative authorities or to the vaccinators themselves. But if (as I imagine) the design is to insure at each place a succession of vaccinations and a perpetual local supply

v. Both measures provide for the prompt vaccination of every unvaccinated person resident in England and Wales, and of all unvaccinated immigrants.

vi. All children born after a certain day are to be vaccinated within three months of birth, according to Bill No. 1; and within four months, according to No. 2. The same penalty as before is to be imposed on recusants, with further penalties, in the latter measure, for continued neglect or refusal, after official warning.

It is needless here to re-state the objections which have been already urged against the limitation of vaccination to so early an age. It is needless again to point out the invalidity of the arguments upon which that limitation is based. If either of these versions of the clause should be pressed, now or at any future time, let us hope that an amendment may be proposed to strike out the words "three" or "four months," and to substitute "one year," as in Germany, or "two years," as in Sweden.

vii. Both measures also propose to raise the fees for public vaccination, from 1s. 6d. and 2s. 6d. respectively, to 2s. 6d. and 3s. 6d.; and another shilling is to be awarded for certification to those medical practitioners who are not public vaccinators.

of lymph, a very brief numerical argument will demonstrate the utter inadequacy of the project. We may suppose that on this scheme there would be 4000 vaccination stations: according to Bill No. 1 there must be at least 2190, and there might be 7000.—(See Dr. Hughes on State Vaccination, p. 12.) The annual births in England and Wales may be stated in round numbers at 600,000; or 150 per annum, on the average, to each station;—that is, three per week. But at least a third of the population will be vaccinated at their residences, or elsewhere than at the "stations," and of the total number born many never live to be vaccinated. Thus the average attendance for vaccination at each station would be less than two per week; and when we recollect that such an average involves a wide range of hebdomadal variation, that children are not born with periodical regularity to suit the plans of official projectors, and that the poor will not bring their children for vaccination in cold or wet weather, it seems inevitable that many more than half the stations, for many more than half the weeks of the year, would be empty and useless; the succession would, of course, be dropped; and the assumed design of the plan would be frustrated.

How often are we reminded of the utter unfitness of speculative writers, however able and learned, to provide against practical difficulties in administration!

This is an approach to a more reasonable "remuneration," to which the doctors will probably offer no objection.*

The provisions of the existing law, with regard to the insusceptibility and the temporary unfitness of subjects for vaccination are confirmed, with some unimportant alterations, in the second Bill.

The first contained a clause (21) directing the medical superintendent of public vaccinations, guided by information to be derived from the Birth Registers (and probably in intervals of his more important occupations), to prosecute all obstinate and unreasonable mothers who do not practically acknowledge the infallibility of Parliament and the Epidemiological Society.

The General Board of Health, however, would commit this hateful duty to the several Boards of Guardians, who will doubtless not increase their popularity by venturing upon its performance.

It is not to be denied, that some defects of the existing law would be remedied by the proposed measures; but the general objection to both, as well as to Acts now in force for the promotion of public vaccination, is—that they treat this subject separately, as distinct from any other sanitary provision, on the piecemeal principle of British legislation; that details are to be defined by Act of Parliament which would be far more properly left to competent authorities; and that laws are proposed to enforce sanitary proceedings without previously constituting and empowering suitable administrative machinery.

§ 18. Now, before showing how a general sanitary organization would apply to the details of State vaccination, it seems desirable to reclaim attention to the objects of the National Vaccine Establishment; objects which, as I have shown, have been neglected in recent legislation, although the operation of

---

* The bait is made the more tempting by the Epidemiological Society, which would empower every *gentleman* to earn sixpence more by persuading the parents to ask for a certificate of successful vaccination!

these Acts has sensibly affected the demand for lymph supplied by that establishment.

There can be no question that (to some extent) the number of applicants for vaccination at the National Institution, and (to a still greater extent) the number of charges of lymph distributed by it, have been influenced by the absence or presence of epidemic small-pox; and this will in a measure explain some of the variations under these heads respectively recorded in different years. Still it is beyond dispute that, while the number of applicants for vaccination for several years past has scarcely exceeded 11,000 per annum, and is now diminishing, the number of charges of lymph distributed annually has slowly but steadily increased; and thus the demand is tending to exhaust the supply.*

That demand was of course very largely augmented during the year (1854) succeeding the enactment of the compulsory measure; and although the demand may not continue to the same inordinate amount as in that exceptional year, we must expect on the whole an increasing pressure upon the resources of the metropolis, unless some measures are adopted by the Legislature to establish similar centres of vaccination in populous districts.† In very dense populations, it is true, where successional vaccination can be maintained under the strict observance of the new law,—the public vaccinators, if not too numerous, may in general be self-dependent for supplies. But the requirements of the Act

* Mr. Ceely.

† In 1832, the number of persons vaccinated by the National Establishment was more than 14,000 (see *Parliamentary Report*, 1833), and this was probably about the average; but in 1839 (the year following the great small-pox mortality) the number of applications at the Metropolitan Institution and stations had increased to 18,659. In 1840, the year of Lord Ellenborough's Act, it was 13,144. For the succeeding thirteen years the average annual number sunk to about 11,500, and is now under 10,000.

With regard to the general distribution of lymph, the changes have been more remarkable. Previously to 1839, the number somewhat exceeded 100,000 per annum: but in that year there were distributed no less than 203,818 charges. In 1840, they amounted to 165,395. For the next thirteen years the annual average was 170,122. But then, again, in 1854, the year following the compulsory enactment, the number of charges distributed was 319,808, or 104,178 in excess of those of the previous year. In 1855, it was 222,532.

in rural and small town districts, under present arrangements, wholly preclude such a result. It appears that weekly vaccinations, even of a limited number of individuals in succession, are altogether impracticable in these less densely-populated districts. The provinces, therefore, have become more directly dependent upon the London Institution for the supply of recent lymph. And there are many valid grounds for doubting the advantage of such absolute dependence. It is very questionable whether the poor of the metropolis alone ought to furnish the *pabulum* of the vaccine disease for the entire population of the kingdom; and whether the purity and efficacy of lymph is best secured by reliance upon a single source in a monster city.

§ 19. These objections may be found to outweigh the probabilities of the National Vaccine Establishment being able adequately to sustain the demands now made upon it; for a reference to its reports shows how wide and vast its operations are in the colonies, the army and navy, the emigrant department, and merchant service.

This is not the place for inquiring whether the alleged diminution in the permanently protective influence of *variola vaccina* be founded in fact; nor, if so, whether it may arise from the careless and imperfect performance of vaccination,* or from defects in the public source and system of supply.† But no one would question the extreme desirableness of such a local organization as would aid in maintaining a general supply of good and effective lymph. And I have now merely to show how completely that and other main objects of a public system of vaccination might be obtained through the medium of the sanitary organization suggested in these Essays.

§ 20. No further special legislation would be required, except

---

* See *Memorial* (1855) *of Epid. Soc.*, pp. 6 and 9 ; also, Mr. Marson's paper, 1853, showing the superiority of continental vaccinations ; also *Medical Times and Gazette*, Jan. 12, 1856.

† See supplementary Note H.

the repeal of certain objectionable provisions of the Compulsory Vaccination Act.

In common with district medical attendance, vaccination ought to be removed from all connexion with the Poor-Law. The unpopular and irrational "three months" limitation should also be abrogated.

The two main objects of an amended system of public vaccination, to be inferred from the preceding remarks, are—(first) the establishment of local institutions for successional vaccination, and for the continual supply of pure and effective lymph, under scientific direction; and (secondly) the inspection of all vaccinated subjects by a third party—a medical referee, holding an office which would preclude all professional rivalry, and whose report would afford to the public that security which the law ought to require.

§ 21. The first of these objects might be attained as follows:— A station, in the proper sense of the term, *i.e.*, an office at which vaccination is most carefully performed, with the purest lymph, and weekly throughout the year if possible; and at which the subjects for vaccination are accurately registered and scientifically inspected;—such a station, I say, could not be maintained by its own operation, and with advantage to the public, in any population of less than 60,000.* A population of that amount, even in crowded districts, would scarcely afford, on the average, more than twenty weekly applicants for gratuitous vaccination. While, during the winter months, the number attending at the station would probably be barely sufficient to keep up a succession of cases, and to perpetuate an unexceptionable form of the disease. A population of even 60,000 might not be always self-dependent for a provision of genuine lymph.

In all other districts, and for all those subjects who are not required to attend from time to time at the central station in

* Mr. Ceely stated this to be his opinion in his communications with the Secretary of State and the Registrar-General in 1853.

order to keep up a succession of lymph, or who do not apply, at their own discretion, to private or public practitioners,—vaccination should be annual, as in continental States; and it should generally be performed in the spring quarter.

In rural districts,—only that portion of the population which surrounds the station within a moderate distance, should be expected to resort to it for vaccination. The remainder would be attended to by the district vaccinators or medical officers, at temporary or tributary stations, or at their own houses, or at the residences of the patients themselves.

§ 22. Now, it should be observed, that the minimum amount of population assumed to be necessary for the maintenance of a permanent station, is very nearly equal to that which, for other reasons, I have estimated as the most suitable to be comprehended in a SANITARY JURISDICTION; and thus my second main object would be secured. For every such sanitary district, it is presumed that an independent OFFICER OF HEALTH, free from the entanglements and responsibilities of private practice, would be appointed. Here, then, we at once possess the proper means for scientific inspection and impartial report. And by this means, also, many of those important functions which the Epidemiological Society would assign to ONE medical Superintendent of Vaccinations, might be easily and thoroughly carried into effect.* Three hundred Officers of Health would effectively promote and superintend the diffusion of vaccination in all parts of England and Wales; while, in any matter requiring superior direction, they might refer to the Circuit Inspectors, hereafter to be suggested, or even to the Council of Health, to which their reports of vaccination would be made.

The central or permanent vaccine station of each sanitary district would be under the special superintendence of the Officer of Health; and he would attend weekly to inspect the vaccinated subjects. If possible, every such station should be identical with the chief public Dispensary, belonging to the same sanitary

* See pp. 5 and 6 of their *Memorial*, 1855.

jurisdiction. At this Dispensary, on the system proposed in the Fourth Essay, there would always be a resident dispenser, who would be precisely the person to act as REGISTRAR OF VACCINATIONS, under the Officer of Health.

§ 23. The medical officer of that visitation district in which the central dispensary might be situated, would naturally hold the office of CHIEF VACCINATOR of the sanitary jurisdiction; while the surgeons of other visitation districts would, on the principle here laid down, be the local vaccinators within their own spheres of duty, unless these were so closely adjacent to the central station as to render some arrangement with it more desirable.

In remoter districts, it might be left either to the proposed sanitary court, or to the Officer of Health, or to the medical officer himself, to appoint one or more temporary places for vaccination as tributary stations, both in times of epidemic small-pox, and at other favourable seasons. But supposing, as I have suggested in the Fourth Essay, that the greater number of sanitary jurisdictions would contain more than one dispensary (and many might require several dispensaries), these would obviously be the places for local vaccination; standing in much the same relation to the central station, rendering similar aid, and making similar returns, as the stationary vaccinators of the National Vaccine Establishment afford to it.

§ 24. All medical officers and practitioners should be required to report, or certify to the Officers of Health of their respective sanitary districts, every vaccination which they may perform; but the parents or guardians of the children so vaccinated should be made responsible for the delivery of the vaccinator's certificate to the Officer of Health. The vaccinator would thus be relieved from further responsibility about the case. The success or non-success of the operation should be determined and registered by the Officer of Health, who would himself, or by deputy, visit the tributary or district dispensaries on the appointed days. If required to call at private houses, he should be remunerated accordingly by the persons thus accommodated. Every child publicly vaccinated, and not brought to the central station or district dispensary for inspection, should be immediately reported to the Officer of Health, who should be empowered to make (or to direct to be made) an inspecting visit to the residence of the patient, at the cost of the parties neglecting or declining to attend at the station.

§ 25. The Registrars of Births—whether themselves medical officers of vaccination districts, or mere Registrars co-operating with the medical officers on an improved local system of registration—might render most important aid in bringing the whole infantile population, by gentle and hortatory measures, under the influence of this invaluable sanitary protection.

In no department of the public health would the orderly co-operation of the three descriptions of sanitary agency mentioned in these Essays, (p. 137 in particular,) be more fully and harmoniously displayed than in the promotion of public vaccination.

NOTE TO p. 375.

1. "'Eighth day after the operation." The Bill of 1854 substituted the seventh day for the eighth. The Epidemiological Society and Mr. Brady still adhere to the eighth day. The last official Bill would confirm the seventh day.

Non nostrum inter vos tantas componere lites.

2. "Nor is any provision made to insure its performance." The Registrar-General has stated his belief that the refusal to grant a certificate would render the practitioner liable to indictment for misdemeanour (see official letter from Mr. Mann, October 6, 1853);—although no opinion is pronounced as to the justice of punishing a private practitioner for not performing a public duty gratuitously.

CHAPTER FIFTH.

The Local Organization of a Civil Medico-Sanitary Service.

§ 1. Having now considered most of those very important duties of investigation, advice, and prevention, which might be performed in extensive sanitary districts, by Officers of Health, independent of private practice, I proceed to make some concluding suggestions on their appointment and organization.

One cannot look forward with hope or satisfaction to a continued exercise of those unrestricted powers of appointment, now used and too often abused by local Boards of Health in the provinces, and by the new District Boards of the metropolis. Reflecting upon the very delicate and difficult responsibilities of this office, —the unusual mental qualities and acquirements which ought to belong to him who holds it,—and the peculiar position and relations, professional and social, in which this new Guardian of the Public Health must find himself,—it is Utopian to expect that all these circumstances, requirements, and qualifications will be fairly weighed and justly estimated by the existing local administrative authorities. There seems no prospect of substantial benefit to the community from forcing the appointment of Health Officers upon reluctant municipalities (as in Sir B. Hall's Metropolitan Act), before the Legislature has settled the position, harmonized the official relations, and defined the rights and duties of the *corps*. In this, as in other matters, Parliament orders an act to be done, without taking the slightest security for its rational, equitable, and efficient performance.

Notwithstanding the loud demand of unemployed doctors for the compulsory institution of this office, it should be recollected that the object of sanitary legislation is not to create places for the medical profession, although the object of organizing that profession is to perfect and consolidate sanitary legislation, and to render sanitary administration effectual.

One sees, indeed, that good appointments may be made under the most defective organization, and one feels it a grateful duty to acknowledge that some very excellent appointments have been made both in London and in provincial towns; but one turns with disgust from the sickening picture which the medical journals have lately drawn of the proceedings in too many of the metropolitan districts;—the encouragement given to a low system of plotting and touting; the prevalence and success of electioneering arts; the triumph of cliques; the utter ignorance of the District Boards on the subject; and the contemptible motives and principles which have been so injudiciously called into operation.

§ 2. Let me rather suggest what might be effected in this matter by superior Sanitary Courts, their powers being defined by wise and comprehensive legislation, and their measures guided by the advice of a properly constituted Council of Health.

The principal difficulty would be felt in the first appointments. The *corps* of district medical officers, from whom the superior officers of health should hereafter be selected, is hardly at present in a state of sufficiently complete organization—perhaps hardly prepared of itself to furnish a sufficient number of the best men for the needs of the country.

For some time, at all events, the choice ought not to be restricted to any existing official class; and the widest opportunity for selection should be afforded. Ultimately, however, the post might be regarded as a step of promotion and reward of meritorious conduct in the office of district medical attendant.*

Some have urged, that a public examination should be instituted, at which all physicians and surgeons of a certain standing might compete for the post. On this scheme, the examiners, we

---

* See Essay IV. p. 286.

may suppose, would be selected by a superior and impartial body (such as a Council of Health) on account of their special and profound knowledge of the literature and science of hygiéne, and their general aptitude for ascertaining the extent of such knowledge in others.

The particular subjects mentioned in the Essay on medical and sanitary education (p. 73), would probably supply the principal matter for such an examination; and this might be held before the medical Faculty and the local administrative authorities of each proposed sanitary jurisdiction; or there might be a place named for the contest of skill in each inspecting circuit.

§ 3. Admitting the vast superiority of some method of the kind to the miserable proceedings now in vogue; I am far from believing that success in a competitive ordeal would constitute the surest and safest test of the higher qualifications for the office. Weight of character, independence of judgment, candour and amenity of disposition, steadiness, patience and accuracy in research, habits of business, and experience in official duties,—all qualifications of the greatest value and importance for a superintending Health Officer,—are not to be elicited by mere competition, at an examination of a day or two, where the ready, the forward, and the theoretical may more easily carry off the prize.*

---

* *Competitive Examinations.*—"There are minds slow, but ample in their operations, cautious and conscientious in every step, reaching eventually the most advanced realizations of science and the boldest stand-points of sagacious practical conjecture, which yet require for their repeated circumambulations of thought, their multifarious combinations and comparisons of view, their continual checks and corrections of incipient opinions, more than any examination, however well conducted, will permit. These men cannot enter the service through a portal open only for a few hurried moments at a time, and through which the agile, ready, and self-possessed, lightly, though perhaps bulkily laden, find it not nearly so difficult to make their way. The strong tendency of admission by competitive examination is to give us rather a clever than an able Civil Service, and especially so, since success in an examination depends quite as much on a capacity for 'cram' as on capacity for knowledge. . . . . . .

"This mode of judgment cannot apply to originality; to general power of intellect; to endurance of effort; to versatility; it can only refer to ACQUISITION."
—*Westminster Review* ("The Civil Service"), vol. vi. 1854, p. 78.

Probably, if all canvassing were prohibited, the testimonials and claims of candidates might be submitted to a well-constituted Sanitary Court,—which, after due consideration, might nominate two or three, from whom the Central Board might select one. The recommendation of the district faculty and the report of the circuit inspector would aid that Board in arriving at a right decision.

§ 4. Although not selected solely from the parochial staff of medical officers, the sanitary superintendent (or Health Officer) would be virtually the head and representative of that staff, and their official connexion with him should be clearly established by law. Removed, as he would be (on the plan submitted in the Fifth Essay), from all professional rivalry with the members of that staff, they might be led to rely upon him as a friendly referee and counsellor, ready to help them in official difficulties and advise them in professional perplexities; yet at hand to warn them of inattention, and to caution them against a negligent or indifferent performance of duty. Whilst, as their official superior, he should be fully empowered to demand from them all the information and assistance which their regular engagements might enable them to afford him in the performance of his own duties.*

§ 5. Some estimate may be expected of the expense of a national organization of Officers of Health.

If, as suggested, new sanitary districts were formed, containing more than 60,000 inhabitants, about three hundred would be required for England and Wales, exclusive of the metropolis. Now the late officer for the City of London received (it is said) 800*l*. a-year, not being prohibited from practising privately. The officer for Liverpool received 750*l*., without permission to practise.

Many more duties and responsibilities are here proposed for

* He would occupy the same relative position to them, as, in the German States, the *Kreis-physicus* does to the *Land-ärzte* or *Armen-ärzte,*—and to the local authorities, as that German officer does to the magistracy—in large towns, the *Stadtsverordneten-Versammlung*, and in districts, the *Land-rath.*—Rönne and Simon, vol. i, pp. 116 and 260.

the Officers of Health than either of those gentlemen fulfilled; so that I assume that less than 700*l.* a-year could now scarcely be thought of by any government as the salary for so arduous and important a post. Thus, the total amount of the annual stipends should not be less than 210,000*l.* But this estimate would provide for the reduction of other items of public expenditure.

The cost of fragmental services in this country is known to be great. There are several kinds of public medical duty paid for separately, which might be performed hereafter, with far greater propriety, by the proposed Officer of Health. I have no means of calculating the cost of these special services. But it will at once appear, that some of the expenses of the witnesses in aid of coroners' inquests would be saved; while a greater number of inspections and examinations (now unwisely dispensed with) would be held without additional expense. There are also important medical duties under the Factory Act, which, for the more perfect security of the labouring population, ought to be performed by persons wholly independent of the local influence of large capitalists and manufacturers. Consultations in difficult cases occurring among the sick poor would also be provided for by the institution of this officer.

§ 6. All the reasons which have been heretofore adduced for charging the salaries of district medical officers upon national funds, apply with tenfold force to those of Officers of Health. It can hardly be necessary to repeat the argument. To charge the cost of this corps upon localities, would be ultimately to defeat the object of its institution, and to disgust the taxed community.

In the Fourth Essay I have estimated the salaries of the parochial medical officers at 200,000*l.* per annum, not including the cost of drugs and workhouse salaries. Another 100,000*l.* should be added for sanitary visitation and preventive duties. Thus, for both these medico-sanitary orders, a total national expenditure of half a million would be required; which, be it recollected, amounts to scarcely more than three per cent. of the cost of our national establishments for war, even in "piping times of peace."

CHAPTER SIXTH.

Circuit Inspection.

§ 1. In the preceding chapters of this Essay, and in the two preceding Essays, I have been occupied, directly and indirectly —that is, sometimes by distinct specification, and sometimes by stating facts which, without comment, are sufficient to suggest important inferences—in sketching a plan for the pedestal and base of the State Column of medico-sanitary organization. The shaft of inspection is now to be added, before we can discuss the substance and form of the capital of central direction.

The necessity for inspection, although occasionally disputed by an ill-informed and obstructive class, may now be viewed as an established postulate in the science of Public Hygiéne. But the exact *status* and the special duties of the inspecting office,—the number of the corps of inspectors, and the extent of their jurisdictions, are questions still wholly unsettled, even in theory.

Some have endeavoured to simplify the project, by proposing to convert the Officer of Health into an Inspector. But few would be bold enough to affirm that the catalogue of duties which I have suggested for the former officer could be performed, however summarily, by fewer than 300 persons throughout the whole of England and Wales; yet 300 would be decidedly too numerous a staff for those still higher and more comprehensive duties of wide observation and comparison, authoritative advice and frequent communication with a central council,—all which would more fully appertain to a small number of Circuit Inspectors, in relation to whom the Health Officers would stand as local deputies. It seems, therefore, essential to any efficient system of public health administration, that such an official order should be interposed between the officers of the Local Boards and the Central Board.

The medical polity of the German States, no less than that of the later Roman Empire, affords valuable precedents for the institution of such an order. Considerable variety, indeed, exists among modern systems. The *Proto-medicus* of Austria and Lombardy seems to exercise a more complete and decisive jurisdiction than is shared by the two grades of *Ober-Präsidenten* and *Medicinal Räthe*, in Prussia.*

A single order of Provincial Inspectors in England should combine the principal functions of the two Prussian ranks. The Medical Inspectors of Ireland, if separated from their Poor-law connexion, and invested with additional local sanitary functions, would represent more correctly the staff which ought to be established in England.

§ 2. The duties of the inspecting office would consist,—partly of some already performed irregularly, inefficiently, and at considerable cost to the nation, by individuals,—and, partly, of those which have never yet been performed at all in this country.

In his sanitary character, the Inspector would naturally control the execution of the duties of the Officers of Health within his circuit. And this would bring all the vital, medical, topographical, and medico-jurisprudential statistics of such a circuit, under his cognizance and revision.

All measures for the prolongation of life, the prevention and relief of sickness, and the improvement of the physical condition of the people, would be subjected to his inquiry, and be aided by his advice. He should have the right of session at each of the proposed Sanitary Courts, and be empowered to examine the records and journals kept by those Boards and their officers. Assisted by the reports of the local officers, he would inspect the administration of medical attendance and the performance of sanitary visitation in each district. Questions of *mala praxis*, or neglect of duty, would most properly come under his consider-

* Rönne and Simon, *supra cit.*, pp. 78, 91.

ation, because he would be still further removed from disturbing associations and local influences than the superintending Officers of Health. To him, in the first place, all appeals would be made by both orders of medico-sanitary officers in his circuit, or should these be made direct to the central Board, they should be referred to him for examination and report. His decisions upon all questions would, of course, be liable to revision or reversal by that council.

§ 3. A most important branch of his duties would be the periodical inspection of all the public hospitals and medical charities within his jurisdiction.

The claims which these institutions have upon the respect and gratitude of the nation have been already mentioned; and the advantages which the public derives from the nominally unpaid services of the Governors and medical officers, have been sufficiently acknowledged. But, inasmuch as they are *public* institutions, professedly undertaking for the State the execution of a great public duty, which must be performed if society is to wear the aspect of Christianity and civilization,—it is but right to demand that they should not escape the consequence of their assumed publicity—namely, responsibility. No quarter should be given to the notion, which sometimes prevails among their honorary medical officers, that these noble establishments are intended for their own special advancement and distinction.

The maintenance of Hospitals by voluntary association and subscriptions, is not incompatible with their responsibility to the State. And such responsibility could be secured only by enforcing the right (and indeed the duty) of Government to inspect their condition and administration. Protests against what some would term the intrusion of an Inspector would be vehement and loud, in direct proportion to the undue influence of private interests and cliques, and the imperfection of management; just in proportion, therefore, to the prevalence of abuses and the necessity for disinterested interference. By whomsoever and howsoever supported and maintained, the State is bound to see that the presumed intentions of the founders and benefactors are carried fully into effect. And it must be recollected, that the vast majority of the subscribers to these Charities are wholly unable to take any active share in the management. They may, therefore, fairly demand the protection of an independent and disinterested authority against the possible caprice of managing Boards, and would probably welcome the intervention of an Inspector, as the means most likely to ensure the greatest amount of benefit to the community, and to the sick poor especially, in the administration of their finances.

Of late years, we have seen "Comparative Statements" of the financial and general management of Hospitals, Infirmaries, and Dispensaries; and the occasional publication of these statements has, doubtless, led to great improvements in their internal regulations. But the results merely show how much more good might be effected, were it made the duty of an Inspector to supply this kind of information—collected with greater accuracy and fulness from all parts—to the managing authorities of every medical charity in his circuit.

§ 4. Those who have meddled at all in the management of English Hospitals and Dispensaries, can testify to the existence of many embarrassments and misunderstandings, which are inseparable from an irresponsible and ill-defined system of administration. Very few, I believe, of our best provincial Infirmaries are, for any length of time, free from collisions between the medical staff and the Board of Managers elected by the subscribers. Either the supposed privileges of the former are invaded, or the powers of the governors are disputed. Some honorary physician or surgeon, feeling that his unpaid services exceed in value the united contributions of a hundred governors, fairly claims to be heard in the direction of affairs. Some resisting governor, on the other hand, recollects the same doctor, when a candidate for the appointment, coming to him hat in hand, and vowing eternal gratitude for the favour of his " vote and interest";—he therefore not unreasonably concludes, that motives, not strictly connected with the "promotion of science and the triumph of humanity," induced the said doctor to incur his professed weight of obligation,—motives, in fact, which place him more or less in the position of a paid officer. The more notional, mazy, and inexplicable are these opposite views—these conceptions and misconceptions—the greater the liability to mutual misunderstanding; and this, as we know, too often practically leads to unseemly strife, turning an institution of mercy and benevolence into something worse than a bear-garden.

How gladly in such circumstances would both parties turn to the unprejudiced counsel and advice of a circuit Inspector, freed from those local relations and class considerations which must disturb the equanimity and bias the judgment of resident managers.

Further, provincial hospitals should be viewed not merely as institutions for the benefit of the sick and maimed poor recommended by subscribing Governors, and for medical instruction to contributing pupils,—but as local centres and sources of scientific information and improvement, especially to established practitioners.

The library of reference, the pathological museum, the sick-wards, the operation-room, and the dead-house, should exist in every hospital, as so many opportunities for renewing those supplies of knowledge, which are too rarely afforded to the toil-worn routinist of a crowded city or a scattered village population. And these sources should be opened to the profession on public grounds, as a matter of right, not of favour or courtesy. But such a degree of publicity is unlikely to be attained, unless regular and systematic inspection by superior officers be made obligatory upon every association of governors and medical volunteers,—in return for the recognition, protection, and freedom from taxation which are so wisely granted by the State.

Any hospital, refusing to admit the visit, or to receive the recommendations of the Inspector, should be placed under the same civil disabilities, which in a former Essay were suggested for refusal to aid in a national registration of sickness.

§ 5. If, however, the Provincial Hospitals and Infirmaries stand in need of inspection, how much more important is it to amend the present system of visitation of hospitals for the insane, and especially "Private Asylums"?

Metropolitan institutions, public and private, for mental disorders, are under the direct superintendence and visitation of the "Commissioners in Lunacy." I do not presume to offer an opinion as to the efficiency or frequency of that visitation within the metropolitan jurisdiction. By those well qualified to judge, it is generally spoken of as judiciously adapted for the attainment of the main objects of State interference,—namely, the protection, humane care, and scientific treatment of the patients; and there seems to be no pretext for suggesting any more decided reform within the limits of that jurisdiction, than a greater frequency of visitation and closeness of inspection, together with the publication of reports, and the transfer of a greater share of responsibility from the proprietors and superintendents to the Commissioners themselves.* These gentlemen would then find full employment in the metropolitan district, which if possible should be identified with the metropolitan Division of the Registrar-General.

The Commissioners (as the accomplished and philanthropic physician to whom I have just referred, writes) have already " much to do besides visitation;" and they might hereafter, with great propriety, form a section of the proposed central Council of Health for the superintendence of hospitals and public curative institutions of every kind; thus assisting in the discharge of functions of general direction and control, which do not at present belong to them, and are not as yet performed by any one.

§ 6. But there are many conclusive reasons for recommending

---

* Dr. Henry Monro, physician to St. Luke's Hospital, who has treated the whole of this subject admirably, and to whose work I am indebted for the above suggestion, recommends a visit once in three or four weeks to all private establishments. —See *Reform of Private Asylums,* pp. 32—44, &c.

an entire change in the visitation of private establishments for the insane, throughout the other ten Divisions of the Registrar-General.

The four annual visits which the Metropolitan Commissioners are required by law to make to every licensed house in England and Wales, are admitted to be quite insufficient to secure the ends of State supervision. The very irregularity and uncertainty of their visits, for which there are obvious and sufficient reasons, is often attended with the disadvantage of an interval of four, five, or even six months. Great changes for the better, perhaps for the worse, may take place in so long an exemption from scientific inspection. It is impossible for any Commissioners to judge accurately and equitably of the comparative state and progress of each among a number of asylums from such rare examinations; neither can the patients derive that comfort or enjoy that sense of protection from these " angels' visits, few and far between," which they might and would do under a better system; nor can the proprietors be relieved, as they ought to be, of the responsibility of deciding upon the question (often one of extreme difficulty and delicacy)—whether a patient should be dismissed or longer detained; nor lastly, can " matters of unavoidable disagreement" between proprietors and patients (or their friends) be arranged speedily and satisfactorily, without the repeated intervention of a superior, impartial, and intelligent authority,—who would act with kindness and discretion, and make it his business to acquire the confidence and respect of both the interested parties.

§ 7. Let no one foster the delusion, that this deficiency of official and scientific inspection, in the case of private provincial asylums, is supplied by the legal visitation of County Magistrates. Let us for a moment suppose the proprietor or superintendent to be not only shrewd and experienced, but sordid and unscrupulous (we may safely admit such a possibility); he would have little difficulty in imposing upon a party of country squires and clergymen, uninstructed in the nature and treatment of mental maladies, even though they might be prompted or seconded by a Medical Visitor, himself not specially qualified for the office, however well instructed in the ordinary duties of his profession. On the other hand, should the views and intentions of the proprietor be of a higher and nobler kind, his scientific efforts would be perpetually liable to be misunderstood, misrepresented, and thwarted by gentlemen who may be humane and intelligent, but who must be unacquainted with the various forms, degrees, and often-changing phenomena of diseases of the nervous system. These gentlemen, it must be also observed, are too often desirous to display their natural acumen and their zeal in the cause of the defenceless and unhappy, and perhaps to exercise their "brief authority,' by fussy meddling and petty dictation about the merest trifles; sometimes even making serious mistakes, and doing no little injury to those whom they wish to befriend.

§ 8. The methods of inspection adopted by these well-meaning Visiting Justices, are rarely calculated to attain their object. Ill-timed and unskilful conferences with the patients, do more to irritate, excite, and even exasperate them, than to promote their welfare and recovery. A highly intelligent, most humane, and long-experienced medical superintendent of an asylum has informed me that his patients are invariably worse—more unhappy and irritable—for some days after the visit of the magistrates.

Then, the medical visitor who accompanies them, who is appointed by them, and who resides in the neighbourhood, cannot be wholly exempt from local prepossessions, or uninfluenced by his patrons. Whatever may be his professional attainments and reputation, he is generally selected on grounds perfectly distinct from his special attention to psychology and mental pathology, or from his practical skill and tact in the treatment of mental disorders, or from his thorough knowledge of the principles of hygiéne—so necessary in the inspection of curative establishments.

§ 9. I am well aware of the improvements and reforms, which have resulted from zealous attacks made within the last few years, by public-spirited and non-professional persons, upon the frightful abuses which have long prevailed in these institutions. I doubt not the humanity or the justice of the great body of English magistrates; but I do not hesitate to affirm, that, on the grounds already mentioned, the provincial system of Asylum Visitation must be condemned as objectionable and inefficient. It neither affords security to the patient against inhumane, unjust, or unscientific treatment, nor is it calculated to secure the cheerful and intelligent co-operation of the proprietor, while it tends to encourage a showy and tricky pretence rather than a real performance of duty.

For this defective system, therefore, it is proposed to substitute a frequent visitation,—not less than twelve times in the year,— by a thoroughly competent Circuit Inspector. He might be always accompanied by one or more of the Visiting Justices, but their interviews with the patients should be under his regulation; and he should be empowered to depute the local Officer of Health to see to the execution of any reforms or changes, in the intervals of his visits, which he may direct. Under such an organization, every difficulty of the case might, I believe, be fully solved and surmounted.

§ 10. Such being the position of the principal functions which might be assigned to a Circuit Inspector, he would be enabled, from the materials placed at his disposal by the Officers of Health, to draw up quarterly Reports of the sanitary condition of his Circuit.

The Government, or a central council, might expect that a Report of this kind would contain information on the following points:—(i.) the vital statistics, reproduction, and mortality of the population; the administration of medical jurisprudence, and the results of forensic inquiry; (ii.) the amount and general nature of sickness among the people, especially their "industrial pathology," and the epidemics, epizöotics, and meteorological phenomena of the period; (iii.) the progress of vaccination and other medical measures of prevention; the state of medical visitation among the poorer classes; the administration of aid in all public Hospitals, Dispensaries, and other sanative institutions; the management of Asylums, and the results of treatment in them; (iv.) the statistics of the medical profession, and the execution of laws for its regulation, or for that of the practice of pharmacy; and (v.) the condition of mortuary interment.* (vi.) He might also aid the Inspectors of Schools, of Prisons, and of Factories and Mines, in reporting upon the health and sanitary regulations of the several establishments under their respective superintendence; and his co-operation would be essential to the Engineering Inspector of the same circuit, in reporting the state of agriculture in its sanitary aspect, the progress of drainage—land and town,—the condition of water-courses and rivers, the supply of water for populous districts, and the execution of ordinary measures of purification and ventilation.

It can hardly be necessary to dilate on the public value and importance of the regular formation of such reports, their transmission to a Government Council or Board, and their circulation, as far as may be deemed expedient, for the information of the public.

§ 11. In considering the requisite number of such inspectors, we are at once reminded that there are *ten* statistical Divisions, besides that of the metropolis, under which the counties of England and Wales have been grouped by the Registrar-General. Each of these divisions, then, might be taken for a circuit, and be furnished with a permanent medico-sanitary Inspector. The average population of each circuit would be from 1,800,000 to 2,000,000; and it would contain about thirty of the proposed sanitary districts, and sixty of the existing Registration districts.

* The proceedings of Burial Boards, if these be not merged (as they ought to be) in the proposed District Sanitary Courts, should be noticed and reported by the Inspector.

The labours of an Inspector in so extensive a jurisdiction would be great and arduous. They would absorb his whole time and attention, and could not be performed unless he were assisted by the proposed local Officers of Health, as his deputies. The amount of his engagements, in the matter of visitation alone, may be roughly estimated by recollecting, that in each provincial Division of the Registrar-General there are, on the average, fourteen Hospitals and Infirmaries, beside Dispensaries and other sanative institutions; also, that private asylums average eight or nine,—and public hospitals for the insane, five,—in each division.* The general hospitals should be inspected quarterly; those for mental disease (at least all private asylums) monthly. On the plan suggested in these pages, there would be thirty Sanitary Courts, at the meetings of which his attendance would be occasionally required. His circuit would also contain about sixty Union Workhouses. More than half his time would be occupied in all these visitations and inspections, leaving barely enough for deliberation and report.

§ 12. Many instances have been given in the course of these Essays, of the waste of official machinery in medico-sanitary administration,—of the fragmentary, expensive, and inefficient distribution of duties among several medical officers employed casually and partially for separate objects. This is particularly observable in the case of Inspectors. The Prisons, the Factories and Mines, the General Register Office, and the General Board of Health, (probably also other departments) have their separate inspecting staffs. Not a few medical duties and sanitary measures have to be superintended in each of these departments, and therefore, I presume that, among the various classes of Inspectors, several physicians and surgeons are to be found.

Now, the distinctly medical portion of their official functions might be transferred to the proposed circuit appointment; and

---

* According to the *Medical Directory of* 1856, there are in England and Wales 138 Provincial Hospitals, 50 Hospitals for the Insane, and 83 Private Asylums beyond the Metropolitan District.—pp. 666—702.

many important public benefits would result from consolidating the chief sanitary duties in each circuit; while other duties, either of general administration, or relating to specialities of management,—to education and moral discipline, to engineering and mathematical calculations, or to the enforcement of regulations,—might with the greatest propriety be left to those other Inspectors now in office or hereafter to be appointed, who do not belong to the medical profession. But I submit that those existing Inspectors, who do belong to that profession, might constitute a considerable portion of the Medical Inspecting Staff now proposed.

The additional cost of completing that staff by a few fresh appointments,—(Officers of Health, whose superior skill and ability have been tested, would make the best Inspectors)—would probably be met by the abolition of a number of petty offices and casual consultations, now charged upon national or local funds; to say nothing of the vast indirect advantage which the community would derive from a complete official machinery for the protection of the Public Health.

"QUOD ADEST, MEMENTO COMPONERE ÆQUUS."

SUPPLEMENTARY NOTES.

A.
See pp. 44 and 53.
NURSES FOR THE SICK POOR.

THE question of Nurses for the Labouring population—in sickness, sporadic or epidemic, in accidents, and in child-birth—is now so fully under consideration, that my brief recommendations on this point (in the Introductory Essay), ought not to appear without some notice of the Nursing Schemes which have lately been projected.

Dr. Sieveking has devoted much praiseworthy attention to the acknowledged necessities of the Sick Poor in this respect, and has proposed a plan for the training and employment of the female inmates of Union Workhouses, as Nurses for the Poor in their own dwellings.

This project has been warmly supported by the Epidemiological Society. It is, however, to be regretted, that its humane and learned originator and promoters were not more practically acquainted with the class out of whom they propose to make Nurses, and that, before promulgating a specific plan, they had not more extensively consulted the Chaplains and Medical Officers of Workhouses.

Even by this time they may have learnt, that the training, habits, notions, and associations of female paupers, as a class (for there are exceptions, of course), are such as to render them most unfit for an employment in which the strictest decency, cleanliness, and morality, with some delicacy of feeling, are essential to the welfare of the patient.

It is also a great mistake to suppose that the very poor ought to be nursed only by those equally low in habits and depressed in circumstances with themselves.

Hours of sickness, tended by superiors, become hours of moral and mental improvement, as well as of physical consolation.

Moreover, we are not explicitly informed how, or by whom, these paupers are to be taught to nurse. In the sick-ward of a workhouse? There the field of observation is too narrow, and proper teachers are wanting.

The project seems to be founded merely on two undeniable facts:—

that the poor want nurses, and that there are, on the average, twenty-three able-bodied female paupers in every Union Workhouse. Now, let us suppose that a few (though the proportion must be small) of these able-bodied inmates are capable of being converted into efficient Nurses—and this I am far from denying,—they ought, for the safe and effectual accomplishment of the object, to be removed from workhouses, and trained elsewhere.

A select few of the younger and more intelligent inmates might, perhaps, be advantageously employed as Assistants to thoroughly-qualified and superior nurses, who ought to be appointed to the sick-wards of every Workhouse. Partial instruction might thus be given. But this is not Dr. Sieveking's plan, nor would it complete the due preparation of a sufficiently numerous *corps* of Nurses.

The series of questions put forth in October, 1854, by the Nursing Scheme Committee of the Epidemiological Society, may, perhaps, have elicited replies which may lead to safer conclusions and more judicious suggestions.

Hospitals afford by far the best opportunities of technical education in nursing, and the complete qualification of every licensed nurse should include attendance for a fixed period as hospital-assistant to the nursing staff. Courses of lectures should also be given to nurse-pupils, on the duties of attendants, and the elements of personal hygiène. Institutions of "Nursing-Sisters" should be multiplied. Every first-class town, or sanitary district, should possess such an Institution, as a centre of supply to the surrounding population.

We have yet to see the results of the remarkable national movement now proceeding out of Miss Nightingale's noble exertions and self-sacrifices at the seat of war. If the Fund to be raised for the training of Nurses under her most able direction, should lead to the formation of a School of Nurses in every principal hospital and infirmary in the kingdom,—all the wants of the labouring classes, and of the sick generally, in this respect, may be adequately supplied.

B.

See p. 193.

SIR G. C. LEWIS'S COMMENTS ON THE PLANS FOR MEDICAL RELIEF LAID BEFORE THE SELECT COMMITTEE IN 1844.

9822. "The result appears to me to be, that, so long as medical relief remains upon its present footing, so long as it is a system of relief connected with other sorts of relief to the poor, and administered by Boards of Guardians from funds furnished by the poor-rate and under the control of the Poor-Law Commissioners, no essential alteration can be made with respect to the mode of obtaining medical relief. If the principle which Mr. Rumsey contends for should be adopted,—if a general system of medical endowment, administered under the control of a central Board of Health, independently of the Poor-Law, should be established,—it is clear that a different mode of obtaining medical attendance might be advantageously substituted; but I confess, with every disposition to devise means of facilitating the procuring of medical relief, and the access of the poor to the medical officers, I am unable to conceive that any material alteration can be made in the existing regulations."

9827. "The practical difficulty in working such a system [as Mr. Guthrie's] will readily occur to the Committee. Suppose a medical man to be appointed one of the three Poor-Law Commissioners, he would be a Commissioner sitting at the Board, and having the same powers, and no greater or less than those of the others. Suppose a case arises as to the amount of salary to a medical officer, the medical Commissioner thinks that the salary should be increased, the two non-medical Commissioners think that it should remain as it is,—what is to be the decision of the Board? Is it to be expected that the two Commissioners should surrender their judgments to that of the third, simply because he is a medical man, and they are not so? So also as to the framing medical regulations; if there is a question as to the framing of a new set of medical regulations, the medical Commissioner takes one view, and the non-medical Commissioners take a different view, is he to over-rule the opinions of his two colleagues, simply because he has a knowledge of medicine? I am unable to understand how a system of that sort can be made to work, unless the control of the medical relief be altogether withdrawn from the department of the Poor-Law Commission, and lodged in different hands,—namely, in a body consisting principally or exclusively of medical men."

9828. (Question.) "If the power were lodged in different hands, do not you think that there would be the possibility of a constant difference of opinion and collision between the two medical superintendents and the Poor-Law Commissioners?"

(Answer.) "I suppose that the possibility of collision would be prevented by the entire separation of the two departments. The supposition that I am making is, that all matters relating to the medical relief of the poor would be transferred to this new body, that they would correspond with Boards of Guardians," [Boards of Health he should have said], "and that all these medical matters would be withdrawn from the cognizance of the Poor-Law Commissioners."

C.

See p. 259.

PRINCIPLES ON WHICH MUTUAL ASSURANCE MIGHT BE APPLIED TO A SELF-PROVISION OF MEDICAL ATTENDANCE BY THE WORKING CLASSES.

1. No Insurance Fund of this nature should be sanctioned or protected by law, or promoted by benevolent persons, to which any labourers or artisans are permitted to contribute, who have not previously insured in a well-regulated Provident or Friendly Society (which does not hold its meetings in a public-house), for a reversionary payment at death, a reversionary annuity in old age, and a weekly allowance in sickness sufficient for the ordinary maintenance of themselves and those dependent upon them.

2. Every such person proposing to insure for the privilege of choosing his own medical attendant, should also be required to have previously provided, by mutual assurance or otherwise, for a supply of dietetic tonics, cordials, and medicines, and perhaps for the attendance of a nurse (the average cost of these requirements in illness being "susceptible of calculation by way of average")—such arrangements to be effected, if possible, by means of legally-authorized local institutions.

3. Those who produce proofs of having made all the above-mentioned provisions, who are not members of public-house clubs, and whose wages, income, or means of living, are duly certified not to exceed a specified rate or amount, proportionate to the number of those dependent on them for support, and to the rate of medical remuneration agreed upon (see 10), might be admitted, with the consent of a fairly-constituted Board, as members of an Insurance Society for the provision of medical attendance, on the following terms:—

4. That every member should be secured the privilege of selecting his medical adviser from among those who are ready to attend on the specified terms; and of changing such adviser as often as he may please.

5. That the contributions of the insurers should be calculated on the same principles as those for a pecuniary allowance during sickness.

The premiums should therefore vary according to the liability of each member to sickness, and be determined by the age, sex, condition of health, place of residence, and occupation of each candidate for admission.

6. That the working classes should be at liberty to insure for their wives and children on the same principles and regulations as for themselves.

7. That the fund so raised should constitute a permanent fund, and the surplus protected by law for future claims, as securely as those of Friendly Societies are at present.

8. That, out of this fund, all those resident practitioners who are appointed to the care of the members, should be remunerated,—each according to the number of cases he may have attended during a given period.

9. That any legally-qualified and resident practitioner, who does not contract (or who engages not to renew any existing contract) with any Benefit or Medical Club, should be permitted to connect his name with the Society,—which, nevertheless, should be nowhere established, unless a majority of such practitioners, residing within the proposed district of its operations, should signify their assent to it.

10. That different tables of insurance contributions should be calculated, to meet different rates of medical remuneration; and that one or more of the latter having been selected by the medical practitioners and Dispensary Committee of a district, the contributions of the working classes would be determined accordingly.

11. Persons who are ill and desirous of joining the Society for the sake of obtaining immediate attendance, should be permitted to do so, on payment of an adequate fine and extra premium.

D.

See pp. 271, 272.

CHARITABLE DISPENSARIES.

Extracts from Evidence taken by Select Committee, in 1844.

9164. "The attendance on Dispensary patients at their own houses, is at present irregular and uncertain. In a few institutions, I am informed that they are regularly visited by the honorary physicians and surgeons. It cannot, however, be expected that any extensive or regular system of home-visiting will be kept up by unpaid officers. In the majority of instances, the ordinary visiting is performed by the paid resident apothecary of the Dispensary; and the honorary officers either do not profess to visit, or they only go to serious cases when requested by the resident apothecary. I firmly believe, although it is difficult to obtain conclusive evidence on this point, that dispensary patients are by no means so thoroughly attended to, or so regularly visited, as the patients of the Union medical officers."

" There are several serious defects in the present mode of dispensing relief. From the number of cases presented to the notice of the physician or surgeon on the morning of his attendance, they are necessarily hurried over, and imperfectly examined. Then the patients are often detained for an inconvenient and injurious length of time; and the regulations for their attendance at the dispensary preclude the possibility of prompt relief in many urgent cases, and often deprive them of the advantage of necessary changes in the treatment of their case. There is also an excessive and unnecessary consumption of drugs, which, however, are always of the best description, and are, in fact, a substitute for regular and frequent attendance."

"Supply the latter, and the former will diminish." . . . . .

9165. . . . . . "The fact is, that the present financial condition of these dispensaries is, in many towns, far from satisfactory. I find from most of the printed Reports that the funds have a steady tendency to diminish, and are only kept up by constant appeals to the benevolent, and an occasional grand effort by the friends of the institution to pay off the balance due to the Treasurer."

2. *Extract from Report of the Huddersfield Infirmary and Dispensary.* 1843.

"The governors are aware that the duty of administering medical assistance to such of the sick poor as are recipients of parochial relief, more immediately belongs to surgeons of unions, and not to the medical officers of infirmaries, whose resources are more appropriately directed to the *prevention* (*not the relief*) of pauperism. They are led to this remark in consequence of the frequent applications of out-patients to this charity who are at the time in receipt of parish relief. If this description of patients consisted merely of accidents and cases requiring operations, or attended with peculiar difficulty, it would be admitted on all hands, that for all such purposes the wards of an infirmary are best calculated; but, exclusive of these instances, there are many who become chargeable to the infirmary, who ought to be more properly placed under the care of the district surgeons, whose province it is to attend to such cases."

3. *The Governors of the Gloucester Dispensary, at their Annual Meeting, in* 1844, *memorialized the Poor-Law Commissioners in the following terms:—*

"That this meeting, feeling that the present system of supplying medicines to the poor materially affects the interests of this Institution, begs to suggest to the Poor-Law Commissioners, the propriety of directing that the medicines for the sick poor be not supplied by the medical officers, but provided by the guardians, at the cost of the Union; and that the Secretary be requested to communicate this to the Poor-Law Commissioners."

E.

See pp. 273, 289.

FRENCH AND BELGIAN SYSTEMS OF OUT-DOOR MEDICAL ATTENDANCE ON THE POOR.

1. *Reformed Administration of Medical Aid and Visitation in Paris.*

The *Moniteur* of Nov. 22, 1853, published an article of which the following is a translation in the Medical Press, Jan. 11, 1853 :—

"An important and salutary innovation in the administration of public aid has been introduced under the direction of the Emperor. The following is a very summary account of the new arrangement. The number of medical attendants at the Bureau de Bienfaisance is fixed at 159; they will be distributed among the twelve arrondissements in proportion to the indigent population. Their services will no longer be gratuitous; they will each receive a salary of 600 francs in the central quarters, and of 1000 francs [some now receive 1200] in those parts such as the *Quartier Popincourt,* the *Invalides, Petit Pologne,* &c., where the indigent circumstances of the population do not give an opportunity of making a practice, while the distance to be traversed increases the labour of visiting. There will also be in each arrondissement paid midwives. The medical attendants will be presented by the Bureau de Bienfaisance, and proposed by the Director of Public Aid; they will be elected for six years and will be capable of re-election. Stations will be appointed in the different quarters, at which patients may consult medical officers, who will be bound to attend at fixed days and hours, and to remain as long as they may be required to give advice. A member of the Bureau de Bienfaisance will be present on each occasion. The medical attendants will visit at their own houses those who may not be able to attend. A register will be opened at the office of each bureau, in which will be inserted the names and residences of all the patients, the date of the commencement of their treatment, and all other necessary information. Patients with acute diseases will be visited at least once a week by an Administrator or Commissioner of Public Aid, who will enter on a schedule such observations as may occur to him, principally with regard to the medical attendance which the patients are receiving. A committee composed of the president or of a vice-president of the bureau, of a governor or commissioner, of the treasurer of the bureau, and one of the medical officers, will meet every week to debate on subjects regarding attendance on the patients, and especially on the visiting lists. They will determine what aid it may be proper to afford in medicine, food, linen, &c., or even in money. In urgent cases, the president may in the intervals advance such aid as is absolutely needed; and of this he shall render an account to the Committee. Persons not enrolled as paupers, such as needy workmen, persons with large families, or those who are in any way very destitute, will be attended at their own houses, either at their own request, or at the requisition of the Mayor or one of the administrators of the bureau in their district, or at the instance of the Director of Public Aid."

2. *French Colonial Medical Aid.*

The Minister of War, Marshal Vaillant, published a report upon the condition of French Algeria, at the end of 1853.

Amongst other matters, he noticed at length the efforts made by to Government for the establishment of institutions of charity and bienfaisance in that colony.

Some of the details are interesting both statistically and as developing the system of French colonization, so widely different from our own, as regards what is left to individual exertion, chance or necessity supply, or is neglected altogether, and what the central government considers as falling within its peculiar province to provide.

After describing the *Banque du pauvre* or Loan Institution, the *Caisses de Secours Mutuelles* or Mutual Aid Societies, and Asylums or Industrial Schools for orphans and deserted children, the Marshal proceeds:—

" I may mention, lastly, as worthy of notice, the system of medical aid established throughout all the remoter parts of the colony by the official assistance of the Government. Each district marked out for colonization has been divided into a number of medical circumscriptions. Every one of these has been provided with its medical attendant, who must be a person furnished with a regular diploma, and to whom a regular salary is allowed by the War Department; together with the expense of a horse, if the extent of his district demands such assistance." This *médecin de colonisation*, as he is termed, is bound to give gratuitous attendance to every indigent person, native or European, within his district, and to provide them also gratuitously with medicines where no regular pharmacy exists. It is his duty also to make regular rounds periodically amongst the population, to vaccinate children, to certify all deaths, and to furnish the administration with all such statistical information as relates to his department and the public health. "This organization," the Report assures us, "is now so perfect, that there is not in Algeria a single locality, where a group of European population is established, which is not now attached to a medical district, and receives in consequence, at least twice a week, the visit of a doctor, and in the case of the poor, gratuitous advice and medicaments."

3.—*Medical care of the Poor in the towns of Belgium.*

All the out-door sick poor are entitled to the attendance of a physician, and to medicines supplied by an appointed apothecary. In some parishes both a physician and surgeon are appointed. The poor when ill must apply first, except in urgent cases, to one of the *maîtres des pauvres*, who gives an order for the doctor. There are from one to four of these *maîtres des pauvres* in every parish; appointed partly by the parochial clergy and partly by the municipality. Both parties must concur in the appointment. The office is honorary, held often for life, as a privilege and a duty. These *maîtres* are much respected, and altogether a contrast, both in principle and practice, to our "relieving officers."

The parishes average about 4000 in population. If the district be more populous, additional medical attendants are employed, beside the regular apothecary. The parish physician makes his report to a Medical Commission, belonging to every large town, and elected by the resident practitioners.

The Government, however, have the right of removing any name from the list of elected Commissioners. But this *veto*, I was informed, is very rarely exercised.

Any defects in the supply of drugs, and other matters affecting the public health, are referred to this local commission. The salaries of the parish physicians are small, and vary both in rate and amount; but the office is esteemed honourable, and sought after by men of the highest standing and qualifications.

These particulars I ascertained at Ghent in 1850.

F.

See p. 298.

EXPULSION OF GREEK PHYSICIANS FROM ROME UNDER THE REPUBLIC.

Learned men have disagreed on this point. The assertion that the Roman Senate influenced by Cato's notions, although after his time, expelled the physicians with other Greek philosophers from Italy, is founded, I believe, on Pliny's statement,*—" Et cum Græcos Italiâ pellerent, diu post Catonem, excepisse medicos."

A very important question to determine first, is the meaning of '*excepisse*.' Sprengel† takes it to mean, that the physicians were specially exempted from the decree of banishment passed upon other Greeks. But the able editor of the *Delphin Classics*,‡—following Brotier—thus paraphrases the disputed passage :—" Nominatim appellasse medicos cum cæteris Græcis urbe pellendos ;" and adds in a note —" *Excipere* hoc loco, non est demere, secernere, vel eximere numero, sed nominatim cavere. Cujus significationis exempla plurima in Jureconsultis occurrunt ; atque in ipso Cic. ad. Q Fratr. I. 1. 'Nominatimque lex exciperet, ut ad templum monumentumque nostrum capere liceret.' "

I may give another instance of this meaning of the verb *excipere*. The important edict of Valentinian and Valens, concerning the medical care of the poor in Rome (most of which I have given as a motto to Essay IV. Part II. p. 238), commences thus :—" Exceptis Portûs Xysti, Virginumque Vestalium, quot regiones Urbis sunt, totidem constituantur Archiatri." This is well known to mean, that a medical superintendent was appointed to the Gymnasium, another to the body of Vestal Virgins, and one to each of the fourteen regions into which Rome was then divided.

If, after this evidence, any one can doubt Pliny's meaning in the word *excepisse*, let him observe the context. Pliny's whole argument is, that the older Romans refused to have anything to do with the foreign doctors, though they had no objection to treat themselves, as Cato did, by the aid of recipe-books of domestic medicine.—'Non rem

---

* *Hist. Nat.* XXIX. c. 8.

† "Als die Römer einst alle Griechen aus Italien vertrieben nahmen sie ausdrücklich die Aerzte von diesem Verbote aus."—*Geschichte der Arzneikunde.* Halle: 1800. Erster Theil. § 113, s. 243.

‡ Regent's Edition. 8vo, 1826, p. 3996.

antiqui *damnabant,* sed artem. Maxime vero quæstum esse immani pretio vitæ *recusabant.* Ideo templum Æsculapii, etiam cum reciperetur is Deus, extra Urbem fecisse, iterumque in Insulâ, traduntur." (Then follows the passage in question.) " Augebo," continues Pliny, "providentiam illorum;" and this promise he endeavours to fulfil, by recommending the study of medicine in the Latin language, and by satirizing the credulity of the Romans of his own time, who were imposed on by practitioners speaking and prescribing in an unintelligible (that is to say, in the Greek) language.

Again, when summing up at the close of the same chapter, he says, " Hæc fuerint dicenda pro senatû illo . . . . . adversus artem;" evidently referring with satisfaction to the decree of banishment.

Sprengel treats the account of the expulsion of the Greek physicians in rather an off-hand manner. " Dass er übrigens sollte die griechischen Aerzte vertrieben haben, ist eine Fabel"! He cites Schulze* in his support. Their objections to the received opinion rest, however, only on negative evidence. They produce no other writer of antiquity to show that the Greek physicians were exempted from the operation of the decree of the Senate, which would have been a remarkable event. That Plutarch names only Carneades and other Greek philosophers as having been banished, is nothing to the point. Probably some of these very philosophers were the identical proscribed doctors. And that we hear of other medical men in professional connexion with famous Romans, at a later period of the Republic, has still less to do with it.

Le Clerc gives us a chapter on the subject; but leaves the matter unsettled. He seems to wish his readers to believe that the doctors were not expelled: but proceeds, in a manner truly characteristic of his nation, to make the best of a misfortune, supposing they were. " Mais quoi qu'il en soit, il ne s'ensuit pas de l'éloignement que Caton et les Romains de ce temps-là pouvoient avoir pour les médecins qu'ils ayent jamais donné un arrêt de banissement contre eux : je ne sache pas du moins, qu'aucun auteur ancien l'ait remarqué. Mais quand cela seroit, que pourroit on inférer de là au désavantage de la Médecine ?" &c. &c.†

The probabilities are, therefore, in my humble opinion, as strongly against the hasty decision of Sprengel and other medical historians, as they are in favour of the correctness of Pliny's simple account of what appears to have been a well-known historical fact.

* *Hist. Med.* p. 432, *seq.*
† *Hist de la Méd.* La Haye, 1729, 4to. Part II., III., c. 2, p. 386.

G.

See p. 317.

Constitution of Councils of Health in France.

Through the kind intervention of Dr. Greenhill, I received the following brief account of the central and local *Conseils d'Hygiène publique*, from Dr. Daremberg of Paris,* who favoured me at the same time with other valuable information on sanitary measures in France.

" Il existe en France un Comité consultatif d'*Hygiène publique*. C'est un Comité supérieur, central et unique.

" Sa composition est complexe. Il y a des membres *effectifs* [acting] recevant un jeton (?) de présence, et des *fonctionnaires* [*ex-officio*] autorisés à assister à des séances.

" Parmi les membres effectifs, au nombre de neuf,—il y a quatre Médecins (dont le Président), un ancien conseiller d'État, un ex-chef de bureau, le directeur de l'École de Pharmacie, un Ingénieur civil et un Architecte. Les membres autorisés sont, un membre du conseil de santé des Armées; l'Inspecteur-général du service de santé de la Marine; un Administrateur des Douanes; le chef de la direction du commerce(?) au Ministère des Affaires Étrangères; un Administrateur des Postes; le Directeur-général de l'Assistance publique; le Secrétaire perpétuel de l'Académie de Médecine; et un Architecte. Le Secrétaire du Comité est médecin et appointé. Ce Comité est institué près le Ministère de l'Agriculture, du Commerce et des Travaux publics.

" Il y a un conseil d'hygiène publique et de Salubrité par *département* et par *arrondissement*, ceux-ci communiquant avec des *commissions cantonales*. Leur existence est plus en puissance que réelle. Cependant ils fonctionnent dans un certain nombre de départements et d'arrondissements. Leur composition est analogue à celle du Comité central. Les Médecins y figurent (?) toujours pour le tiers ou le quart. Il y a aussi des pharmaciens-chimistes, un vétérinaire, des ingénieurs, des architectes et des notables. Les membres de ces conseils sont nommés par les préfets des départements.

" Ces conseils sont purement consultatifs; ils n'ont aucun droit d'initiative et aucun pouvoir exécutif."

The real local administrative authorities are the *Préfets* and *Sous-Préfets*, with certain legal, medical, and scientific officers.

* The illegibility of some words in the manuscript must be my excuse for any errors in transcribing.

H.

See p. 389.

Mr. Estlin and the National Vaccine Board.

It was the opinion of the late Mr. Estlin, of Bristol, a surgeon of great experience, close observation, and calm judgment, that the supply of vaccine lymph had considerably deteriorated. His own philanthropic efforts, during the alarming prevalence of small-pox in 1838-9, in renewing an appeal to the original source, and in distributing the lymph so procured (at a Gloucestershire dairy) very extensively in the West of England and in America,—excited general and deep interest at the time. He even induced the National Vaccine Board to employ the new virus, which appeared to himself and others who used it, to produce vesicles better marked and developed, and attended with more constitutional disturbance, than those produced by the old (and in his view, effete) stock of lymph.

The National Vaccine Board, however, asserted at that time, as they have always done, their complete satisfaction with the lymph resulting from their own successional vaccinations. Their Report, in the same year, evinced their tendency to exaggerate the perfection of their supply.

After stating their regret that any anxiety should have been expressed to recur to the disease of the cow;—" We have," said they, " the opportunities of bearing our most ample testimony to the continuance of the efficiency of the original vaccine lymph introduced by Dr. Jenner, through nearly a million of subjects successively, of whom many thousands have been exposed, with entire impunity, to small-pox in its most malignant form."

This was too much for Mr. Estlin, and he vented his disapprobation in the following severe but fair piece of criticism :*—

" Now it is only forty years since the introduction of vaccination, and however numerous may be the subjects that have been vaccinated at one time from the same individual, the stock of matter at present employed at the National Vaccine Establishment, can only have passed through 2080 subjects, even supposing that lymph for subsequent vaccination had been taken every seven days from a fresh subject, without any interruption, from the time when Dr. Jenner first sent it to London.

* *London Medical Gazette*, vol. xxiii. p. 864.

In order that it should pass through a million subjects, the lapse of 19,230 years and ten months would be required.

"In periods of general alarm, to what extent it may be justifiable to have recourse to the *pious fraud* of strong and not very accurate statements, for the purpose of calming the public mind, I am not casuist enough to determine; my preference, however, is for truth and correctness at all times; and I cannot but think it a matter of regret, on the present occasion, that an official document should have emanated from the National Vaccine Establishment of England, attested by the name of the learned President of the Royal College of Physicians, and destined to be circulated, not only throughout our own kingdom, but in countries where great attention is paid to the accuracy of medical statistics, so expressed, as to refer the origin of vaccination to such a remote period as thirteen thousand years before the beginning of the world."

THE END.

PUBLIC HEALTH IN AMERICA

An Arno Press Collection

Ackerknecht, Erwin H[einz]. **Malaria In the Upper Mississippi Valley: 1760-1900.** 1945

Bowditch, Henry I[ngersoll]. **Consumption In New England Or, Locality One of Its Chief Causes** and **Is Consumption Contagious, Or Communicated By One Person to Another In Any Manner?** 1862/1864. Two Vols. in One.

Buck, Albert H[enry] (Editor). **A Treatise On Hygiene and Public Health.** 1879. Two Vols.

Boston Medical Commission. **The Sanitary Condition of Boston:** The Report of a Medical Commission. 1875

Budd, William. **Typhoid Fever:** Its Nature, Mode of Spreading, and Prevention. 1931

Chapin, Charles V[alue]. **A Report On State Public Health Work,** Based On a Survey of State Boards of Health: Made Under the Direction of the Council on Health and Public Instruction of the American Medical Association. [1915]

Davis, Michael M[arks], Jr. and Andrew R[obert] Warner. **Dispensaries:** Their Management and Development. 1918

Dublin, Louis I[srael] and Alfred J. Lotka. **The Money Value of a Man.** 1930

Dunglison, Robley. **Human Health.** 1844

Emerson, Haven. **Local Health Units for the Nation.** 1945

Emerson, Haven. **A Monograph On the Epidemic of Poliomyelitis (Infantile Paralysis) In New York City In 1916.** 1917

Fish, Hamilton. **Report of the Select Committee of the Senate of the United States On the Sickness and Mortality On Board Emigrant Ships.** 1854

Frost, Wade Hampton. **The Papers of Wade Hampton Frost, M.D.:** A Contribution to Epidemiological Method. 1941

Gardner, Mary Sewall. **Public Health Nursing.** 1916

Greenwood, Major. **Epidemics and Crowd Diseases:** An Introduction to the Study of Epidemiology. 1935

Greenwood, Major. **Medical Statistics From Graunt to Farr.** 1948

Hartley, Robert M. **An Historical, Scientific and Practical Essay On Milk, As an Article of Human Sustenance:** With a Consideration of the Effects Consequent Upon the Unnatural Methods of Producing It for the Supply of Large Cities. 1842

Hill, Hibbert Winslow. **The New Public Health.** 1916

Knopf, S. Adolphus. **Tuberculosis As a Disease of the Masses & How To Combat It.** 1908

MacNutt, J[oseph] Scott. **A Manual for Health Officers.** 1915

Richards, Ellen H. [Swallow]. **Euthenics:** The Science of Controllable Environment. 1910

Richardson, Joseph G[ibbons]. **Long Life and How To Reach It.** 1886

Rumsey, Henry Wyldbore. **Essays On State Medicine.** 1856

Shryock, Richard Harrison. **National Tuberculosis Association 1904-1954:** A Study of the Voluntary Health Movement In the United States. 1957

Simon, John. **Filth-Diseases and Their Prevention.** 1876

Sternberg, George M[iller]. **Sanitary Lessons of the War and Other Papers.** 1912

Straus, Lina Gutherz. **Disease In Milk:** The Remedy Pasteurization. The Life Work of Nathan Straus. 1917

Wanklyn, J[ames] Alfred and Ernest Theophron Chapman. **Water Analysis:** A Practical Treatise on the Examination of Potable Water. 1884

Whipple, George C. **State Sanitation:** A Review of the Work of the Massachusetts State Board of Health. 1917. Two Vols. in One.

Selections From Public Health Reports and Papers Presented at the Meetings of the American Public Health Association (1873-1883). 1977

Selections From Public Health Reports and Papers Presented at the Meetings of the American Public Health Association (1884-1907). 1977

Animalcular and Cryptogamic Theories On the Origins of Fevers. 1977

The Carrier State. 1977

Clean Water and the Health of the Cities. 1977

The First American Medical Association Reports On Public Hygiene In American Cities. 1977

Selections from the Health-Education Series. 1977

Health In the Southern United States. 1977

Health In the Twentieth Century. 1977

The Health of Women and Children. 1977

Minutes and Proceedings from the First, Second, Third and Fourth National Quarantine and Sanitary Conventions. 1977. Four Vols. in Two.

Selections from the Journal of the Massachusetts Association of Boards of Health (1891-1904). 1977

Sewering the Cities. 1977

Smallpox In Colonial America. 1977

Yellow Fever Studies. 1977